Vestibular Rehabilitation

Contemporary Perspectives in Rehabilitation

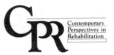

Steven L. Wolf, PhD, FAPTA, Editor-in-Chief

Vestibular Rehabilitation

Susan J. Herdman, PhD, PT
Professor and Director of Vestibular Rehabilitation
Department of Otolaryngology
University of Miami
School of Medicine
Miami, Florida

 F. A. DAVIS COMPANY • Philadelphia

F. A. Davis Company
1915 Arch Street
Philadelphia, PA 19103

Printed in the United States of America

Last digit indicates print number: 10 9 8 7 6 5 4 3 2

Senior Allied Health Editor: Jean-François Vilain
Senior Allied Health Developmental Editor: Ralph Zickgraf
Production Editor: Crystal S. McNichol

As new scientific information becomes available through basic and clinical research, recommended treatments and drug therapies undergo changes. The author(s) and publisher have done everything possible to make this book accurate, up to date, and in accord with accepted standards at the time of publication. The authors, editors, and publisher are not responsible for errors or omissions or for consequences from application of the book, and make no warranty, expressed or implied, in regard to the contents of the book. Any practice described in this book should be applied by the reader in accordance with professional standards of care used in regard to the unique circumstances that may apply in each situation. The reader is advised always to check product information (package inserts) for changes and new information regarding dose and contraindications before administering any drug. Caution is especially urged when using new or infrequently ordered drugs.

Vestibular rehabilitation / Susan J. Herdman.
   p. cm. — (Contemporary perspectives in rehabilitation)
  Includes bibliographical references and index.
  ISBN 0-8036-4624-0 (hardback : alk. paper)
  1. Vestibular apparatus—Diseases. 2. Vestibular apparatus—Diseases—Treatment. 3. Vestibular apparatus—Diseases—Exercise therapy. I. Herdman, Susan. II. Series.
  [DNLM: 1. Vestibular Diseases—rehabilitation. WV 255 V5836 1994]
RF260.V4725 1994
617.8′82—dc20
DNLM/DLC
for Library of Congress   93-23544
                                                                    CIP

This book is dedicated to the memory of my father, William E. Herdman.

Foreword

As scientists and clinicians we sometime marvel at how an apparently small and innocuous system of ossicles and semicircular canals, deeply embedded within the petrous portions of temporal cortical bone, can have such an intricate and profound influence on our ability to exist in an ever-changing environment. Yet as students and users of rehabilitation procedures, we spend little time learning about the complexities of the vestibular system. We know that intimate ties exist between the vestibular apparatus, our sense of "dizziness," and postural stability. Despite this knowledge, the use of exercise within a rehabilitative context is relatively new, and many health-related professionals are naive about both the rationales inherent in exercise protocols and their potential benefit as an adjunct to surgical or pharmacologic interventions. With these realities in mind, Susan Herdman, an experienced physical therapist with extensive clinical and research experience in vestibular system pathology, has assembled an expert team of researchers and clinicians to help fill the gaps in our knowledge of vestibular system pathophysiology and rehabilitative treatment options.

All the contributors are sensitive to the fact that few texts addressing this topic have been geared to the varied needs of rehabilitation personnel. Accordingly, this book is written with both student and clinician in mind. Dr. Herdman has carefully grouped the chapters into four sections covering, respectively: fundamentals, medical assessment, medical management, and rehabilitation. In this manner all readers can follow a logical progression from fundamental physiology to pathophysiologic occurrences following deafferentation, inflammatory disease, or trauma. Medical assessment issues are presented to acquaint (or reacquaint) the reader with typical methods for quantifying vestibular function and addressing concurrent auditory problems. The section on medical management offers rehabilitation providers insight into how physicians decide on pharmacologic or surgical interventions and medical treatments (including treatment of disorders related to migraine). Most important, and in keeping with the underlying philosophy of the Contemporary Perspectives in Rehabilitation series, several of these contributions contain case studies presented in a decision-making format so that the reader can "think along" with the clinician/author. This approach is most obvious in the remarkably comprehensive yet diversified section on rehabilitation assessment and management. The six chapters in this section, while filled with valuable clinical information, also challenge the clinician or student to think logically and deductively as master clinicians write about their treatment approaches to vestibular hypofunction, bilateral vestibular loss, benign paroxysmal positional vertigo, and vestibular pathology among traumatic brain-injured patients and in children with vestibular disorders. These contributions are heavily documented and offer many opportunities for applying the clinical experience bestowed in each chapter with case-study formats.

At the risk of flaunting the excellence embodied in this text, I can say unequivocally that this text is unparalleled in its breadth of content and sensitivity to the needs of its diversified readership. If the process of absorbing the context and fresh ideas in this very special but important area of rehabilitation spawns new ideas or yields treatment insights, this labor of love will have been well worth the many hours spent in its delivery.

Steven L. Wolf, PhD, FAPTA
Series Editor

Preface

Management of patients with vestibular disorders is a formidable problem. Dizziness and balance problems account for 5 to 10 percent of all physician visits and affect 40 percent of people over the age of 40. Dizziness is the number one reason for physician visits by people over the age of 65. One of the difficulties in managing these patients is that the term "dizzy" is used to mean a variety of sensations, from vertigo to disequilibrium to lightheadedness. Dizziness, therefore, can be due to any of a myriad of problems including vestibular pathology, drug interactions, orthostatic hypotension, anxiety, and somatosensory loss in the lower extremities.

Identifying dizziness due to vestibular pathology is not always easy. Although vertigo is sometimes considered to be a marker for a vestibular deficit, patients can have severe vestibular dysfunction without vertigo. Furthermore, although we assess the health of the vestibular system by measuring the vestibulo-ocular reflex, this measurement gauges only the function of the horizontal canals and not that of the vertical canals or otoliths. This means that patients may have vestibular problems that cannot be measured. Attempts to isolate the function of the vestibulospinal system also have had limited success. Although patients with vestibular deficits may have difficulty maintaining their balance when both visual and somatosensory cues are altered, patients with nonvestibular balance disorders have similar difficulties.

Treatment of patients with vestibular problems also has been difficult. Sixty years ago, Dandy treated vertigo by performing bilateral vestibular nerve sections. He knew that vestibular deficits resulted in vertigo and believed that the loss of vestibular inputs would have no effect on a person's function. Fifteen years ago, patients with vertigo were given drugs, placed on bedrest, and often told they would have to "learn to live with it."

Today, management of the patient with a vestibular problem is more sophisticated. Although surgical management is still primarily ablative, care is taken to limit the surgical destruction of the inner ear, and the results of these procedures are carefully studied. Medical management recognizes that the use of vestibular suppressant medications may not be appropriate in all patients and that prolonged use in certain patients may actually delay recovery. New medical treatments have been developed for a variety of vestibular disorders.

The use of exercises as a treatment modality is the third approach that is now used extensively for patients with vestibular deficits. Although Cawthorne and Cooksey introduced the use of exercises as a treatment for patients with vestibular disorders in the 1940s, it is only in the last few years that physical therapists have become interested in treating this common and complicated patient population. Originally, this interest was due to an increased awareness of the importance of the vestibular system in balance control; now, it reflects the added awareness that many patients with vestibular deficits can be treated for the vestibular problem itself.

This text provides a thorough introduction of vestibular disorders to rehabilitation students and is a comprehensive resource for clinicians treating patients with vestibular dysfunction. Chapters on vestibular anatomy and physiology, vestibular adaptation, and the role of the vestibular system in postural control provide the basis for understanding how the normal vestibular system functions. The main concern in this book, however, is the assessment of patients with vestibular disorders and the development of different treatments. Because a diagnosis often is not available in patients with complaints of vertigo and disequilibrium, the assessment and identification of problems and goals become even more critical. The intent of the book is to provide the information necessary to enable the student to understand and the clinician to make appropriate decisions about the use of exercises for patients with vestibular lesions. The book is suitable for the therapist who has extensive experience with the dizzy patient, those therapists who are just beginning to work with these patients, and students who are contemplating working with such patients. Physical therapists who may find this book of interest include those in general hospital settings, private practice, or rehabilitation centers. Because vestibular disorders can be due to a variety of problems including viral infection, head trauma, motor vehicle accidents, stroke and aging, all physical therapists should find this book useful. In addition, this book should be a useful resource to occupational therapists, audiologists, otolaryngology nurses, and otolaryngologists.

Susan J. Herdman

Acknowledgments

In addition to those who actually set words to paper, many people contributed to this book. First are the patients with vestibular and other balance disorders, whose experiences with vertigo and with the process of diagnosis and treatment are the basis for this book. Second, I would like to thank all my colleagues at Johns Hopkins, including those who wrote individual chapters. I have enjoyed working with them very much. Third, I am grateful to the reviewers, whose critical reading and careful suggestions helped shape the text: Robert Baloh, MD (UCLA School of Medicine); Emily Keshner, EdD, PT (University of Illinois at Chicago); Susan B. O'Sullivan, MS, RPT (University of Lowell); Anne Shumway-Cook, PhD, PT (Northwestern Hospital, Seattle); and Robert A. Whipple, MAPT (Balance and Gait Enhancement Laboratory, University of Connecticut Health Center). Finally, I would like to acknowledge those who are responsible for my becoming a physical therapist, especially Dorothy Baethke, E. Jane Carlin, and Eugene Michels.

Contributors

Diane F. Borello-France, MS, PT
Clinical Specialist, Balance Disorders
University of Pittsburgh Medical Center
School of Health and Rehabilitation
  Sciences
Clinical Assistant Professor
Department of Physical Therapy
University of Pittsburgh
Pittsburgh, Pennsylvania

Ian S. Curthoys, PhD
Psychology Department
University of Sydney
Sydney, Australia

**Georgia A. DeGangi, PhD, OTR,
  FAOTA**
Director
Cecil and Ida Green Research and
  Training Institute
Reginald S. Lourie Center for Infants
  and Young Children and
Ivymount School
Rockville, Maryland

M. Cara Erskine, MEd
Department of Otolaryngology — Head
  and Neck Surgery
Assistant Professor
Audiology and Speech Pathology
The Johns Hopkins Hospital
Baltimore, Maryland

M. Fetter, MD
Department of Neurology
Eberhard-Karls University
Tubingen, Germany

Timothy C. Hain, MD
Associate Professor of Neurology and
  Otolaryngology
Northwestern University School of
  Medicine
Chicago, Illinois

G. Michael Halmagyi, MD
Neurology Department
Royal Prince Alfred Hospital
Sydney, Australia

Susan J. Herdman, PhD, PT
Professor and Director of Vestibular
  Rehabilitation
Department of Otolaryngology
University of Miami
School of Medicine
Miami, Florida

Michael A. Hillman, MD
Clinical Assistant Professor of Neurology
University of Wisconsin
Madison, Wisconsin
Director of the Vestibular Testing Center
Marshfield Clinic
Marshfield, Wisconsin

Vicente Honrubia, MD, DMSc
Professor
Division of Head and Neck Surgery
UCLA School of Medicine
Los Angeles, California

Fay B. Horak, PhD, PT
Senior Scientist
R.S. Dow Neurological Sciences Institute
Good Samaritan Hospital and Medical
  Center
Portland, Oregon

Emily A. Keshner, EdD, PT
Research Associate and Professor
Northwestern University School of
  Medicine
Chicago, Illinois

R. John Leigh, MD
Staff Neurologist
V.A. Medical Center
Professor
Departments of Neurology and
  Biomedical Engineering
Case Western Reserve University
Cleveland, Ohio

Douglas E. Mattox, MD
Professor and Director
Division of Otolaryngology — Head and
  Neck Surgery
University of Maryland Medical Center
Baltimore, Maryland

Mary McCandless Goodin, MEd, OTR
Occupational Therapist
Reginald S. Lourie Center for Infants
  and Young Children and
Ivymount School
Rockville, Maryland

James A. Sharpe, MD, FRCPC
Professor and Head of Neurology
University of Toronto
Director
The Toronto Hospital Neurological
  Center
Toronto, Ontario, Canada

Hiroshi Shimizu, MD
Associate Professor Emeritus
Department of Otolaryngology — Head
  and Neck Surgery
The Johns Hopkins Hospital
Baltimore, Maryland

Anne Shumway-Cook, PhD, PT
Research Coordinator
Department of Physical Therapy

Northwest Hospital
Seattle, Washington

Charlotte L. Shupert, PhD
Assistant Scientist
R.S. Dow Neurological Sciences Institute
Good Samaritan Hospital and Medical
  Center
Portland, Oregon

Ronald J. Tusa, MD, PhD
Professor and Director of the Dizziness
  and Balance Center
Department of Otolaryngology
University of Miami School of Medicine
Miami, Florida

Susan L. Whitney, PhD, PT, ATC
Assistant Professor
Departments of Physical Therapy and
  Otolaryngology
School of Health and Rehabilitation
  Sciences
University of Pittsburgh
Pittsburgh, Pennsylvania

Shirley Wietlisbach, MS, OT
Clinical Occupational Therapist and
Research Assistant
Reginald S. Lourie Center for Infants
  and Young Children and
Ivymount School
Rockville, Maryland

David S. Zee, MD
Professor of Neurology and
  Otolaryngology — Head and Neck
  Surgery
Johns Hopkins Hospital
Baltimore, Maryland

Contents

SECTION IV: Rehabilitation Assessment and Management

Chapter 18 Treatment of Vestibular Deficits in Children with
Developmental Disorders   360
Georgia A. DeGangi, PhD, OTR, FAOTA
Mary McCandless Goodin, MEd, OTR
Shirley Wietlisbach, MS, OTR

SECTION I

Fundamentals

CHAPTER 1

Anatomy and Physiology of the Normal Vestibular System

Timothy C. Hain, MD
Michael A. Hillman, MD

PURPOSE OF THE VESTIBULAR SYSTEM

The human vestibular system is made up of three components: a peripheral sensory apparatus, a central processor, and a mechanism for motor output (Fig. 1–1). The peripheral apparatus consists of a set of motion sensors that send information to the central nervous system, specifically the vestibular nucleus complex and the cerebellum, about head angular velocity, linear acceleration, and orientation of the head with respect to the gravitational axis. The central nervous system processes these signals and combines them with other sensory information to estimate head orientation. The output of the central vestibular system goes to the ocular muscles and spinal cord to serve two important reflexes, the *vestibulo-ocular reflex* (VOR) and the *vestibulospinal reflex* (VSR). The VOR generates eye movements that enable clear vision while the head is in motion. The VSR generates compensatory body movement to maintain head and postural stability, thereby preventing falls. The performance of the VOR and VSR are monitored by the central nervous system and readjusted as needed by an adaptive processor.

From a rehabilitation perspective, it is crucially important to realize that there are multiple fail-safe mechanisms closely integrated into these reflexes. The capability for repair and adaptation is so remarkable that after removal of half of the peripheral vestibular system, such as by a unilateral vestibular nerve section, finding clinical evidence of vestibular dysfunction is often quite difficult. The ability of central mechanisms to use vision, proprioception, auditory input, tactile input, or cognitive knowledge regarding an impending movement allows vestibular responses to be based on a richly textured, multimodal sensory array. With these general philosophic considerations in mind, the purpose of this chapter is to describe the anatomy and the physiologic responses of the vestibular system, paying particular attention to aspects relevant to rehabilitation. We proceed from the peripheral to central structures and conclude with a

Sensory Input   **Central Processing**   **Motor Output**

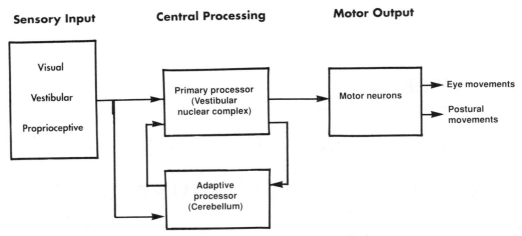

FIGURE 1–1. The organization of the vestibular system.

discussion of "higher-level" problems in vestibular physiology, which are relevant to rehabilitation.

PERIPHERAL SENSORY APPARATUS

Figure 1–2 illustrates the peripheral vestibular system in relation to the ear. The peripheral vestibular system includes the membranous and bony labyrinths and the motion sensors of the vestibular system, the hair cells. The peripheral vestibular system lies within the inner ear, which is bordered laterally by the air-filled middle ear, and

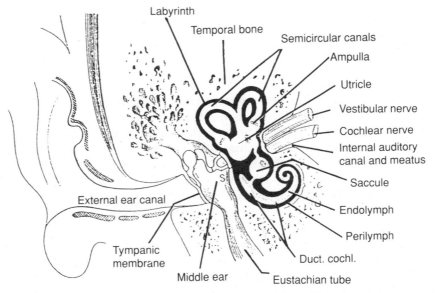

FIGURE 1–2. Anatomy of the peripheral vestibular system.

medially by temporal bone. Note that for the sake of clarity Figure 1–2 shows only two of the three semicircular canals.

Bony Labyrinth

The *bony labyrinth* (Fig. 1–3) consists of three semicircular canals and a central chamber called the *vestibule*. On Figure 1–2, the bony labyrinth is designated as the "labyrinth." The bony labyrinth is filled with perilymphatic fluid that has a similar chemistry to cerebrospinal fluid (high Na:K ratio). Perilymphatic fluid communicates via the cochlear aqueduct (not shown) with cerebrospinal fluid in the subarachnoid space.

Membranous Labyrinth

The membranous labyrinths are suspended within the bony labyrinths by fluid and supportive connective tissue. They contain five sensory organs, which are the membranous portions of the three semicircular canals and the two otolith organs, the utricle and saccule. One end of each semicircular canal is widened in diameter to form an ampulla.

The membranous labyrinths are filled with endolymphatic fluid (see Fig. 1–3). In contrast to perilymph, the electrolyte composition of endolymph resembles intracellular fluid (high K:Na ratio). Under normal circumstances, no communication exists between the endolymph and perilymph compartments.

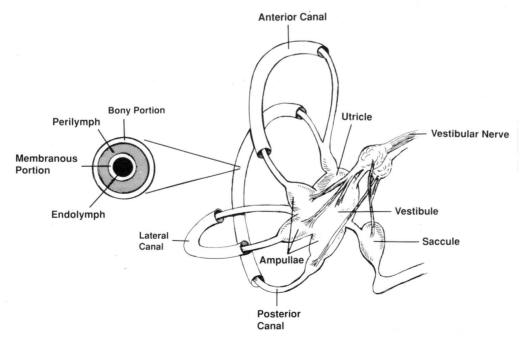

FIGURE 1–3. The membranous and bony labyrinths. The inset illustrates the perilymphatic and endolymphatic fluid compartments.

Hair Cells

Specialized hair cells suspended in each ampulla and otolith organ are biologic sensors that convert displacement due to head motion into neural firing (Fig. 1–4). The hair cells of the ampullae rest on a tuft of blood vessels, nerve fibers, and supporting tissue, called the *crista ampullaris*. The hair cells of the saccule and utricle, the maculae, are located on the medial wall of the saccule and the floor of the utricle. Each hair cell is innervated by an afferent neuron. When hairs are bent toward the longest process of the hair cell, firing rate increases in the neuron and the vestibular nerve is excited (see Fig. 1–4A). A gelatinous membrane called the *cupula* overlies each crista. The cupula causes endolymphatic flow associated with head motion to be coupled to the hair cells (see Fig. 1–4B). Similar membranes overlie the otolithic maculae.

These otolithic membranes contain calcium carbonate crystals called *otoconia* and, therefore, have substantially more mass than the cupulae (Fig. 1–5). The increased mass of the otolithic membrane causes the maculae to be sensitive to gravity. In contrast, the cupulae have the same density as the surrounding endolymphatic fluid and are insensitive to gravity.

Vascular Supply

The labyrinthine artery supplies the peripheral vestibular system (Fig. 1–6, and see Fig. 1–11). The labyrinthine artery has a variable origin. Most often it is a branch of the anterior-inferior cerebellar artery (AICA), but occasionally it is a direct branch of the

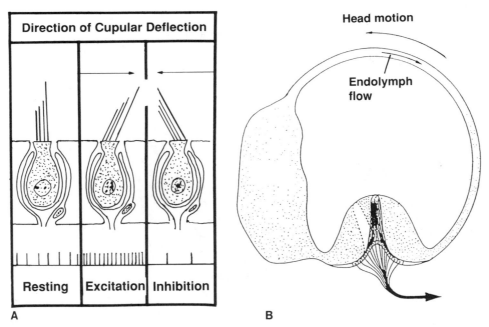

FIGURE 1–4. Effects of head rotation on the semicircular canals. (*A*) The direction from which hair cells are deflected determines whether or not hair-cell discharge frequency increases or decreases. (*B*) Endolymph flow and cupular deflection in response to head motion. (From Bach-Y-Rita, P, Collins, CC, and Hyde, JE [eds]: The Control of Eye Movements. Academic Press, New York, 1971. ©1971 IEEE, with permission.)

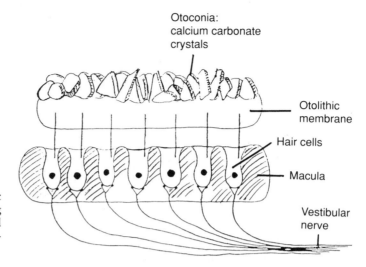

FIGURE 1–5. The otolithic macula and its overlying membrane. (From Baloh and Honrubia,[2] p 4, with permission.)

basilar artery. Upon entering the inner ear, the labyrinthine artery divides into the anterior vestibular artery and the common cochlear artery. The anterior vestibular artery supplies the vestibular nerve, most of the utricle, and the ampullae of the lateral and anterior semicircular canals. The common cochlear artery divides into a main branch, the main cochlear artery, and the vestibulocochlear artery. The main cochlear artery supplies the cochlea. The vestibulocochlear artery supplies part of the cochlea, the ampulla of the posterior semicircular canal, and the inferior part of the saccule.

The labyrinth has no collateral anastomotic network and is highly susceptible to ischemia. Only 15 seconds of selective blood flow cessation is needed to abolish auditory nerve excitability.[3,4]

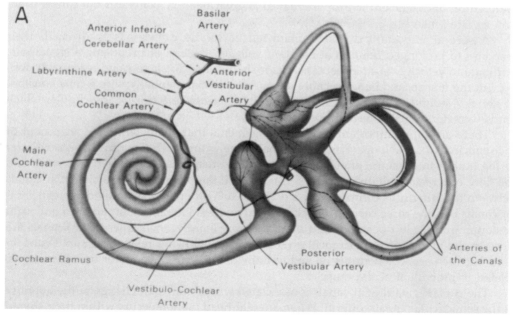

FIGURE 1–6. The arterial supply of the labyrinth. (From Schuknecht,[5] with permission.)

The hair cells of the canals and otoliths convert the mechanical energy generated by head motion into neural discharges directed to specific areas of the brain stem and the cerebellum. By virtue of their orientation, the canals and otolith organs are able to respond selectively to head motion in particular directions. By virtue of differences in the mechanics, the canals are able to respond to velocity and the otoliths to acceleration.

Semicircular Canals

The semicircular canals provide sensory input about head *velocity*, which enables the VOR to generate an eye movement that matches the velocity of the head movement. The result is that the eye remains still in space during head motion, enabling clear vision. Neural firing in the vestibular nerve is proportional to head velocity over the range of frequencies in which the head commonly moves (0.5 to 7 Hz). In engineering terms, the canals are *rate sensors*.

This fact poses a significant problem: How do the hair cells of the semicircular canals, which are activated by displacement, produce sensory input proportional to velocity? The labyrinth must contain a method of converting head velocity into displacement. Certain biophysical properties of the semicircular canal loops accomplish the conversion.[6] The membranous canal loops have very thin walls and a small-diameter lumen relative to the radius of the loop curvature. These characteristics make viscous drag on the endolymph very powerful. Viscosity is essentially fluidic friction and causes endolymph motion to be slowed down, in a way similar to how honey slowly runs down the side of a jar. In a frictionless system, for a step of constant rotational velocity, endolymph displacement would be proportional to the product of velocity times time. The viscosity creates resistance to endolymph displacement, causing rapid damping of displacement. In approximate mathematic terms, the viscosity puts a differential operator into the displacement equation, so that displacement becomes proportional to head velocity. Because of these considerations, over the usual frequencies of head movement, endolymph displacement is proportional to angular head velocity and the canals function as rate sensors.

A second important dynamic characteristic to the canals has to do with their response to prolonged rotation at constant velocity. Instead of producing a signal proportional to velocity, as a perfect rate sensor should, the canals respond reasonably well only in the first second or so, because output decays exponentially with a time constant of about 7 seconds. This behavior is owing to a springlike action of the cupula, which tends to restore it to its resting position.[4]

There are three important spatial arrangements that characterize the alignment of the semicircular canal loops. First, each canal plane within each labyrinth is *perpendicular* to the other canal planes, analogous to the spatial relationship between two walls and the floor of a rectangular room (Fig. 1–7). Second, the planes of the semicircular canals between the labyrinths conform very closely to each other. The six individual semicircular canals become three *coplanar* pairs: (1) right and left lateral, (2) left anterior and right posterior, and (3) left posterior and right anterior. Thirdly, the planes of the canals are close to the planes of the extraocular muscles, thus allowing relatively simple connections between sensory neurons related to individual canals, and motor output neurons, related to individual ocular muscles.

The coplanar pairing of canals is associated with a *push-pull* change in the quantity of the semicircular canals' output. When angular head motion occurs within their shared

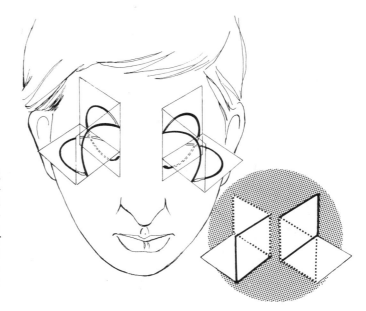

FIGURE 1–7. The spatial arrangement of the semicircular canals. The canals on each side are mutually perpendicular, paired with conjugate canals on the opposite side of the head, and closely aligned with the optimal pulling directions of the extraocular muscles.

plane, the endolymph of the coplanar pair is displaced in opposite directions, with respect to their ampullae, and neural firing increases in one vestibular nerve and decreases on the opposite side. For the lateral canals, displacement of the cupula toward the ampulla (ampullopetal flow) is excitatory, while for the vertical canals, displacement of the cupula away from the ampulla (ampullofugal flow) is excitatory.

There are three advantages to the push-pull arrangement of coplanar pairing. First, pairing provides *sensory redundancy*. If disease affects the semicircular canals' input from one member of a pair (as in vestibular neuronitis), the central nervous system will still receive vestibular information about head velocity within that plane from the contralateral member of the coplanar pair. Second, such a pairing allows the brain to ignore changes in neural firing that occur on both sides simultaneously, such as might occur owing to changes in body temperature or chemistry. These changes are not related to head motion and are *common mode noise*. The engineering term for this desirable characteristic is *common mode rejection*. Third, as will be discussed in a later section, a push-pull configuration assists in compensation for sensor overload.

Otoliths

The otoliths register forces related to linear acceleration (Fig. 1–8). They respond both to linear head motion and to static tilt with respect to the gravitational axis. The function of the otoliths is illustrated by the situation of a passenger in a commercial jet. During flight at a constant velocity, we have no sense that we are traveling at 300 miles per hour. However, in the process of taking off and ascending to cruising altitude, we sense the *change in velocity* (acceleration) as well as the *tilt* of the plane on ascent. The otoliths therefore differ from the semicircular canals in two basic ways: they respond to linear motion instead of angular motion, and they respond to acceleration rather than to velocity.[6]

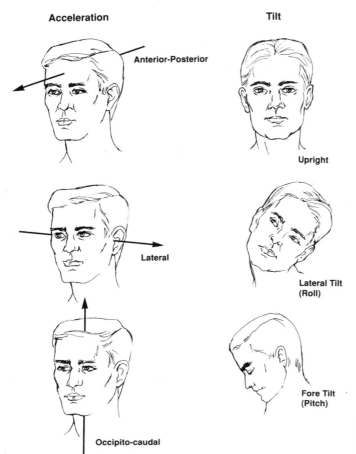

Acceleration

Anterior-Posterior

Lateral

Occipito-caudal

Tilt

Upright

Lateral Tilt
(Roll)

Fore Tilt
(Pitch)

FIGURE 1-8. The otoliths register linear acceleration and static tilt.

The otoliths have a simpler task to perform than the canals. Unlike the canals, which must convert head velocity into displacement to properly activate the hair cells of the cristae, the otoliths need no special hydrodynamic system. Exquisite sensitivity to gravity and linear acceleration is obtained by incorporating the mass of the otoconia into the otolithic membrane (see Fig. 1–5). As force equals mass times acceleration, by incorporating a large mass, a given acceleration produces enough shearing force to make the otoliths extremely sensitive (the term "shearing force" refers to force that is directed perpendicularly to the processes of the hair cells).

Like the canals, the otoliths are arranged to respond to motion in all three dimensions (Fig. 1–9). However, unlike the canals, which have one sensory organ per axis of angular motion, there are only two sensory organs for three axes of linear motion. In an upright individual, the saccule is vertical (parasagittal), while the utricle is horizontally oriented (near the plane of the lateral semicircular canals). In this posture, the saccule can sense linear acceleration in its plane, which includes the acceleration oriented along the occipitocaudal axis and also linear motion along the anterior-posterior axis. The utricle senses acceleration in its plane, which includes lateral accelerations along the interaural axis, as well anterior-posterior motion.

Because earth's gravitational field is a linear acceleration field, on earth, the otoliths register tilt. For example, as the head is tilted laterally (which is also called *roll* [see Fig.

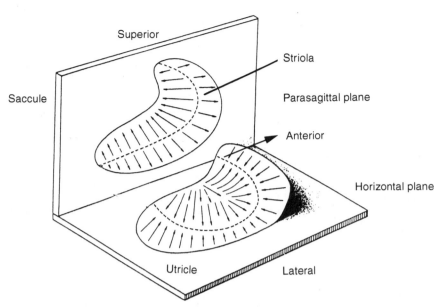

FIGURE 1–9. Geometry of the otoliths. This schematic diagram shows only orientation; the saccule is actually inferior to the utricle. (From Barber and Stockwell,[7] with permission.)

1–8]), shear force is exerted on the utricle, causing excitation, while shear force is lessened on the saccule. Similar changes occur when the head is tilted forward or backward (called *pitch*). Because linear acceleration can come from two sources, earth's gravitational field and linear motion, there is a sensor ambiguity problem. We discuss strategies that the central nervous system might use to solve this problem in Section VI.

In the otoliths, as in the canals, there is a push-pull arrangement of sensors; but in addition to splitting the sensors across sides of the head, the push-pull processing arrangement for the otoliths is also incorporated into geometry of the otolithic membranes. Within each otolithic macula, a curving zone, the *striola*, separates the direction of hair-cell polarization on each side. Consequently, head tilt results in increased afferent discharge from one part of a macula, while reducing the afferent discharge from another portion of the same macula.

THE VESTIBULAR NERVE

Vestibular nerve fibers are the afferent projections from the bipolar neurons of Scarpa's (vestibular) ganglion. The vestibular nerve transmits afferent signals from the labyrinths along its course through the internal auditory canal (IAC). In addition to the vestibular nerve, the IAC also contains the cochlear nerve (hearing); the facial nerve; the nervus intermedius (a branch of the facial nerve that carries sensation); and the labyrinthine artery. The IAC travels through the petrous portion of the temporal bone to open into the posterior fossa at the level of the pons. The vestibular nerve enters the brain stem at the pontomedullary junction. Because the vestibular nerve is interposed between the labyrinth and the brain stem, some authors consider this nerve a peripheral structure, whereas others consider it a central structure.

There are two patterns of firing in vestibular afferent neurons. *Regular afferents* usually have a tonic rate and little variability in interspike intervals. *Irregular afferents* often show no firing at rest, and when stimulated by head motion, develop highly variable interspike intervals.[8] Regular afferents appear to be the most important type for the VOR, as irregular afferents can be ablated in experimental animals without much change in the VOR. However, irregular afferents may be important for the VSR.

Regular afferents of the monkey have tonic firing rates of about 90 spikes/sec, and sensitivity to head velocity of about 0.5 spikes/deg/sec.[9,10] We can speculate about what happens immediately after a sudden change in head velocity. Humans can easily move their heads at velocities exceeding 300 deg/sec. As noted previously, the semicircular canals are connected in push-pull, so that one side is always being inhibited while the other is being excited. Given the sensitivity and tonic rate noted earlier, the vestibular nerve, which is being inhibited, should be driven to a firing rate of 0 spikes/sec, for head velocities of only 180 deg/sec! In other words, head velocities greater than 180 deg/sec may be unquantifiable by half of the vestibular system. This cutoff behavior has been advanced as the explanation for Ewald's second law, which says that responses to rotations that excite a canal are greater than for rotation that inhibits a canal.[11,12] Cutoff behavior may explain why patients with unilateral vestibular loss avoid head motion toward the side of their lesion. More will be said about this in Section VI where we discuss how the central nervous system may compensate for overload.

CENTRAL PROCESSING OF VESTIBULAR INPUT

There are two main targets for vestibular input from primary afferents, namely the vestibular nuclear complex and the cerebellum (see Fig. 1-1). The vestibular nuclear complex is the primary processor of vestibular input, and it implements direct, fast connections between incoming afferent information and motor output neurons. The cerebellum is the adaptive processor—it monitors vestibular performance and keeps it "tuned up." At both locations, vestibular sensory input is processed in association with somatosensory and visual sensory input.

Vestibular Nucleus

The vestibular nuclear complex consists of four "major" nuclei (superior, medial, lateral, and descending) and at least seven "minor" nuclei (Fig. 1-10). This large structure, located primarily within the pons, also extends caudally into the medulla. The superior and medial vestibular nuclei are relays for the VOR. The medial vestibular nucleus is also involved in vestibulospinal reflexes and coordinates head and eye movements that occur together. The lateral vestibular nucleus is the principal nucleus for the vestibulospinal reflex. The descending nucleus is connected to all of the other nuclei and the cerebellum, but it has no primary outflow of its own. The vestibular nuclei are laced together via a system of commissures, which for the most part are mutually inhibitory. The commissures allow information to be shared between the two sides of the brain stem and implement the push-pull pairing of canals discussed earlier.

In the vestibular nuclear complex, processing of the vestibular sensory input occurs concurrently with the processing of extravestibular sensory information (proprioceptive,

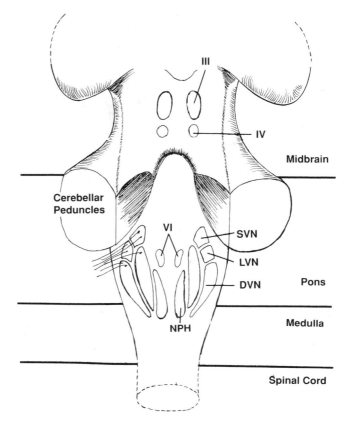

FIGURE 1–10. The vestibular nuclear complex. This section shows the brain stem with the cerebellum removed. DVN = descending vestibular nucleus; LVN = lateral vestibular nucleus; NPH = nucleus prepositus hypoglossi; III = oculomotor nucleus (inferior oblique muscle and medial, superior, and inferior rectus muscles); IV = trochlear nucleus (superior oblique muscle); VI = abducens nucleus (lateral rectus). The medial vestibular nucleus (MVN), not shown, lies between the NPH and the DVN.

visual, tactile, and auditory). Extensive connections between the vestibular nuclear complex, cerebellum, ocular motor nuclei, and brain stem reticular activating systems are required to formulate appropriate efferent signals to the VOR and VSR effector organs, the extraocular and skeletal muscles.

Vascular Supply

The *vertebro-basilar arterial system* provides the vascular supply for both the peripheral and central vestibular system (Fig. 1–11). The posterior-inferior cerebellar arteries (PICA) branch off of the vertebral arteries. They supply the surface of the inferior portions of the cerebellar hemispheres, as well as the dorsolateral medulla, which includes the inferior aspects of the vestibular nuclear complex. The *basilar artery* is the principal artery of the pons. The basilar artery supplies central vestibular structures via perforator branches, which penetrate the medial pons; short circumferential branches, which supply the anterolateral aspect of the pons; and long circumferential branches, which supply the dorsolateral pons. The AICA supplies both the peripheral vestibular system via the labyrinthine artery, as well as the ventrolateral cerebellum and the lateral tegmentum of the lower two thirds of the pons. Recognizable clinical syndromes with vestibular components may appear after occlusions of the basilar artery, the labyrinthine artery, the AICA, and the PICA.

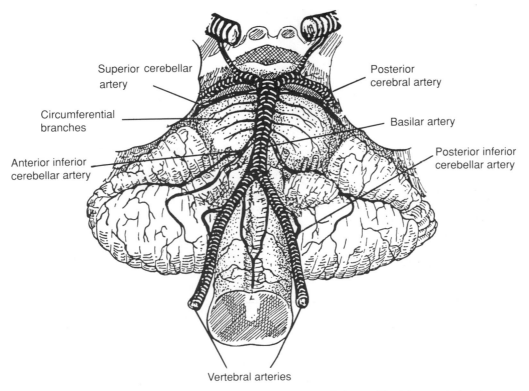

FIGURE 1-11. The vertebrobasilar system. (From Osborne,[13] with permission.)

Cerebellum

The cerebellum is a major recipient of outflow from the vestibular nucleus complex and is also a major source of input itself. Although not required for vestibular reflexes, when the cerebellum is removed, vestibular reflexes become uncalibrated and ineffective. Originally, the vestibulocerebellum was defined as the portions of the cerebellum that received direct input from the primary vestibular afferents. We now understand that most parts of the cerebellar vermis (midline) respond to vestibular stimulation. The cerebellar projections to the vestibular nuclear complex have an inhibitory influence on the vestibular nuclear complex.

The cerebellar flocculus adjusts and maintains the gain of the VOR.[14] Lesions of the flocculus reduce the ability of experimental animals to adapt to disorders that reduce or increase the gain of the VOR. Patients with *cerebellar degenerations* or the *Arnold-Chiari malformation* typically have floccular disorders.

The cerebellar nodulus adjusts the duration of VOR responses and is also involved with processing of otolith input. Patients with lesions of the cerebellar nodulus, such as patients with medulloblastoma, show gait ataxia and often have nystagmus that is strongly affected by the position of the head with respect to the gravitational axis.

Lesions of the anterior-superior vermis of the cerebellum affect the VSR and cause a profound gait ataxia with truncal instability. These patients are unable to use sensory input from their lower extremities to stabilize their posture. These lesions commonly are related to excessive alcohol intake and thiamine deficiency.

Neural Integrator

Thus far, we have discussed processing of velocity signals from the canals or acceleration signals from the otoliths. These signals are not suitable for driving the ocular motor neurons, which need a neural signal-encoding eye position. The transformation of velocity to position is accomplished by a brain stem structure called the *neural integrator*. The location of the neural integrator has been identified only recently. The nucleus prepositus hypoglossi, located just below the medial vestibular nucleus, appears to provide this function for the oculomotor system.[15] Although a similar structure must exist for the vestibulospinal system, the location of the VSR neural integrator is presently unknown.

MOTOR OUTPUT OF THE VESTIBULAR SYSTEM NEURONS

Output for the Vestibulo-ocular Reflex

The output neurons of the VOR are the motor neurons of the ocular motor nuclei, which drive the extraocular muscles. The extraocular muscles are arranged in pairs, which are oriented in planes that are very close to those of the canals. This geometric arrangement enables a single pair of canals to be connected predominantly to a single pair of extraocular muscles. The result is conjugate movements of the eyes in the same plane as head motion.

There are two white matter tracts that carry output from the vestibular nuclear complex to the ocular motor nuclei. The ascending tract of Deiters carries output from the vestibular nucleus to the ipsilateral abducens nucleus (lateral rectus) during the horizontal VOR. All other VOR-related output to the ocular motor nuclei is transmitted by the medial longitudinal fasciculus (Fig. 1–12).

Output for the Vestibulospinal Reflex

The output neurons of the VSR are the anterior horn cells of the spinal cord gray matter, which drive skeletal muscle. However, the connection between the vestibular nuclear complex and the motor neurons is more complicated than for the VOR. The VSR has a much more difficult task than the VOR, because there are multiple strategies that can be used to prevent falls that involve entirely different motor synergies. For example, when shoved from behind, one's center of gravity might become displaced anteriorly. To restore "balance," one might: (1) plantarflex at the ankles, (2) take a step, (3) grab for support, or (4) use some combination of all three activities. The VSR also has to adjust limb motion appropriately for the position of the head on the body (see the frame of reference problem discussed in Section VII), and must also use otolith input to a greater extent than does the VOR.

There are three major white matter pathways that connect the vestibular nucleus to the anterior horn cells of the spinal cord. The lateral vestibulospinal tract originates from the ipsilateral lateral vestibular nucleus, which receives the majority of its input from the otoliths and the cerebellum (see Fig. 1–12). This pathway generates antigravity postural motor activity, primarily in the lower extremities, in response to the head position

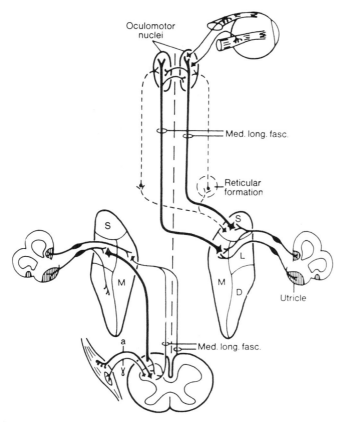

FIGURE 1–12. The vestibulo-ocular and vestibulospinal reflex arcs. S, L, M, and D indicate the superior, lateral, medial, and descending vestibular nuclei. The lateral vestibulospinal and medial vestibulospinal tracts are shown as heavy and light lines, respectively, beginning in the lateral vestibular nucleus, respectively. (From Brodal,[16] with permission.)

changes that occur with respect to gravity. The medial vestibulospinal tract originates from the contralateral medial, superior, and descending vestibular nuclei (see Fig. 1–12) and mediates ongoing postural changes in response to semicircular canal sensory input (angular head motion). The medial vestibulospinal tract descends only through the cervical spinal cord in the medial longitudinal fasciculus and activates cervical axial musculature.

The reticulospinal tract receives sensory input from all of the vestibular nuclei, as well as all of the other sensory and motor systems involved with maintaining balance. This projection has both crossed and uncrossed components and is very highly collateralized. As a result, the reticulospinal tract through the entire extent of the spinal cord is poorly defined but is probably involved in most balance reflex motor actions, including postural adjustments made to extravestibular sensory input (auditory, visual, and tactile stimuli).

VESTIBULAR REFLEXES

The sensory, central, and motor output components to the vestibular system have been described. We will now outline their combination into the VOR and the VSR.

The Vestibulo-ocular Reflex

The purpose of the VOR is to maintain stable vision during head motion. As an example, let us examine the sequence of events that occurs as a result of lateral head rotation to the right.

1. When the head turns to the right, endolymphatic flow deflects the cupulae to the left (see Fig. 1–4B).
2. The discharge rate from hair cells in the right crista increases in proportion to the velocity of the head motion, whereas the discharge rate from hair cells in the left lateral crista decreases (Fig. 1–4A).
3. These changes in firing rate are transmitted along the vestibular nerve and influence the discharge of the neurons of the medial vestibular nucleus.
4. Excitatory impulses are transmitted via white matter tracts in the brain stem to the oculomotor nuclei that activate the right (ipsilateral) medial rectus and the left (contralateral) lateral rectus. Inhibitory impulses are also transmitted to their antagonists.
5. Simultaneous contraction of the left lateral rectus and right medial rectus muscles and relaxation of the left medial rectus and right lateral rectus occurs, resulting in lateral compensatory eye movements toward the left.

The Vestibulospinal Reflex

The purpose of the VSR is to stabilize the head and body. Unlike the VOR, there is no single VSR but rather an assemblage of several reflexes that are dependent on the sensory and motor context. VSRs include the vestibulocollic reflex and tonic and dynamic labyrinthine reflexes. As an example of a VSR, let us examine the sequence of events involved in generating a tonic labyrinthine reflex.

1. When the head is tilted to one side, both the canals and otoliths are stimulated.
2. The vestibular nerve and vestibular nucleus are activated as described for the VOR.
3. Impulses are transmitted via the vestibulospinal tracts to the spinal cord.
4. Extensor activity is induced on the side to which the head is inclined, and flexor activity is induced on the opposite side.
5. The maintained limb position is derived from the otoliths.

HIGHER-LEVEL PROBLEMS IN VESTIBULAR PROCESSING

In this section, we identify some of the more sophisticated aspects of central vestibular processing, which are especially apt to be disrupted by disease, and for this reason are especially relevant to rehabilitation. The underlying theme, repeated throughout, is the multimodal nature of the vestibular system. Over and over we will see a need to resolve multiple, partially redundant sensory inputs and to produce a motor signal distributed to multiple, highly redundant motor output mechanisms.

Velocity Storage

How good does the VOR have to be? To keep the eye still in space while the head is moving, the velocity of eyes should be exactly opposite to head movement. When this happens, the ratio of eye movement to head movement amplitude, called the *gain*, equals − 1. To maintain normal vision, retinal image motion must be less than 2 deg/sec. For example, for a head velocity of 100 deg/sec, which is easily produced by an ordinary head movement, the gain of the VOR must be 98 percent accurate, because any greater error would cause vision to be obscured.

The normal VOR can deliver this high standard of performance only for brief head movements. In other words, the VOR is compensatory for high-frequency head motion but is not compensatory for low-frequency head motion. This fact can be most easily seen by considering the response of the semicircular canals to a sustained head movement, which has a constant velocity. The canals respond by producing an exponentially decaying change in neural firing in the vestibular nerve. The *time constant* of the exponential is about 7 seconds, that is, the firing rate decays to 32 percent of the initial amount in 7 seconds. Ideally, the time constant should be infinite, which would be associated with no response decline. Apparently, a time constant of 7 seconds is not long enough because the central nervous system goes to the trouble to perseverate the response and replace the peripheral time constant of 7 seconds with a central time constant of about 20 seconds. The preserveration is provided via a brain stem structure called the *velocity storage mechanism*.[17]

The velocity storage mechanism is used as a repository for information about head velocity derived from several kinds of motion sensors. During rotation in the light, the vestibular nucleus is supplied with *retinal slip* information. Retinal slip is the difference between eye velocity and head velocity. Retinal slip can drive the velocity storage mechanism and keep vestibular-related responses going even after vestibular afferent information decays away. The vestibular system also uses somatosensory and otolithic information to drive the velocity storage mechanism.[18] This example shows how the vestibular system resolves multiple, partially redundant sensory inputs.

Compensation for Overload

A second problem related to an imperfection in sensors is the response to high-velocity head movement. Humans can easily move their heads at velocities exceeding 300 deg/sec. For example, while driving in the car, if one hears a horn to the side, the head may rapidly rotate to visualize the problem and potentially avoid an impending collision. Similarly, during certain sports (e.g., racquet ball), head velocity and acceleration reach high levels. One must be able to see during these sorts of activities, but the vestibular nerve is not well suited to transmission of high-velocity signals. The reason is the cutoff behavior discussed in Section V. High-velocity head movement may cause the nerve on the inhibited side to be driven to a firing rate of 0.

In this instance, the vestibular system must depend on the excited side, which is wired in "push-pull" with the inhibited side. The inhibited side can only be driven to 0 spikes/sec, but the side being excited can be driven to much higher levels. Thus, the push-pull arrangement takes care of part of the overload problem. Note, however, that patients with unilateral vestibular loss do not have this mechanism available to deal with the overload problem and commonly are disturbed by rapid head motion toward the side of their lesion.

Sensor Ambiguity

Sensory input from the otoliths is intrinsically ambiguous, as the same pattern of otolith activation can be produced by either a linear acceleration or a tilt. In the absence of other information, we have no method of deciding whether we are being whisked off along an axis or if the whole room just tilted. Canal information may not be that useful in resolving the ambiguity, because one might be rotating *and* tilting at the same time. These sorts of problems are graphically demonstrated in subway cars and airplanes, which can both tilt and/or translate briskly.

Outside of moving vehicles, vision and tactile sensation can be used to decide what is happening. As long as one does not have to make a quick decision, these senses may be perfectly adequate. However, remember that visual input takes 80 msec to get to the vestibular nucleus, and that tactile input must be considered in the context of joint position and intrinsic neural transmission delays between the point of contact and the vestibular nuclear complex.

Another strategy that the brain can use to separate tilt from linear acceleration is *filtering*. In most instances, tilts are prolonged, while linear accelerations are brief. Neural filters that pass low and high frequencies can be used to tell one from the other. Nevertheless, in humans, evolution apparently has decided that the ambiguity problem is not worth solving. Otolith-ocular reflexes appropriate to compensate for linear acceleration or tilt do exist in darkness but are extremely weak in normal humans.[19] Stronger otolith-ocular reflexes are generally only seen in the light when vision is available to solve the ambiguity problem. Sensory ambiguity becomes most problematic for patients who have multiple sensory deficits because they cannot use other senses to formulate appropriate vestibulospinal responses.

Motion Sickness

An instructive illustration of how the brain routinely processes multiple channels of sensory information simultaneously is found in the *space motion sickness syndrome*. About 50 percent of Space Shuttle astronauts experience space motion sickness during the initial 24 to 72 hours of orbital flight. We currently think that space motion sickness is due to otolith-tilt translation.[20] The otoliths normally function in the context of a gravitational field, so that at any moment the total force acting on the otoliths is the vector sum of the force due to gravity and the force due to linear acceleration of the head, and the central nervous system expects linear acceleration to be mainly related to tilt. Linear acceleration due to gravity is usually much greater than that due to acceleration of the head. When outside of earth's gravitational field, such as is the situation for astronauts in outer space, the only source of linear acceleration is that due to head acceleration. In susceptible individuals, the central nervous system continues to interpret linear acceleration as being primarily related to tilt, which is now untrue, causing the motion sickness syndrome.[20,21]

Repair

Thus far, we have described some of the problems posed by the limitations of the vestibular sensor apparatus and the constraints of physics. In normal individuals, these problems can be satisfactorily resolved by relying on redundancy of sensory input and central signal processing. In addition to these intrinsic problems, there are also extrinsic problems that are related to ongoing changes in sensory apparatus, central processing capabilities, and motor output channels. Because being able to see while one's head is moving and avoiding falls is so important to survival, the *repair facility* of the vestibular system must be considered as an integral part of its physiology, and for this reason, it is our final topic.

Adaptive plasticity for peripheral vestibular lesions is dealt with elsewhere in this volume. Suffice it to say that repair is amazingly competent, even enabling the vestibular system to adapt to peculiar sensory situations requiring a reversal of the VOR.[22] However, one should consider the high degree of *context dependency* to the repair of peripheral vestibular lesions. Adaptations learned within one sensory context may not work within another. For example, a patient who can stabilize gaze on a target with the head upright may not be able to do so when making the same head movements from a supine posture. Experimentally, in the cat, VOR gain adaptations can be produced that depend on the orientation of the head.[23] Similarly, when the VOR of cats is trained using head movements of low frequency, no training effect is seen at high frequencies.[24]

Another type of context dependency relates to the VSRs, and has to do with the difference in reference frames between the head and body. Because the head can move on the body, information about how the head is moving may be rotated with respect to the body. For example, consider the situation when the head is turned 90 degrees to the right. In this situation, the coronal plane of the head is aligned with the sagittal plane of the body, and motor synergies intended to prevent a fall for a given vestibular input must also be rotated by 90 degrees. For example, patients with vestibular impairment who undergo gait training in which all procedures are performed only in a particular head posture (such as upright) may show little improvement in natural situations where the head assumes other postures, such as looking down at one's feet. Little is understood about the physiology of context dependency.

Repair of central lesions is much more limited than that available for peripheral lesions; this is the Achilles' heel of the vestibular apparatus. Symptoms caused by central lesions last much longer than symptoms due to peripheral vestibular problems. The reason for this vulnerability is not difficult to understand. To use an analogy, if your television breaks down, you can take it to the repair shop and get it fixed. If, however, your television is broken and the repair shop is closed, you have a much bigger problem. The cerebellum fulfills the role of the repair shop for the vestibular system. When there are cerebellar lesions, or lesions in the pathways to and from the cerebellum, symptoms of vestibular dysfunction can be profound and permanent. Clinicians use this reasoning when they attempt to separate peripheral from central vestibular lesions. A spontaneous nystagmus, which persists over several weeks, is generally caused by a central lesion, because a peripheral nystagmus can be repaired by an intact brain stem and cerebellum.

SUMMARY

The vestibular system is an old and sophisticated human control system. Accurate processing of sensory input about rapid head and postural motion is difficult, as well as critical to survival. Not surprisingly, the body uses multiple, partially redundant sensory inputs and motor outputs, combined with a competent central repair capability. The system as a whole can withstand and adapt to major amounts of peripheral vestibular dysfunction. The Achilles' heel of the vestibular system is a relative inability to repair central vestibular dysfunction.

REFERENCES

1. Bach-Y-Rita, P, Collins, CC, and Hyde, JE (eds): The Control of Eye Movements. Academic Press, New York, 1971.
2. Baloh, RW and Honrubia, V: Clinical Neurophysiology of the Vestibular System. FA Davis, Philadelphia, 1990.
3. Ledoux, A: Les canaux semi-circulares Etude electrophysiologique: Contribution a l'effort d'uniformisation des epreuves vestibulaires. Essai d'interpretation de la semiologie vestibulaire. Acta Oto-Rhino-Laryngol, Belgica. 12:109, 1958.
4. Perlman, HB, Kimura, RS, and Fernandez, C: Experiments on temporary obstruction of the internal auditory artery. Laryngoscope 69:591, 1959.
5. Schuknecht, HF: Pathology of the Ear. Harvard University Press, Cambridge, Massachusetts, 1974.
6. Wilson, VJ and Jones, MJ: Mammalian Vestibular Physiology. Plenum Press, New York, 1979.
7. Barber, HO and Stockwell, CW: Manual of Electronystagmography. CV Mosby, St. Louis, 1976.
8. Goldberg, JM and Fernandez, C: Physiology of peripheral neurons innervating semicircular canals of the squirrel monkey. I. Resting discharge and response to constant angular acceleration. J Neurophysiol 34:634, 1971.
9. Fernandez, C and Goldberg, JM: Physiology of peripheral neurons innervating semicircular canals of the squirrel monkey. II. Response to sinusoidal stimulation and dynamics of the peripheral vestibular system. J Neurophysiol 34:661, 1971.
10. Miles, FA and Braitman, DJ: Long term adaptive changes in primate vestibulo-ocular reflex. II. Electrophysiological observations and semicircular canal primary afferents. J Neurophysiol 43:1426, 1980.
11. Baloh, RW, Honrubia, V, and Konrad HR: Ewald's second law re-evaluated. Acta Otolaryngol 83:474, 1977.
12. Ewald, R: Physiologische Untersuchungen ueber das endorgan des nervus octavus. Bergmann, Wiesbaden, 1892.
13. Osborne, AG: Introduction to Cerebral Angiography. Harper & Row, New York, 1980.
14. Robinson, DA: Adaptive gain control of the vestibulo-ocular reflex by the cerebellum. J Neurophysiol 39:995, 1976.
15. Cannon, SC and Robinson, DA: Loss of the neural integrator of the oculomotor system from brain stem lesions in the monkey. J Neurophysiol 57:1383, 1987.
16. Brodal, A: Neurological Anatomy in Relation to Clinical Medicine, ed 3. Oxford University Press, New York, 1981.
17. Raphan, T, Matsuo, V, and Cohen, B: Velocity storage in the vestibulo-ocular reflex arc (VOR). Exp Brain Res 35:229, 1979.
18. Hain, TC: A model of the nystagmus induced by off-vertical axis rotation. Biological Cybernetics 54:337, 1986.
19. Israel, I and Berthoz, A: Contribution of the otoliths to the calculation of linear displacement. J Neurophysiol 62:247, 1989.
20. Parker, DE, et al: Otolith tilt-translation reinterpretation following prolonged weightlessness: Implications for preflight training. Aviat Space Environ Med 56:601, 1985.
21. Oman, CM, et al: MIT/Canadian vestibular experiments on the spacelab-1 mission: 4. Space motion sickness: Symptoms, stimuli and predictability. Exp Brain Res 64:316, 1986.
22. Gonshor, A and Melvill Jones, G: Extreme vestibulo-ocular adaptation induced by prolonged optical reversal of vision. J Physiol (Lond) 256:381, 1976.
23. Baker, J, Wickland, C, and Peterson, B: Dependence of cat vestibulo-ocular reflex direction adaptation on animal orientation during adaptation and rotation in darkness. Brain Res 408:339, 1987.
24. Godeaux, E, Halleux, J, and Gobert, C: Adaptive change of the vestibulo-ocular reflex in the cat: The effects of a long-term frequency selective procedure. Exp Brain Res 49:28, 1983.

CHAPTER 2

Role of the Vestibular System in Postural Control

Fay B. Horak, PhD, PT
Charlotte L. Shupert, PhD

One of the most important tasks of the human postural control system is that of balancing the body over the small base of support provided by the feet. As a sensor of gravity, the vestibular system is one of the nervous system's most important tools in controlling posture. The vestibular system is *both a sensory and a motor system*. As a sensory system, the vestibular system provides the central nervous system (CNS) with information about the position and motion of the head and the direction of gravity. The CNS uses this information, together with information from other sensory systems, to construct a picture (sometimes called a "model" or "schema" or an "internal representation" or "map") of the position and movement of the entire body and the surrounding environment. In addition to providing sensory information, the vestibular system also contributes directly to motor control. The CNS uses descending motor pathways that receive vestibular and other types of information to control static head and body positions and to coordinate postural movements.

Because the vestibular system is both a sensory and a motor system, it plays many different roles in postural control. In this chapter we explore the four most important roles (Fig. 2–1). First, we discuss the role of the vestibular system in the sensation and perception of position and motion. Second, we discuss its role in orienting the head and body to vertical, including the static alignment of the head and body and the selection of appropriate sensory cues for postural orientation in different sensory environments. These two roles are primarily sensory in nature; the vestibular system provides the sensory information about head motion and position and the direction of gravity that the CNS needs to carry out these functions. Third, we discuss the role of the vestibular system in controlling the position of the body's center of mass, both for static positions and dynamic movements; and fourth, we discuss its role in stabilizing the head during postural movements. These two roles involve motor aspects of the vestibular system.

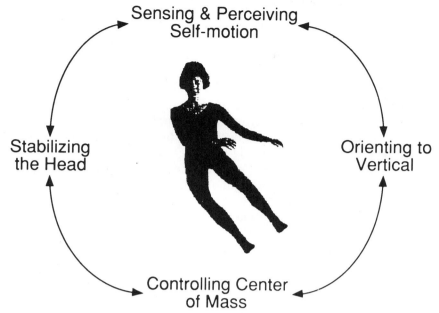

FIGURE 2–1. Four important roles of the vestibular system in postural control. The vestibular system interacts with other sensory and motor systems to accomplish tasks like maintaining equilibrium and body alignment on an unstable surface.

SENSING AND PERCEIVING POSITION AND MOTION

The vestibular system provides information about the movement of the head and its position with respect to gravity and other inertial forces (like those generated by moving vehicles). Therefore, this system contributes important information to the sensation and perception of the motion and position of the body as a whole. The vestibular system consists of two types of motion sensors, the *semicircular canals* and the *otoliths*. The canals sense rotational movement of the head. Rotational movements in the sagittal and frontal planes are detected by the vertical (anterior and posterior) canals. The horizontal canals are sensitive to motions in the horizontal plane. The largest head motions during quiet stance and walking or running occur in the sagittal (anterior-posterior) plane. Frontal plane (side to side) and horizontal plane (as if to shake the head "no") movements also occur, but they are smaller.[1] Information from all three sets of canals contributes directly to the perception of self-motion.

In contrast to the canals, which sense rotational motion, the *otoliths* sense linear accelerations. Vertical linear accelerations of the head, like the head translations generated during deep knee bends, are sensed by the *saccular otoliths*. Horizontal linear accelerations, like the translations of the head generated during walking forward, are sensed by the *utricular otoliths*. The otolith organs also provide information about the direction of gravity. Gravity, which is also a linear acceleration, produces an otolith signal that changes systematically as the head is tilted. The CNS uses this signal to determine head alignment with respect to gravitational vertical.

As important as good vestibular function is for determining the position and motion of the body, vestibular information by itself is not enough. First, the vestibular system can only provide information about head movements and not the position or movement of any of the other body segments. Second, vestibular information about head movements can be amibiguous. A signal from the vertical canals indicating anterior head rotation can be produced by the head flexing on the neck or by the body flexing at the waist, but the vestibular system alone cannot distinguish between the two. In addition to these problems, the vestibular system is not equally sensitive to the entire range of possible head movements. The semicircular canals are most sensitive to faster head movements, such as those that occur at heel strike during gait or as a result of a sudden trip or slip.[2-4] The canals respond poorly to slower head movements, such as the slow drifting movements that occur during quiet stance. The otolith organs can signal tilts with respect to gravity and slow, drifting movements, but only when these movements are linear, rather than rotational.[5-8]

To clarify the ambiguities inherent in vestibular information and to get good sensory information about the entire range of possible head and body movements, the CNS relies on information from all available sensory systems. Each sensory system contributes a different important kind of information about body position and motion to the CNS, and each sensory system is most sensitive to particular types of motion.[9-14] The *visual system* signals the position and movement of the head with respect to surrounding objects. The visual system can provide the CNS with the information necessary to determine whether a signal from the otoliths corresponds to a tilt with respect to gravity or a linear translation of the head. The visual system also provides information about the direction of vertical, because walls and door frames are typically aligned vertically, parallel to gravity. The visual system provides good information about slow movements or static tilts of the head with respect to the visual environment.[11,15,16]

In contrast to vision, the *somatosensory system* provides information about the position and motion of the body with respect to its support surface and about the position and motion of body segments with respect to each other. For example, somatosensory information can help the CNS distinguish whether a head rotation signal from the vertical canals is owing to motion of the head on the neck or owing to flexion of the body at the waist. The somatosensory system can also provide information about how body segments are aligned with respect to each other and the support surface by providing information about muscle stretch and joint position at the ankle or more proximal joints. The somatosensory system is particularly sensitive to fast movements, like those generated by sudden perturbations of joint positions.[17]

The contribution of each sensory system to the sensation of self-motion has been demonstrated experimentally by stimulating the individual sensory systems. Electrical stimulation of the vestibular nerve by means of current passed through electrodes placed on the skin over the mastoid bone produces sensations of self-motion or tilt in humans by mimicking the vestibular signals that would be generated by an actual head movement.[18,19] Similar results can be achieved by presenting subjects with large moving visual scenes (Fig. 2-2).[11,16,20-22] When the head is moved, the image of the entire visual scene moves in the opposite direction. When subjects watch a large moving visual scene, the CNS often misinterprets the visual stimulus, and the observers feel self-motion in the opposite direction. Vibrating tendons in the neck and legs, which stimulate somatosensory motion detectors, can also give rise to sensations of body motion.[9,23,24]

The perception of self-motion and orientation depends on more than sensory cues alone, however. What the subject predicts and knows about the sensory environment or what the subject has experienced in the past (sometimes called the subject's "central

FIGURE 2–2. Visual information can be used to determine how the body is moving. In this and all subsequent stick figures, the asterisk corresponds to the position of the body's center of mass, which is located about 2 cm in front of the spinal column at the level of the pelvis. As the body sways forward (*B*) visual objects placed in front of the subject loom toward the observer. If visual objects are moved toward a stationary observer (*C*), the observer can experience an illusion of forward sway (*dotted arrow*), especially in cases of vestibular loss.

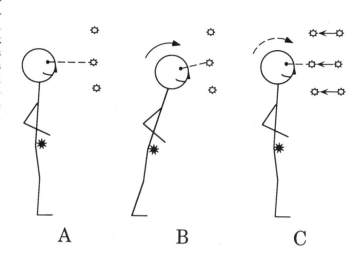

A   B   C

set'') can contribute powerfully to how sensory signals are interpreted.[25] For example, imagine two cars stopped next to each other at a traffic light. If one car moves forward slightly, the driver of the second car may step on the brake, mistakenly believing that his or her car has rolled backward. This illusion is very powerful, because cars often do roll backward when stopped, as most drivers know. The "central set" of the driver is to expect his or her car to move, and so the driver accepts the visual motion cue, despite the fact that both the vestibular and somatosensory systems indicate that the driver has not moved. This phenomenon has also been demonstrated in the laboratory. Subjects seated in a stationary chair who observe a large moving visual scene may perceive either chair motion or visual scene motion, depending on whether they are asked to concentrate on visual or somatosensory cues.[26] This observation is particularly interesting because these illusions of motion occur despite the fact that the vestibular system is signaling no motion in either case.

Given the vestibular system's important role in the sensation of self-motion, it is not surprising that patients with vestibular disorders often have abnormal perceptions of self-motion. Patients may report that they feel themselves spinning or rocking or that the room appears to spin around them. These sensations may be associated with particular head positions, depending on the disorder. Patients may adopt leaning postures while insisting that they feel themselves aligned vertically, indicating that self-motion perception and automatic postural responses may be independent of each other to some degree. Patients with profound losses of vestibular function have difficulty determining how they are moving in environments lacking good visual and somatosensory orientation cues, such as walking at night on a sandy beach or swimming in muddy water.

In summary, the vestibular system, along with other sensory systems, provides the CNS with the information about body motion and position with respect to vertical that is critical for sensing and perceiving self-motion. No sensory system alone provides all of the necessary information for sensing motion of the whole body; each sensory system contributes different and necessary information. In the next section, we explore how sensory information is used by the CNS to align the body to vertical, and how the CNS selects sensory information for body orientation in different environments.

ORIENTING THE BODY TO VERTICAL

Keeping the body properly aligned parallel to gravity and directly over the feet is one of the most important goals of the postural control system. The vestibular system, which can detect the direction of gravity, plays a very important role in maintaining the orientation of the whole body to vertical. Because the term "orientation" also includes the alignment of body segments other than the head with respect to each other and with respect to vertical, other sensory systems contribute to body orientation as well. In this section, we discuss the role of the vestibular system in the orientation of the head and body to vertical and how the nervous system selects appropriate sensory information for orientation in different sensory environments.

Postural Alignment

Spinal radiographs and fluoroscopy have revealed that most vertebrates hold the cervical spine parallel to gravitational vertical.[27] The vestibular system, which signals the direction of gravity, plays an important, but not exclusive, role in the head and body alignment in animals. Unilateral vestibular lesions in animals result in head and body tilts toward the lesioned side.[27] These head and body tilts are most severe and longest lasting in lower species.[28,29] The amount of asymmetric posturing gradually diminishes over time, and the return to normal postural alignment has been considered a sign of vestibular compensation.[30]

The vestibular system also plays an important role in the alignment of the head and body with respect to gravity in humans. Galvanic stimulation of the vestibular system results in tonic head tilts and weight shifts in normal humans.[18,19] The effect of unilateral vestibular lesions on postural alignment is more variable and more short-lived in humans than in animals, however. Humans with sudden loss of vestibular function on one side can also show lateral flexion of the head to the side of the loss during the acute phase of the lesion.[29] Bilateral loss of vestibular function may be associated with a forward head position.[31] Altered postural alignment, sometimes associated with excessive muscle tension and pain, especially in the neck, is a familiar problem for patients with vestibular dysfunction.[32]

In addition to head tilts, the entire body seems to shift, temporarily, to the side of vestibular loss. Patients with unilateral vestibular lesions shift their weight to the side of their lesions and then regain normal weight distribution over the course of several weeks.[33] Fukuda[34] developed a stepping-in-place test to document the asymmetry and gradual compensation that follow unilateral vestibular loss. In this test, subjects attempt to step in place with eyes closed, and patients with unilateral losses typically rotate slowly toward the side of the lesion. Patients with bilateral vestibular loss have also been reported to shift their weight forward or backward.[35]

One hypothetic explanation for the altered postural alignment of patients with vestibular deficits is that the vestibular lesion has resulted in an altered internal map of body orientation in space. Gurfinkel and colleagues[12] have suggested that the CNS constructs a model or internal map of the direction of gravity based on vestibular and other sensory information and that the CNS aligns the body according to this map. In patients with vestibular disorders, the internal map may be faulty, resulting in faulty body or head alignment. Vestibular information also contributes to another important internal map, the map of "stability limits," and vestibular pathology may lead to defects in this internal map as well. A human standing with feet planted on the ground may sway forward or backward a small amount (about 4 degrees backward and about 8 degrees forward) without losing balance and taking a step. The boundaries of the area over which an individual may safely sway are called the *stability limits*.[36] The actual stability limits for any individual in any situation are determined by biomechanical constraints, such as the firmness and size of the base of support, and by neuromuscular constraints, such as strength and swiftness of muscle responses.[37] Vestibular pathology might result in a poor match between a patient's actual stability limits and the internal map of those limits. The internal map could be smaller or larger than the actual stability limits, or the map could be poorly aligned with respect to gravity. As a result, patients may align themselves near the edges of their actual stability limits. Because visual and somatosensory information may substitute for vestibular information, alignment may be normal in patients with well-compensated vestibular losses, but may be very abnormal in patients with deficits in multiple sensory systems. Figure 2–3 shows a patient with bilateral loss of vestibular function, peripheral neuropathy, and cataracts, who aligns herself near her backward limits of stability in stance.

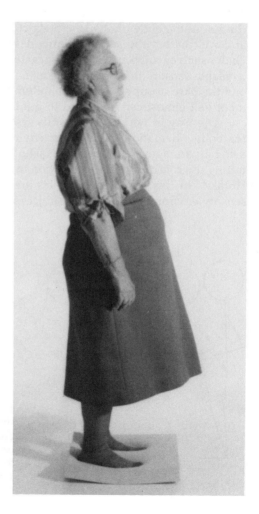

FIGURE 2–3. Elderly woman with loss of vestibular function, peripheral neuropathy, and cataracts who aligns herself near her backward limits of stability. In this photograph, she is standing on a compliant foam pad, which decreases her ability to use somatosensory cues for orientation.

Selecting Sensory Information

The studies of abnormal body alignment resulting from vestibular lesions show that the vestibular system plays an important role in the orientation of the body in space. The fact that normal alignment can be recovered with time even following bilateral vestibular loss, however, also argues that vestibular information is not the only source of sensory information that can be used for orientation. Visual and proprioceptive information also contribute to body alignment, as experiments with large, moving visual surrounds and tendon vibrations have shown.[16,20-23] Whether and how vestibular or other sensory information is used for orientation depends, in part, on the sensory information available in the environment.

Under normal conditions (i.e., a stable support surface and well-lighted visual environment), orientation information from all three sensory modalities is available and is congruent; that is, all three modalities yield similar estimates of body position and motion. There are, however, many environmental conditions in which the sensory orientation references are not congruent with each other. For example, when the support surface is compliant (like mud, sand, or a raft floating on water) or uneven (like a ramp or rocky ground), the position of the ankle joint and other somatosensory and proprioceptive information from the feet and legs may bear little relationship to the orientation of the rest of the body; that is, the body could be aligned parallel to the direction of gravity and well within the stability limits despite large amounts of ankle motion (Fig. 2–4). Under such circumstances, it is critical that the nervous system be able to extract from the available sensory information the actual orientation of the body with respect to gravity and the base of support, because failure to align the body properly in a gravity environment will almost certainly lead to a fall.

The way in which the nervous system selects the appropriate sensory information for body orientation in different environments has been investigated experimentally using a paradigm developed by Nashner and his colleagues.[38-40] A similar protocol for testing the role of sensory interaction in balance was developed by Shumway-Cook and Horak.[41] In this paradigm, subjects are asked to stand quietly in each of six different sensory environments, and the subject's postural sway is measured. In the first environ-

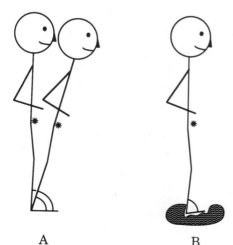

A   B

FIGURE 2–4. When subjects stand on a flat, firm support (A), ankle flexion corresponds to a forward body position. When the support surface is compliant or tilted, however, (B), ankle flexion can correspond to an upright or even backward body position. Thus, vestibular information is more important for postural control in (B) than in (A).

ment, the subject's support surface and visual surround are fixed to the earth, and the subject stands with eyes open; the second is the same, but the subject stands with eyes closed. This part of the test is equivalent to the standard Romberg test used in clinical evaluations of standing balance.

In the remaining four environments, either the support surface or the visual surround or both are moved in proportion to the subject's postural sway. This type of stimulation is referred to as "sway-referencing" (Fig. 2–5). By sway-referencing the support surface and/or the visual surround, the normal sensory feedback relationships between the different sensory systems can be disrupted. For example, when the support surface is sway-referenced, somatosensory information from the ankle joints correlates poorly with the position of the body. Support surface sway-referencing can be mimicked by placing the subject on compliant foam, and visual sway-referencing can be mimicked by placing a striped dome over the subject's head.[41] Vestibular information gives a more accurate estimate of body position and motion under these circumstances, and the CNS should rely more heavily on vestibular information for orientation.

Figure 2–6 shows how normal subjects react when exposed to such altered sensory environments. Normal subjects sway a small amount even under normal circumstances (condition 1), and this sway increases slightly when visual information is removed by eye closure (condition 2). Although sway increases slightly more when either the visual surround alone (condition 3) or the support surface (condition 4) alone is sway-referenced, subjects are still able to select useful sensory information from the sources available and maintain body orientation with respect to gravity. Even when the support surface is sway-referenced and visual information is eliminated by eye closure (condition 5) or altered by sway-referencing (condition 6), normal subjects are able to use vestibular cues to orient the body, albeit somewhat less efficiently. This is not surprising; conditions 5 and 6 are similar to walking on uneven surfaces in poorly lit environments (Fig. 2–7), swimming in murky water, or standing in the cabin of a ship, which are all tasks that normal persons can do without great difficulty.

Patients with clinically diagnosed vestibular disorders have also been tested using the same paradigm.[38–41] One of the most important findings from these studies is that not all patients with vestibular disorders respond in the same way. Patients identified in Figure 2–6 as "type I" lost all sense of orientation and fell in conditions 5 and 6, in which orientation information from both the surface and vision has been altered, and the

FIGURE 2–5. "Sway-referencing" the subject's support surface and visual surround interferes with the ability to use somatosensory and visual information to orient the body to vertical. In (A), the subject stands aligned to vertical, and the center of mass projects directly over the foot. In (B), the subject has swayed forward, resulting in a toe-down rotation of the platform and a forward rotation of the visual surround. Although the ankle angle and the position of the head with respect to the visual surround have not changed, the center of mass is now in front of the foot, and the subject is in imminent danger of a fall. Normal subjects can detect this forward sway using vestibular information and avoid a fall, but patients with vestibular losses have difficulty doing so.

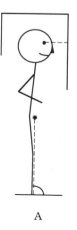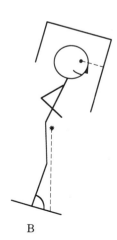

A   B

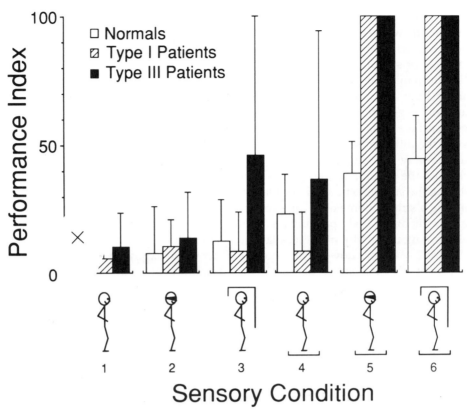

FIGURE 2–6. Median postural sway (as a percentage of the maximum sway possible without a fall) and 95th percentile limits for normal subjects and two groups of vestibular patients in six different sensory conditions. Stick figures along the abscissa show the sensory information available in each condition. Blindfold indicates eyes closed; a box around the feet indicates that the platform was sway-referenced; and a box around the head indicates a sway-referenced visual surround.

subject is forced to rely more heavily on vestibular information. One should note, however, that these patients performed as well as normal persons in conditions 1 to 4, in which at least one unaltered source of sensory information was available to them. In conditions 5 and 6, however, these patients appear to use vestibular information that is missing or abnormal. This pattern of results is typical of patients with long-standing, well-compensated bilateral losses of peripheral vestibular function. The fact that patients with well-compensated vestibular losses can use visual or somatosensory information to orient the body limits the sensitivity and specificity of the standard Romberg test as a test of vestibular function.[42]

In contrast to the type I patients, type III patients, who had uncompensated vestibular disorders, showed increased sway in conditions 3 to 6 (see Fig. 2–6). That is, they had difficulty with orientation whenever somatosensory information was altered or not available. Why type III patients have difficulty orienting in conditions 3 and 4, which have normal somatosensory and visual information (respectively), is not clear. They probably have chosen to orient their bodies to visual or support surface references that correspond poorly to gravity. Some investigators have hypothesized that some humans are predisposed to "weight" (i.e., to rely more heavily on) sensory information from a

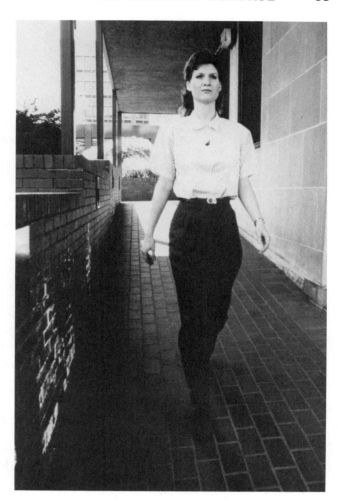

FIGURE 2-7. Walking in a poorly lighted environment on an uneven surface like a ramp puts demands on vestibular information for postural control.

particular source, like vision or somatosensation,[14,26] particularly when vestibular cues to orientation are unreliable. Incomplete CNS adaptation to a vestibular lesion may also be a factor. This pattern of results is typical of patients in the acute stages of vestibular lesions. Patients who undergo postural testing shortly after surgery to destroy vestibular function on one side perform similarly to patients in type III.[43] However, as these patients recover and the CNS adapts to the vestibular loss, their results come to resemble those of type I patients, and many eventually return to normal sensory orientation for postural control.

In summary, these studies show that vestibular information for body orientation is most important in environments that lack good somatosensory or visual cues for orientation. Patients attempting to rely on faulty or missing vestibular information in these environments may align themselves poorly and fall. However, they may also choose another source of orientation information, regardless of its usefulness, when vestibular information is bad or missing. Figure 2-8A shows a healthy child who maintains a normal orientation with respect to gravitational vertical despite standing on a tilted surface. Figure 2-8B shows a child with abnormal vestibular function who appears to rely most heavily on surface information for orientation; he maintains a perpendicular

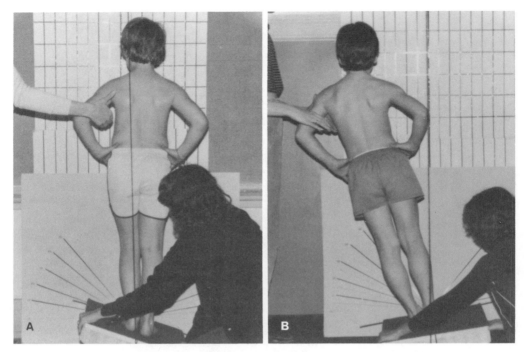

FIGURE 2–8. (*A*) Child with normal vestibular function orienting head and body with respect to gravity while surface is tipped and eyes are closed. (*B*) Child with absent vestibular function orienting head and body with respect to the tipped surface while eyes are closed.

orientation to his tilted support surface. If the support surface is orthogonal with respect to gravity, this strategy may work fairly well. However, when the support surface is tilted, as it is in Figure 2–8, this strategy works poorly.

Although the subject shown in Figure 2–8*B* chooses somatosensory information for orientation, other vestibular patients behave as if they rely most heavily on vision for orientation and sway or fall when attempting to stand near large moving objects (like buses or cars). These patients appear to misinterpret the movement of external objects as self-motion in the opposite direction. As a result, they may throw themselves into disequilibrium as they attempt to maintain a constant orientation with reference to the moving visual object. Thus, vestibular patients may either align themselves with a faulty vestibular estimate of the direction of gravity or may align themselves with an estimate of the direction of gravity from another sensory system.

CONTROLLING CENTER OF BODY MASS

The previous sections described how the vestibular system detects the position and motion of the head and how this sensory information is used for postural orientation. This section will describe how motor output from the vestibular system contributes to static body positions and dynamic postural movements that help subserve the postural goal of maintaining equilibrium or controlling the center of body mass within its limits of stability. We know from anatomic studies that motor output pathways leave the central vestibular nuclei and descend in the spinal cord, where they terminate on the neurons that activate neck, trunk, and limb muscles. However, the functional significance of the descending vestibular system for the control of orientation and equilibrium in alert intact humans and animals is still poorly understood. Nevertheless, there is evidence that vestibular signals probably play a variety of roles, including tonically activating antigravity (extensor) muscles, triggering postural responses, contributing to the selection of appropriate postural strategies for the environmental conditions, and coordinating head and trunk movements.

Orientation and equilibrium represent two distinct postural goals. To accomplish some tasks, greater priority must be placed on achieving a specific postural orientation, at the cost of postural equilibrium. For example, an experienced soccer or volleyball player may make contact with a ball even though making contact requires falling to the ground. Other tasks require equilibrium at the cost of postural orientation. For example, balancing across a wire may require rapid hip flexions and extensions to maintain equilibrium. In this task, trunk orientation with respect to vertical is sacrificed to achieve the goal of equilibrium. The way in which the CNS achieves the trade-off between control of orientation and control of equilibrium in postural tasks is not well understood. Both static positions and dynamic movements require a system that prioritizes behavioral goals and uses all the sensory information available to effectively and efficiently control the limbs and trunk to achieve both orientation and equilibrium.

Role in Static Positions

Magnus[44] was the first to investigate the role of descending vestibulospinal pathways in the control of static body position, and he used decerebrate animals to isolate the vestibulospinal system from other higher motor centers. He described reflexive movements of the limbs elicited by different head positions in decerebrate cats, and these descriptions were later refined and modified by Roberts.[45,46] Placing the head in different positions with respect to gravity and with respect to the body modifies activity in both the vestibular end organs and neck afferents (muscle spindles, joint receptors, etc.), which in turn affect limb muscle activity through the vestibulospinal (VSR) and cervicospinal (CSR) reflex pathways (see Chapter 1). To determine the role of the vestibular system alone, decerebrate animals are tilted in the dark with the head fixed to the trunk. To determine the role of neck afferents alone, the heads of decerebrate animals are held in a fixed position with reference to gravity, and the body is tilted with respect to the head. The combined effect of CSR and VSR can be examined by tilting both the head with respect to gravity and the neck with respect to the trunk.

In these experiments, Roberts[46] found that VSR and CSR seem to oppose each other in their effect on limb musculature. These effects are illustrated in Figure 2–9, which shows the nine different head and neck postures used in his experiment and their resulting effects on limb position. Normal neutral stance is shown in the center panel of Figure 2–9. When the cat's head and body were tilted nose-up (stimulating the vestibular system alone), forelimb flexion was observed (Fig. 2–9, column 1, middle panel). When the cat's body was elevated to produce nose-up cervical stimulation alone, forelimb extension was observed (Fig. 2–9, column 2, top panel). When the two reflexes were evoked simultaneously, limb position did not change (column 1, top panel), presumably because the two reflexes canceled each other.

Magnus[44] hypothesized that the functional effect of this observed reflex cancellation is to permit the head to move independently with respect to the body without altering

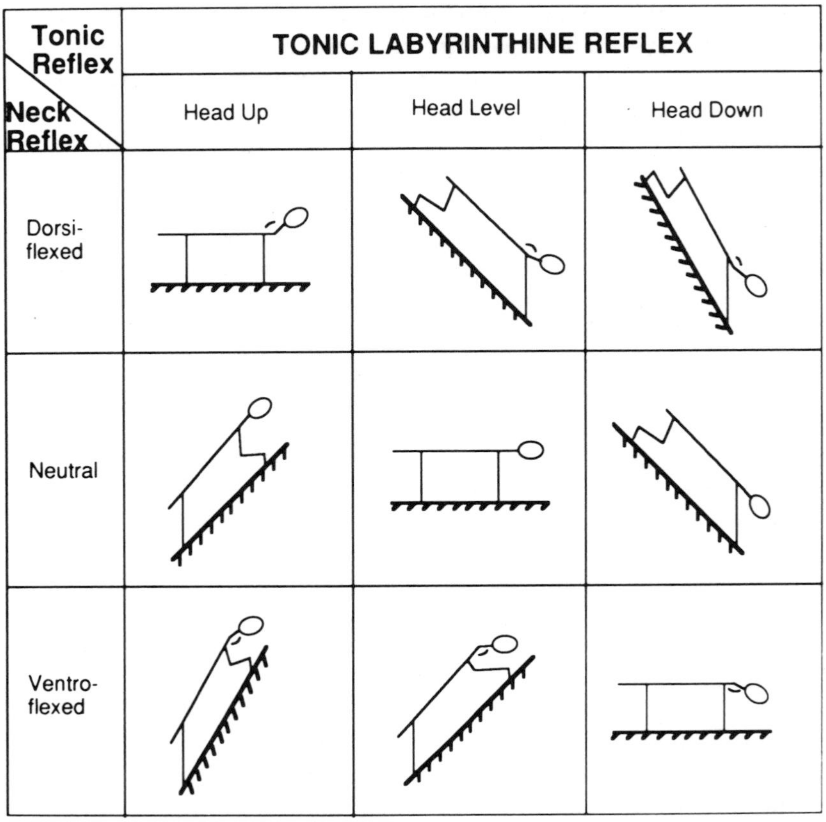

Tonic Reflex / Neck Reflex	TONIC LABYRINTHINE REFLEX		
	Head Up	Head Level	Head Down
Dorsi-flexed			
Neutral			
Ventro-flexed			

FIGURE 2–9. Effects of tonic neck and labyrinthine reflexes in the forelimbs and hindlimbs of decerebrate cats. (Adapted from Roberts.[46])

limb muscle activity. Roberts[45] later proposed a second hypothesis: Simultaneous head and neck tilts would probably occur during stance on uneven or inclined surfaces, and the interaction of the CSR and VSR in these cases would produce the appropriate pattern of tonic limb muscle activity for stabilizing the trunk in a constant horizontal position with respect to gravity. So, no matter what the orientation of the head and body, the combined action of the vestibular and cervical reflexes would always evoke extension of the downhill limbs and flexion of the uphill limbs.

Subsequent studies attempting to quantify the effects of VSR and CSR by recording electromyographic activity in triceps and biceps in decerebrate cats do not all confirm Robert's findings, however. Some experimenters find little modulation of triceps with head movements in the pitch plane[47] and others[48-50] find limb activation in the opposite direction to that predicted by Roberts. Studies in intact, behaving animals, while quite limited, also fail to confirm Roberts's hypothesis. Intact cats trained to stand freely on a tilted platform recently have been found to show a stereotyped postural strategy in which projection of the center of mass on the support surface and limb orientation with respect to vertical varied minimally with surface tilt angle.[51] Rather than stabilizing the trunk in space as suggested by Roberts, intact cats seem to maintain the orientation of their trunks parallel to the tilted surface and stabilize center of body mass and limb orientation with respect to gravity.

Thus, while static VSR and CSR may be seen in decerebrate animals, they may not play a dominant role in static body postures in intact animals. Also, although the effects of tonic labyrinthine or neck reflexes may be observed very early in development or in cases of brain injury, they have not been conclusively demonstrated in intact human subjects. In healthy adults, the stretch reflex of the soleus muscle becomes more excitable when the head is placed in different positions with respect to gravity. However, unlike Roberts's decerebrate cats, who increased forelimb or hindlimb extension when the head was tilted with respect to gravity, human ankle extensors are *less* excitable when the head is out of normal position with respect to gravity that is, when the subject is supine or prone.[52] Also, the excitability of ankle extensors is suppressed by foot support in standing subjects. Thus, static postures in intact animals and humans are probably dominated by proprioceptive inputs from the limbs and/or movement patterns programmed at a higher level of the nervous system, rather than vestibular and neck reflexes.[53-55]

Role in Automatic Postural Responses

TRIGGERING AUTOMATIC POSTURAL RESPONSES

If balance is disturbed in a standing human, limb muscles are activated at short latencies to restore equilibrium. Because the latencies of these muscle activations are shorter than a voluntary reaction time and because they restore equilibrium, they are called *automatic postural responses*. A great deal of research has been devoted to determining the role of the vestibular system in automatic postural responses. As noted earlier, direct vestibulospinal pathways from both the canals and the otoliths that could convey automatic postural responses to perturbations in stance have been identified anatomically. Both cats and humans respond to sudden drops with short latency ankle extensor activations (50 to 100 msec in cats; 80 to 200 msec in humans). These muscle responses are present with eyes closed, so they are not likely to be a result of visual stimulation. These responses are missing in patients with absent vestibular function, but survive procedures in animals that eliminate the canals but spare the otoliths. The magnitude of the responses is also proportional to head acceleration, all of which suggests a vestibular, and, more specifically, an otolith, origin.[56-59]

Quick displacements directly to the head during stance also result in muscle activations in the neck (45 msec), trunk (85 msec), thigh (90 msec), and ankle (70 msec).[60-63] These responses are absent in patients with adult-onset vestibular loss, suggesting a vestibular origin. However, adults who lost vestibular function as infants may show normal patterns of response to these head perturbations, suggesting that cervicospinal responses may adaptively compensate for the loss of vestibular input early in life.[63]

Another way to investigate the role of the vestibular system in triggering postural limb responses is to stimulate the vestibular system electrically delivering low-level (<2 mA) electric currents to the labyrinths through electrodes on the mastoid processes.[18,19,64-66] Galvanic stimulation reliably elicits activity in ankle muscles at latencies of about 100 msec. These responses are typically absent or abnormal in patients with vestibular nerve sections, which supports a vestibular origin.[67,68] Postural responses to electrical stimulation can be enhanced when subjects stand on a sway-referenced surface that provides poor somatosensory feedback for orientation, indicating that the role of the vestibular system in triggering automatic postural responses is increased when somatosensory information for postural control is unreliable.[18]

While studies of postural responses to electrical stimulation of the vestibular system have shown that the vestibular system can play an important role in automatic postural responses, they also show that the nervous system takes both vestibular and somatosensory information into account when organizing these responses. The direction of body sway and the corresponding muscle activations induced by galvanic stimulation is modulated by the position of the head on the trunk. With the head facing forward, sway is typically lateral, because the galvanic current simulates the vestibular signal that would result if the body swayed to the side of the stimulated ear. If the head is turned on the trunk so that the stimulated ear is placed forward or backward, sway is increased in the anterior-posterior plane.[18] This observation suggests that information about head position from neck receptors is combined with vestibular information to trigger an appropriate postural response regardless of head position with respect to the body.[18] When the head and lower limbs are aligned forward but the trunk is aligned differently, postural responses to galvanic stimulation are appropriate to alignment of the head and feet regardless of trunk alignment.[69] Thus, equilibrium control centers use information about body position and motion derived from proprioceptive afferents from many body segments, not just the neck, in combination with vestibular information to produce an accurate picture of body sway and appropriate postural responses.[70]

Because limb muscles are activated in response to disturbances in head position and galvanic stimulation, investigators have hypothesized that vestibulospinal mechanisms may also play a role in automatic postural responses to stand perturbations induced at the feet by movable platforms.[71,72] Two types of platform perturbations have been used to test this hypothesis, backward or forward translations, which induce forward or backward sway, respectively, and platform rotations, which induce ankle dorsiflexion or plantarflexion (Fig. 2–10). Platform translations result in activation of the stretched ankle muscles which occur at 80 to 100 msec following the onset of platform movement and act to restore the body to initial position. It does not appear, however, that vestibular inputs contribute a great deal to these responses. Human subjects and cats with complete absence of vestibular function can respond to surface translations using automatic postural responses with normal latencies and patterns, even when vision is not present.[38,73–76] Proprioceptive information from stretched muscles appears to be sufficient for recovery from platform translations. This conclusion is supported by the finding

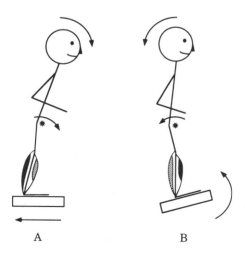

A   B

FIGURE 2–10. Platform translations and rotations. In (A), backward horizontal translation of the platform results in stretch of ankle plantarflexors (*solid*) and forward sway of the body. Medium latency activation of ankle plantarflexors and other muscles restores equilibrium in response to backward platform translations. In (B), however, toe-up rotation of the platform, which also results in stretch of ankle plantarflexors, results in backward sway of the body. For toe-up platform rotations, medium latency activation of the shortened ankle dorsiflexors (*solid*) restores equilibrium. The central nervous system relies more heavily on vestibular information for postural control for platform rotations.

that automatic postural responses to surface translations are delayed when proprioceptive inputs are disrupted by sway-referencing of the surface or eliminated with pressure cuffs at the thigh or in peripheral neuropathy.[77-79] Finally, relatively large head accelerations are required to produce relatively weak responses in the limbs, and the head accelerations that occur in response to platform translations are quite small.[61-63] Therefore VSR probably do not play a large role in the recovery of equilibrium following platform translations.

In contrast to responses to translations, responses to platform rotations may rely much more heavily on vestibular mechanisms. Platform rotations produce ankle dorsiflexion or plantarflexion, stretching muscles in the lower leg, but they do not produce corresponding forward or backward body sway. Responses to platform rotations consist of two parts. First to occur is a response in the stretched ankle muscle at 70 to 100 msec, which is probably triggered by proprioceptive inputs[60,71,72,79-81] and which could, if unopposed, actually destabilize the body. Slightly later a stabilizing response occurs in the shortened ankle muscle (at 100 to 120 msec), and this response is probably more dependent on vestibular and visual inputs. Patients with bilateral and unilateral loss of the vestibular system have reduced magnitudes and delayed latencies of this stabilizing response.[72] The ability to adaptively reduce the magnitude of the destabilizing response to repeated surface tilts is impaired in some patients with loss of vestibular function.[38] The cause of this failure to adapt could either be because vestibular information is required to trigger the adaptive process or because patients with absent vestibular function become hypersensitive to proprioceptive information.[82]

These studies, as do many others, suggest that the role of the vestibular system's automatic postural responses increases when proprioceptive information about body sway is lacking or inaccurate, and they also suggest that accurate, efficient recovery of equilibrium following stance perturbation requires a close interaction of vestibular and somatosensory information. This hypothesis is supported by studies that show that the magnitude of responses to head perturbations increases when subjects stand on compliant or moving surfaces.[61,62,80] Further, responses to peripheral vestibular stimuli are stronger in cats suspended by hammocks than in cats who support themselves on their legs. Cats suspended in hammocks have no access to proprioceptive information about body position, and are thus more dependent on vestibular stimulation.[83]

SELECTION OF POSTURAL STRATEGIES

Not all postural tasks require the same type of movement for the recovery of equilibrium, and different automatic postural responses are triggered in different situations. These different responses have different muscle activation patterns, different body movements, and different joint forces, and are called *postural control synergies* or *strategies*.[18] Normal subjects typically use either an "ankle strategy" or a "hip strategy" to move the body center of mass without moving the feet (Fig. 2–11).[84] An ankle strategy is used by most subjects recovering from body sway when standing on a firm, flat support surface. The body sways roughly as an inverted pendulum by exerting force around the ankle joints. A hip strategy is typically used on narrow (beamlike) or compliant support surfaces, or when center of mass position must be corrected quickly and consists of rapid body motions about the hip joints that transmit shear (horizontal) forces to the support surface. There is evidence that these postural control strategies are centrally programmed and can be combined depending on biomechanical conditions, subject expectations, and prior experience. For example, normal subjects typically show a mixed ankle and hip

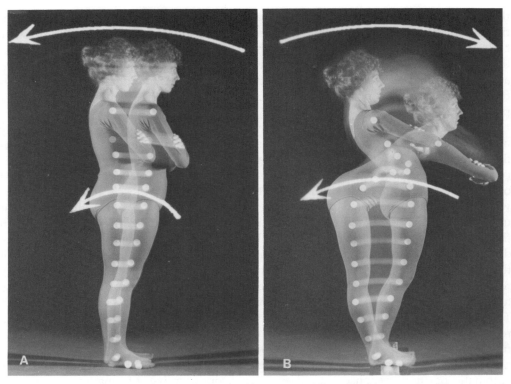

FIGURE 2–11. Normal subject using an ankle strategy (*A*) and a hip strategy (*B*) to control postural sway. Arrows at the hips show direction of corrective center of mass (COM) movement. Arrows at the heads show direction of corrective head movement. The relationship between vestibular and somatosensory information is different for ankle (*A*) and hip (*B*) strategy. In (*A*), a subject recovers from forward sway using ankle strategy, and ankle extension corresponds to backward movement of the center of mass and backward pitch of the head. In (*B*), the subject recovers using hip strategy. Ankle extension and backward movement of the COM now correspond to forward movement of the head and trunk. (Reprinted from PHYSICAL THERAPY, 67:1881, 1987, with the permission of the American Physical Therapy Association.)

strategy when responding to a translation of a 10-cm beam for the first time, or when responding to translations of a flat surface for the first time after responding to a series of beam trials.[85]

Vestibular information does not seem to be essential for initiation or execution of a normal ankle strategy, since subjects with complete absence of vestibular function show normal kinematic and electromyogram patterns associated with an ankle strategy.[31,75,76] In contrast, vestibular information seems to be critical for the hip strategy, since patients with loss of vestibular function do not execute a hip strategy, even when required by the task.[73,75,76] However, it does not appear to be the case that this is because hip strategy responses are triggered by vestibular signals exclusively. Studies of head motion prior to the initiation of hip strategy response do not reveal large head motions that would trigger a vestibularly driven postural control response.[31] Nevertheless, the finding that subjects with vestibular loss cannot execute hip strategy is consistent with reports of poor performance in tasks such as one foot stand, heel/toe walking, and beam balancing in patients with loss of vestibular function.[86–88] Proprioceptive information from the feet seems to be critical for the ankle strategy but not for the hip, as subjects with loss of somatosensory information from the surface owing to ankle ischemia or peripheral neuropathy use a hip strategy when an ankle strategy would be more efficient.[73]

Why is vestibular information critical for a hip strategy and proprioceptive information for an ankle strategy? An important difference between the ankle and the hip strategy is that the head moves in the opposite direction from the center of body mass in the ankle and hip strategies. When a subject is swaying about the ankles, backward movement of the center of mass is associated with vestibular and visual information, signaling backward pitch of the head. Thus, in ankle strategy, somatosensory information indicating backward movement of the center of mass (ankle extension) corresponds with vestibular and visual information indicating backward movement of the head. When a subject sways about the hips, however, backward motion of the center of mass (ankle extension) is associated with vestibular and visual information, signaling forward pitch of the head (see Fig. 2–11A and B). For hip strategy, somatosensory information about center of mass motion and information from the head senses correspond in an entirely different way. Proper execution of ankle strategy may not require good vestibular information because, for ankle strategy, vestibular information and somatosensory information are somewhat redundant. In contrast, execution of hip strategy may require a complete complement of sensory information, because the somatosensory and vestibular systems provide very different and important types of information, both of which may be required for an accurate internal representation of body movement.

Vestibular information may also be necessary for hip strategy because it plays a predictive, rather than a feedback, role. If sensory feedback about body movement indicates that somatosensory and vestibular information about body movement correspond badly in a particular task or environment, the CNS may automatically switch to hip strategy. Patients who lack vestibular information may not be able to detect when somatosensory and vestibular signals are at odds and may therefore be unable to switch to hip strategy. Alternatively, vestibular loss patients may be unable to execute hip strategy because hip strategy may require good stabilization of the head with respect to gravity, which is likely to be faulty in patients lacking vestibular information.

If vestibular information is necessary for execution of the hip strategy, why do some patients with pathology of the vestibular system habitually use hip movements to control center of mass position?[39,75] Some patients with vertigo and ataxia consistent with vestibular dysfunction but normal horizontal VOR function (i.e., who have damaged, but not destroyed, vestibular systems) rely on hip sway for postural movements.[32,39,75,89] Preliminary results suggest that some vestibular patients who show hip sway use a coordinated pattern of active hip motions similar to hip strategy in normal people. Others appear to generate large ankle forces that result in hip sway because the patients exert no control over their trunks. Coordination of head and trunk motions are abnormal in both types of patients (see below).

There are several possible explanations for an overreliance on hip sway in some patients with vestibular disorders. (1) As a result of disease or damage, the vestibular system in these patients may become hyperresponsive and automatically trigger a hip strategy. (2) The hyperresponsive vestibular system may overestimate the velocity of head motion signals during body sway, and the CNS may respond to small perturbations as though they were much bigger. (3) The vestibular dysfunction may impair patients' ability to interpret somatosensory input from feet, so they may perform similarly to patients with somatosensory loss and use hip strategy. (4) The abnormal vestibular information may contribute to abnormal internal perception of stability limits, so patients may behave as if small disturbances in stance push them beyond their stability limits.

Patients who perceive themselves to be in a different relation to their stability limits than they actually are may show inappropriate postural movement strategies in response to destabilization.[32,89] For example, some patients may not take a step necessary to recover equilibrium in response to a displacement of center of body mass outside their limits of stability because they perceive themselves to be well within their stability limits. In contrast, other patients may make exaggerated postural responses to small perturbations well within their limits of stability because they perceive themselves to be at their limits of stability and therefore at risk for a fall. The type of response may depend both on the type of vestibular dysfunction and the requirements of the task.

In summary, vestibular information is used, with information from other senses, to construct internal maps of the limits of stability, which, in turn, affect body alignment and recovery from postural disturbances. The information provided by the vestibular system and its relationship to information from the other senses changes depending on the movement strategy used in controlling equilibrium. We have hypothesized that postural strategies are specific prescriptions for mapping interactions among sensory and motor elements of the postural system, that is, a method for solving a sensorimotor problem. Individuals need a variety of different movement strategies to choose from depending on current, past, and expected environmental conditions and task constraints. Although the vestibular system may not be prescribing the details of the coordinated motor pattern for postural movements, it seems to be intimately involved in the appropriate selection of movement strategies.

DEVELOPMENT OF MOTOR COORDINATION

Consistent with the concept that the vestibular system does not shape the details of coordinated postural patterns, intact vestibular function does not appear to be crucial for the normal development of many aspects of motor coordination. Deaf children who sustain complete or partial loss of vestibular function within the first year of life score within or above normal limits in tests of interlimb coordination such as kicking, walking, running, skipping, hopping, and fine coordination of the hands.[87,90,91] Clinical measures of balance function, such as duration of one-foot standing and ability to walk on a balance beam, however, are affected by loss of vestibular function. These tasks are difficult because one-foot stance and balance beams compromise the patient's ability to use somatosensory information to control posture. However, these tasks also require hip strategy for center of mass control, which is usually abnormal in patients with absent vestibular function.[73,75,76]

STABILIZING THE HEAD

The use of visual and vestibular information for the control of posture is complicated by the fact that these sense organs are located in the inertially unstable head. Because the center of gravity of the head is located above its axis of rotation, any movement of the body will result in head motion. Uncontrolled head motion complicates the use of vestibular information to make estimates of body motion and position. Also, if the range of head motions exceeds that which can be compensated for by the vestibulo-ocular reflex, blurred vision could result. For these reasons, investigators have suggested that the nervous system might stabilize the head with respect to gravity during postural control, either to simplify the interpretation of vestibular information or to facilitate gaze

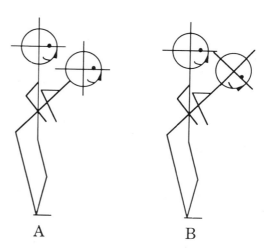

FIGURE 2–12. Alternative strategies for control of head position during postural movements. Example is given for a subject using hip strategy to control center of mass. Head is stabilized with respect to gravity in (A), and head is stabilized with respect to trunk in (B).

A   B

stabilization (Fig. 2–12A).[92,93] In the absence of good information about gravity from the vestibular system, or in an attempt to simplify the coordination of head and trunk movements, it also has been suggested that the nervous system might stabilize the head with respect to the trunk (Fig. 2–12B).[92]

While there is some movement of the head in space during most locomotor tasks, the position of the head with respect to gravity is held relatively constant, despite the large movements of the body that can occur during tasks like hopping or running.[93–95] In these studies, neck muscle activity was not recorded, so it is difficult to know whether head position was being actively stabilized by the CNS. Head position does appear to be controlled actively during recovery from some types of postural disturbances. Normal subjects respond to fast translations and rotations of a large, rigid surface with neck muscle activations.[72,96] Neck muscle activations are also observed in normal subjects using hip strategy.[76] In these studies, the neck muscle activations occurred prior to any large change in head position, and so the activations appear to be a result of an anticipatory control strategy. These muscle activations prevent the large tilts of the head with respect to gravity that could occur during the large trunk movements characteristic of a hip strategy.

To determine the role of the vestibular system in maintaining head position with respect to gravity, the control of head position has also been studied in patients with vestibular loss.[31,76,97,98] During tasks like walking and running, patients with profound vestibular loss show variability in head position with respect to gravity. Profound loss of vestibular function has little effect on the control of head position in patients using ankle strategy to respond to platform translations, but both the control of the position of the center of mass and the control of head position are abnormal in vestibular-loss patients in situations that require hip strategy.[75,76] As discussed earlier, some vestibular patients with ataxia and vertigo, who have not lost vestibular function, tend to rely on hip sway to control posture, and the control of head position is also abnormal in these patients. They fail to activate neck muscles in anticipation of their hip movements and, as a result, they control head position with respect to gravity poorly.[75]

The findings of these studies are fairly clear. The head appears to be approximately stabilized, with respect to gravity, for a wide range of movement tasks. The vestibular system plays an important role in this head stabilization. In contrast, the vestibular system appears to be less important for the control of the position of the center of mass, especially when good somatosensory cues about body position are available. These observations are consistent with the hypothesis that the distal-to-proximal muscle activations that control the center of mass are triggered by somatosensory information from the feet and legs, and that the neck and trunk muscle activations that control head position are triggered by vestibular mechanisms.[3,4,93]

SUMMARY

The vestibular system plays many potential roles in postural control. The role it plays in any given postural task will depend both·on the nature of the task and on the environmental conditions. When the stabilization of the head is critical for good performance, the vestibular system assumes a very important role. Likewise, when somatosensory (and, to a lesser degree, visual) information is not available, vestibular information for postural control assumes a dominant role. Table 2–1 suggests some tasks and conditions in which vestibular information for postural control is important and some balance abnormalities that suggest a vestibular disorder.

Consider, for example, a task and a set of environmental conditions that occur frequently in clinical examinations of postural control: the patient sits, with eyes closed, on a tilted board (see Fig. 2–1). This task is appropriate to test the ability of the patient to use vestibular information for the control of posture because visual and somatosensory cues for orientation are poor, and normal subjects typically stabilize their heads with respect to gravity while executing such tasks. When asked to perform this task, patients who have recently lost vestibular function will demonstrate abnormalities in the use of vestibular information in each of its four roles. First, they will have difficulty perceiving and reporting when their bodies or heads are oriented to gravity. Second, they will orient head and body position poorly to gravity, showing tilts rather than upright orientations. Third, if the board is tipped suddenly, they may not be able to recover balance; and fourth, head position with respect to gravity will vary a great deal as they attempt to recover from the perturbation.

TABLE 2–1 Roles of the Vestibular System in Postural Control

Role of the Vestibular System	Clinical Assessment	Findings Suggestive of Vestibular Disorder
Sensing and perceiving self-motion	Patient performs head motions and/or positions in different planes	Patient reports abnormal sensations of motion and/or vertigo
Orienting to vertical	Patient stands on inclined surface	Trunk oriented to support surface instead of gravity
	Patient stands on foam with eyes closed	Patient falls or sway increases markedly
Controlling center of mass	Patient stands or walks on a beam	Patient is not able to use hip strategy to control center of mass and falls
Stabilizing the head	Patient leans or is tilted	Head not stabilized with respect to vertical

Unfortunately, the assessment of vestibular function in a clinical setting is not so straightforward in patients with partial losses of vestibular function or in those whose vestibular losses are well compensated. What one observes in these patients is often not the primary action of the vestibular system but the result of the body's attempt to compensate for the loss. For example, vestibular patients often have difficulty with stiffness in the neck and shoulders. Assuming, however, that this neck stiffness is a primary result of vestibular activation of tonic neck reflexes would be a mistake. The stiffness may be the result of an increase in gain in the cervicocollic system or a change in strategy; if the head can no longer be aligned to gravity because the direction of gravity cannot be detected, the CNS may choose to stabilize the head to the trunk. Alternatively, the neck stiffness could be a result of voluntary attempts to stabilize head position to limit vertigo or oscillopsia.

Although we once assumed that the abnormal balance of patients with vestibular disorders was the simple and necessary consequence of the loss of vestibular reflexes, we now know that the role of the vestibular system in the control of posture is much more complex. In addition to providing (together with vision and somatosensation) the sensory information necessary for orientation and balance, the vestibular system also interacts with the parts of the CNS responsible for expectation and learning. Although automatic and rapid, postural control is also flexible and capable of adaptation to many different sensory environments and musculoskeletal constraints. The role of the vestibular system in postural control will not be fully appreciated until we better understand the complex and multifaceted nature of postural control itself.

REFERENCES

1. Grossman, GE, et al: Frequency and velocity of rotational head perturbations during locomotion. Exp Brain Res 70:470, 1988.
2. Winters, JM and Peles, JD: Neck muscle activity and 3-D head kinematics during quasi-static and dynamic tracking movements. In Winters, JM and Woo, SLY (eds): Multiple Muscle Systems: Biomechanics and Movement Organization. Springer Verlag, New York, 1990, p 461.
3. Keshner, E and Peterson, B: Mechanisms of human head stabilization during random sinusoidal rotations. Soc Neurosci Abstr 14:1235, 1988.
4. Keshner, E and Peterson, B: Frequency and velocity characteristics of head, neck and trunk during normal locomotion. Soc Neurosci Abstr 15:1200, 1989.
5. Barmack, NH: A comparison of the horizontal and vertical vestibulo-ocular reflexes of the rabbit. J Physiol (Lond) 314:547, 1981.
6. Van der Steen, J and Collewijn, H: Ocular stability in the horizontal, frontal, and sagittal planes in the rabbit. Exp Brain Res 56:263, 1984.
7. Pettorossi, V, Errico, P, and Santarelli, R: Contribution of the maculo-ocular reflex to gaze stability in the rabbit. Exp Brain Res 83:366, 1991.
8. Nashner, L, et al: Organization of posture controls: An analysis of sensory and mechanical constraints. In Allum, JHJ and Hulliger, M (eds): Progress in Brain Research, Vol 80: Afferent Control of Posture and Locomotion. Elsevier, Amsterdam, 1989, p 411.
9. Lackner, JR: Some mechanisms underlying sensory and postural stability in man. In Held, R, Leibowitz, HW, and Teuber, HL (eds): Handbook of Sensory Physiology. Springer Verlag, New York, 1978, p 806.
10. Stoffregen, TA and Riccio, GE: An ecological theory of orientation and the vestibular system. Psychol Rev 95:3, 1988.
11. Lestienne, F, Soechting, J, and Berthoz, A: Postural readjustments induced by linear motion of visual scenes. Exp Brain Res 28:363, 1977.
12. Gurfinkel, VS, et al: Body scheme in the control of postural activity. In Gurfinkel, VS, et al (eds): Stance and Motion: Facts and Theories. Plenum Press, New York, 1988, p 185.
13. Xerri, C, et al: Synergistic interactions and functional working range of the visual and vestibular systems in postural control: Neural correlates. In Pompeiano, O and Allum, JHJ (eds): Progress in Brain Research, Vol 76: Vestibulospinal Control of Posture and Locomotion. Elsevier, Amsterdam, 1988, p 193.
14. Zacharias, G and Young, L: Influence of combined visual and vestibular cues on human perception and control of horizontal rotation. Exp Brain Res 41:159, 1981.

15. Mauritz, KH, et al: Frequency characteristics of postural sway in response to self-induced and conflicting visual stimulation. Pfluegers Arch Ges Physiol 335:37, 1975.
16. van Asten, W, Gielen, C, and Denier van der Gon, J: Postural adjustments induced by simulated motion of differently structured environments. Exp Brain Res 73:371, 1988.
17. Matthews, PBC: Mammalian Muscle Receptors and their Central Actions. Arnold, London, 1972.
18. Nashner, L and Wolfson, P: Influence of head position and proprioceptive cues on short latency postural reflexes evoked by galvanic stimulation of the human labyrinth. Brain Res 67:255, 1974.
19. Magnusson, M, Johansson, R, and Wiklund, J: Galvanically induced body sway in the anterior-posterior plane. Acta Otolaryngol (Stockh) 110:11, 1990.
20. Dichgans, J and Brandt, T: Visual-vestibular interaction: Effects on self-motion perception and postural control. In Held, R, Leibowitz, H, and Teuber, HL (eds): Handbook of Sensory Physiology, Vol VIII: Perception. Springer Verlag, Berlin, 1978, p 755.
21. Howard, I: Human Visual Orientation. John Wiley & Sons, Ltd, Chichester, 1982.
22. Stoffregen, T: Flow structure versus retinal location in the optical control of stance. J Exp Psych: Hum Perc Perf 11:554, 1985.
23. Pyykko, I, et al: Vibration-induced body sway. In Claussen, C and Kirtane, M (eds): Computers in Neurootologic Diagnosis. Werner Rudat, 1983, p 139.
24. Johansson, R, Magnusson, M, and Akesson, M: Identification of human postural dynamics. IEEE Trans Biomed Eng 35:858, 1988.
25. von Holst, E and Mittelstaedt, H: Das Raefferenzprinzip. Naturwissenschaften 37:464, 1957.
26. Mergner, Y and Becker, W: Perception of horizontal self-rotation: Multisensory and cognitive aspects. In Warren, R and Wertheim, A (eds): Perception and Control of Self-Motion. Lawrence Erlbaum, New Jersey, 1990, p 219.
27. de Waele, C, et al: Vestibular control of skeletal geometry. In Amblard, B, Berthoz, A, and Clarac, F (eds): Posture and Gait: Development, Adaptation and Modulation. Elsevier, Amsterdam, 1988, p 423.
28. Dow, RS: The effects of unilateral and bilateral labyrinthectomy in monkey, baboon, and chimpanzee. Am J Physiol 121:392, 1938.
29. Schaefer, K and Meyer, D: Compensation of vestibular lesions. In Kornhuber, H (ed): Handbook of Sensory Physiology, Vol VI: The Vestibular System, Part 2: Psychophysics, Applied Aspects, and General Interpretation. Springer Verlag, Berlin, 1978, p 463.
30. Precht, W: Recovery of some vestibuloocular and vestibulospinal functions following unilateral labyrinthectomy. In Freund, HJ, et al (eds): Progress in Brain Research, Vol 64: The Oculomotor and Skeletomotor Systems: Differences and Similarities. Elsevier, Amsterdam, 1986, pp 381–389.
31. Shupert, C, et al: Coordination of the head and body in standing posture in normals and patients with bilaterally reduced vestibular function. Soc Neurosci Abstr 13:352, 1987.
32. Shumway-Cook, A and Horak, FB: Rehabilitation strategies for patients with vestibular deficits. In Arenberg, IK and Smith, DB (eds): Neurologic Clinics, Vol 8: Diagnostic Neurotology. WB Saunders, Philadelphia, 1990, p 441.
33. Takemori, S, Ida, M, and Umezu, H: Vestibular training after sudden loss of vestibular functions. Otorhinolaryngology 47:76, 1985.
34. Fukuda, T: The stepping test: Two phases of the labyrinthine reflex. Acta Otolaryngol (Stockh) 50:95, 1959.
35. Norre, M: Treatment of unilateral vestibular hypofunction. In Oosterveld, W (ed): Otoneurology. John Wiley and Sons, Chichester, 1984, p 24.
36. McCollum, G and Leen, TK: Form and exploration of mechanical stability limits in erect stance. J Motor Behav 21:225, 1989.
37. Shumway-Cook, A and McCollum, G: Assessment and treatment of balance deficits. In Montgomery, P and Connolly, B (eds): Motor Control and Physical Therapy: Theoretical Framework and Practical Applications. Chattanooga Corporation, Chattanooga, 1990, pp 123–141.
38. Nashner, L, Black, FO, and Wall, C, III: Adaptation to altered support and visual conditions during stance: Patients with vestibular deficits. J Neurosci 5:536, 1982.
39. Black, F and Nashner, L: Vestibulospinal control differs in patients with reduced and distorted vestibular function. Acta Otolaryngol 406:110, 1984.
40. Black, FO, et al: Abnormal postural control associated with peripheral vestibular disorders. In Pompeiano, O and Allum, JHJ (eds): Progress in Brain Research, Vol 76: Vestibulospinal Control of Posture and Locomotion. Elsevier, Amsterdam, 1988, p 263.
41. Shumway-Cook, A and Horak, FB: Assessing the influence of sensory interaction on balance. Phys Ther 66:1548, 1986.
42. Black, FO, Wall, C, III, and O'Leary, D: Computerized screening of the human vestibulospinal system. Ann Otol Rhinol Laryngol 87:853, 1978.
43. Black, FO, et al: Effects of unilateral loss of vestibular function on the vestibulo-ocular reflex and postural control. Ann Otol Rhinol Laryngol 98:884, 1989.
44. Magnus, R: In Van Harreveld, A (ed): Body Posture. New Delhi, Amerind, 1988. (Original published by Springer Verlag, Berlin, 1924).
45. Roberts, TDM: Reflex balance. Nature 244:56, 1973.

46. Roberts, TDM: Neurophysiology of Postural Mechanisms. Butterworths, London, 1967.
47. Wilson, VJ, et al: Spatial organization of neck and vestibular reflexes acting on the forelimbs of the decerebrate cat. J Neurophys 55:514, 1986.
48. Anderson, JH, Soechting, JF, and Terzuolo, CA: Dynamic relations between natural vestibular inputs and activity of forelimb extensor muscles in the decerebrate cat: I. Motor output during sinusoidal linear accelerations. Brain Res 120:1, 1977.
49. Anderson, JH, Soechting, JF, and Terzuolo, CA: Dynamic relations between natural vestibular inputs and activity of forelimb extensor muscles in the decerebrate cat: II. Motor output during rotations in the horizontal plane. Brain Res 120:17, 1977.
50. Soechting, JF, Anderson, JH, and Berthoz, A: Dynamic relations between natural vestibular inputs and activity of forelimb extensor muscles in the decerebrate cat: III. Motor output during rotations in the vertical plane. Brain Res 120:35, 1977.
51. Lacquaniti, F, et al: The control of limb geometry in cat posture. J Physiol 426:177, 1990.
52. Chan, CWY and Kearney, RE: Influence of static tilts on soleus motoneuron excitability in man. Neurosci Lett 33:333, 1982.
53. Macpherson, JM, Horak, FB, and Dunbar, DC: Stance dependence of automatic postural adjustments in humans. Exp Brain Res 78:557, 1989.
54. Massion, J, et al: Axial synergies under microgravity conditions. Exp Brain Res 656:854–856, 1992.
55. Bernstein, N: The Coordination and Regulation of Movement. Pergamon Press, London, 1967.
56. Melvill-Jones, G and Watt, DGD: Muscular control of landing from unexpected falls in man. J Physiol (Lond) 219:729, 1971.
57. Greenwood, R and Hopkins, A: Landing from an unexpected fall and a voluntary step. Brain 99:375, 1976.
58. Watt, DGD: Effect of vertical linear acceleration on H-reflex in decerebrate cat: I. Transient stimuli. J Neurophys 45:644, 1981.
59. Lacour, M, Xerri, C, and Hugon, M: Muscle responses and monosynaptic reflexes in falling monkey: Role of the vestibular system. J Physiol Paris 74:427, 1978.
60. Dietz, V, Horstmann, GA, and Berger, W: Interlimb coordination of leg-muscle activation during perturbation of stance in humans. J Neurophysiol 62:680, 1989.
61. Shupert, C, et al: Short latency postural responses to head/neck perturbations. Soc Neurosci Abstr 15:397, 1989.
62. Shupert, C, et al: Automatic responses to head/neck perturbations. In Brandt, T, et al (eds): Disorders of Posture and Gait. George Thieme Verlag, Stuttgart, 1990, p 177.
63. Horak, F, et al: Vestibular-somatosensory interaction in rapid responses to head perturbations. In Tomko, D and Guedry, F (eds): Annals of the New York Academy of Science: Sensing and Controlling Motion: Vestibular and Somatosensory Function, in press.
64. Folkerts, JF and Njiokiktjien, CJ: The influence of L-dopa on the postural regulation of Parkinson patients. Agressologie 13:19, 1972.
65. Coats, AC: The sinusoidal galvanic body-sway response. Acta Otolaryngol (Stockh) 74:155, 1972.
66. Kots, YM: Descending reflex influences during the organization of voluntary movement. In Evarts, EV (ed): The Organization of Voluntary Mechanisms: Neurophysiological Mechanisms. Plenum Press, New York, 1977, p 181.
67. Tokita, T, et al: Diagnosis of otolith and semicircular-canal lesions by galvanic nystagmus and spinal reflexes. In Graham, M and Kemink, J (eds): The Vestibular System: Neurophysiologic and Clinical Research. Raven, New York, 1987, p 305.
68. Watanabe, Y, et al: Clinical evaluation of vestibular-somatosensory interactions using galvanic body sway test. In Graham, M and Kemink, J (eds): The Vestibular System: Neurophysiologic and Clinical Research. Raven, New York, 1987, p 393.
69. Lund, S and Broberg, C: Effects of different head positions on postural sway in man induced by a reproducible vestibular error signal. Acta Physiol Scand 117:307, 1983.
70. Gurfinkel, VS, Lipshits, MI, and Popov, KY: Is the stretch reflex the main mechanism in the system or regulation of the vertical posture of man? Biofizika 19:744, 1974.
71. Allum, JHJ and Pfaltz, CR: Visual and vestibular contributions to pitch sway stabilization in the ankle muscles of normals and patients with bilateral peripheral vestibular deficits. Exp Brain Res 58:82, 1985.
72. Keshner, E, Allum, J, and Pfaltz, C: Postural coactivation and adaptation in the sway-stabilizing responses of normals and patients with bilateral vestibular deficits. Exp Brain Res 69:77, 1987.
73. Horak, R, Diener, H, and Nashner, L: Postural strategies associated with somatosensory and vestibular loss. Exp Brain Res 82:167, 1991.
74. Thomson, DB, et al: Bilateral labyrinthectomy in the cat: Motor behavior and quiet stance parameters. Exp Brain Res 85:364, 1991.
75. Shupert, C, Horak, FB, and Black, FO: The effect of peripheral vestibular disorders on head-trunk coordination during postural sway in humans. In Berthoz, A, Graf, W, and Vidal, P (eds): The Head-Neck Sensory Motor System: Evolution, Development, Neuronal Mechanisms and Disorders. Oxford University Press, New York, 1991, p 607.
76. Shupert, C, et al: Coordination of the head and body in response to support surface translations in normals

and patients with bilaterally reduced vestibular function. In Amblard, B, Berthoz, A and Clarac, F (eds): Posture and Gait: Development, Adaptation, and Modulation. Elsevier, Amsterdam, 1988, p 281.

77. Diener, HC, et al: The significance of proprioception on postural stabilization as assessed by ischemia. Brain Res 296:103, 1984.

78. Mauritz, KH, Dietz, V, and Haller, M: Balancing as a clinical test in the differential diagnosis of sensory-motor disorders. J Neurol Neurosurg Psychiatry 43:407, 1980.

79. Nashner, L: Fixed patterns of rapid postural responses among leg muscles during stance. Exp Brain Res 30:59, 1977.

80. Diener, HC, et al: Stabilization of human posture during induced oscillations of the body. Exp Brain Res 45:126, 1982.

81. Nashner, L and McCollum, G: The organization of human postural movements: A formal basis and experimental synthesis. Behav Brain Sci 8:135, 1985.

82. Horak, FB: Comparison of cerebellar and vestibular loss on scaling of postural responses. In Brandt, T, et al (eds): Disorders of Posture and Gait. George Thieme Verlag, Stuttgart, 1990, p 370.

83. Kasper, J, et al: Influence of standing on vestibular neuronal activity in awake cats. Exp Neurol 92:37, 1986.

84. Horak, FB and Nashner, L: Central programming of postural movements: Adaptation to altered support surface configurations. J Neurophysiol 55:1369, 1986.

85. McCollum, G, Horak, F, and Nashner, L: Parsimony in neural calculations for postural movements. In Bloedel, J, Dichgans, J, and Precht, W (eds): Cerebellar Functions. Springer-Verlag, Berlin, 1984, p 52.

86. Horak, FB, et al: Vestibular function and motor proficiency in children with hearing impairments and in learning disabled children with motor impairments. Dev Med Child Neurol 30:64, 1988.

87. Kaga, K, Suzuki, J, and Marsh RR: Influence of labyrinthine hypoactivity on gross motor development of infants. Ann NY Acad Sci 374:412, 1981.

88. Fregly, A: Vestibular ataxia and its measurement in man. In Kornhuber, H (ed): Handbook of Sensory Physiology, Vol VI: The Vestibular System, Part 2: Psychophysics, Applied Aspects, and General Interpretation. Springer-Verlag, Berlin, 1974, p 321.

89. Shumway-Cook, A and Horak, FB: Vestibular rehabilitation: An exercise approach to managing symptoms of vestibular dysfunction. Semin Hearing 10:196, 1989.

90. Shumway-Cook, A, Horak, FB, and Black, FO: Critical examination of vestibular function in motor-impaired learning disabled children. Int J Ped Otorhinolaryngol 14:21, 1988.

91. Crowe, TK and Horak, FB: Motor proficiency associated with vestibular deficits in children with hearing impairments. Phys Ther 68:1493, 1988.

92. Nashner, L: Strategies for organization of human posture. In Igarashi, M and Black, FO (eds): Vestibular and Visual Control on Posture and Locomotor Equilibrium. Basel, Karger, 1985, p 1.

93. Pozzo, T, Berthoz, A, and Lefort, L: Head stabilization during various locomotor tasks in humans: I. Normal subjects. Exp Brain Res 82:97, 1990.

94. Grossman, G, et al: Performance of the human vestibuloocular reflex during locomotion. J Neurophys 62:264, 1989.

95. Assaiante, C and Amblard, B: Head-trunk coordination and locomotor equilibrium in 3- to 8-year-old children. In Berthoz, A, Graf, W, and Vidal, PP, (eds): The Head-Neck Sensory Motor System. Oxford University Press, New York, 1991, p 121.

96. Keshner, E, Woollacott, M, and Debu, B: Neck, trunk and limb muscle responses during postural perturbations in humans. Exp Brain Res 75:455, 1988.

97. Grossman, G and Leigh, RJ: Instability of gaze during locomotion in patients with deficient vestibular function. Ann Neurol 27:528, 1990.

98. Pozzo, T, et al: Head stabilization during various locomotor tasks in humans: II. Patients with bilateral peripheral vestibular deficits. Exp Brain Res 85:208, 1991.

CHAPTER **3**

Postural Abnormalities in Vestibular Disorders

Emily A. Keshner, EdD, PT

The vestibular system is considered to play an integral role in the control of posture and balance. Much of the evidence for this conclusion has, in fact, relied on findings of postural disorders in patients with vestibular abnormalities.[1] Both clinical and experimental observations have shown that along with symptoms of vertigo, past pointing, and nystagmus, equilibrium disturbances are one of the major complaints of patients with partial or total destruction of the vestibular labyrinths.[2] Despite these fairly consistent symptoms, examination of any one patient with postural abnormalities arising from damage to the vestibular system could yield an uncertain diagnosis.[2,3] Most diagnoses are based on subjective complaints, and patient descriptions of symptom might differ. One person might experience a perception of the world spinning about, whereas another might complain of imbalance and falling. Both, however, could have the same vestibular pathology.[3] Since the process of central nervous compensation proceeds over a lengthy period of time, patients also can have different symptoms when they finally arrive at a clinic, although suffering a similar deficit.

The question for the clinician and the clinical investigator is whether any one compensatory strategy is more efficient or effective for the population of patients with a vestibular deficit. If one strategy is better, then a systematic approach to treatment could be followed. To determine the effectiveness of the compensation, however, we must first determine how to reliably indicate whether the patient is suffering from postural dyscontrol and whether vestibular dysfunction is responsible for the symptoms. In this chapter, some of the methods available for testing postural disorders that are associated with vestibular pathology are briefly discussed. Then postural behaviors that have been quantified and associated with specific vestibular pathologies will be described. Finally, the issue of how the postural system compensates for loss or damage to vestibular signals is discussed.

EXAMINING THE VESTIBULOSPINAL SYSTEM

The majority of vestibular disorders are diagnosed through examinations of the vestibulo-ocular system. Tests of vestibulo-ocular integrity and vestibulospinal function may not be correlated, however.[3] First, the well-defined loop of the vestibulo-ocular reflex (VOR) does not, in any way, reveal the integrity of the more complex vestibulospinal pathways that are intimately involved in the control of posture and balance. Second, tests of the VOR are commonly performed in the plane of the horizontal semicircular canals, whereas vestibulospinal reflexes are dependent on inputs from the vertical semicircular canals and the otoliths. A number of tests of the vestibulospinal system are available to the clinician, and some of the problems inherent in each method of testing will be discussed in this chapter. Table 3–1 summarizes the advantages and disadvantages of the tests discussed here.

Advantages and Limitations of Clinical Tests

TESTS OF QUIET STANCE

Traditional clinical examinations of vestibulospinal function include tests of self-localization, such as the Romberg test.[4] Initially, Romberg's test of instability was based on a population of patients with proprioceptive loss from tabes dorsalis who were unable to stand with feet together and eyes closed. The Romberg test is insensitive for detection of chronic unilateral labyrinthine impairment, however, and it is highly variable even within a subject.[5] Modifying the test by having the patient stand in a tandem heel-to-toe position (sharpened or tandem Romberg) has made the test more sensitive,[2] probably

TABLE 3–1 Advantages and Disadvantages of Clinical
Tests of Postural Instability

	Static Tests	
	Advantages	Disadvantages
Romberg	Easily performed in clinic	Qualitative
		Does not test adaptive responses
Stabilometry	Quantitative	Requires a force platform
	Can manipulate sensory inputs	Intersegmental shifts confound results
		Does not test adaptive responses
	Dynamic Tests	
Stepping tests	Easily performed in clinic	Does not test adaptive responses
	Can be quantified	Has not been shown to be reliable
Tiltboards	Easily performed in clinic	Qualitative
	Requires adaptation to external forces	Amplitude and application of force is not controlled
Posturography	Quantitative	Requires a posture platform
	Requires adaptation to external forces	
	Can manipulate sensory signals	

because of the narrowed base of support. Even so, tests of quiet stance fail to measure the adaptive components of the postural response that are essential to dynamic balance during most daily activities.[6]

Tests of quiet stance may indicate the severity of a balance problem because patients with vestibular system damage will demonstrate increased sway and falling when the base of support is constrained during quiet standing. Conclusions about the neural processes contributing to postural imbalance are severely limited, however. The effect of altered proprioceptive and cutaneous information on low-frequency sway stabilization cannot be determined by tests of quiet standing. Changing velocity of the visual field is a significant parameter controlling body sway during quiet standing,[6] but simple removal of vision does not alter the temporal or spatial organization of the automatic postural reactions.[7] Furthermore, behavioral measures as to how often a subject falls or to which direction he or she deviates do not convey information about the motor and sensory mechanisms that may be involved in postural control.[8,9] Thus, attempting to assess the integrity of the vestibular system through a test of quiet standing opens the door to many confounding variables and is far from specific to the vestibulospinal disorders that may produce a postural deficit.[10,11] Despite these limitations, the concept of deviation from the vertical during quiet standing continues to underlie most clinical testing of vestibular dysfunction.

STABILOMETRY

Stabilometry is a clinical tool that measures anterior-posterior and lateral excursions of the body in subjects standing quietly on a force platform, usually over time.[12-14] During that time, the subject stands quietly on a force plate, and the excursion of the center of gravity is measured across several conditions that can include eyes open, eyes closed, and eyes closed with head extension. Attempts to stress the vestibulospinal system have been incorporated into this system of measurement by altering signals from other sensory pathways. For example, adding a layer of foam rubber to the base of support to make somatosensory inputs less effective[15] or placing the subjects within a visually controlled environment to modify visual feedback.[16] This attempt to quantify the classical Romberg test has made the measurement of postural sway during quiet standing more objective, but the mechanisms contributing to the observation of increased sway still cannot be identified. One problem is that changing the position of the body parts (either randomly or through experimenter directive) could shift the center of pressure without affecting the stability of the subject.[12] In general, because the sensory apparatus of the vestibular system is most responsive to changes in acceleration and orientation in space[17] and because patients with vestibular deficits tend to have normal Romberg signs, tests of quiet standing on a stabilometer are not compelling measures of vestibulospinal function.

TILTBOARDS

Tilt reactions, or reflexes opposing bodily displacement, traditionally were evoked through a lateral tilt or anterior-posterior tilt of the supporting surface about a horizontal axis.[18-20] On tilting the base of support, the reaction to regain a stable equilibrium occurred by moving the body against the angular momentum and repositioning the center of gravity within the vertical projection of its base of support.[18-21] These reactions have also been elicited in the clinic by simply pushing the patient at the shoulder girdle.

Problems with the accuracy of this test are threefold. First, because the tilt reactions are measured by observational techniques, later voluntary responses (greater than 150 msec) rather than automatic postural reactions are being evaluated. Second, the response pattern alters if the force is applied directly to the trunk rather than to the support surface. Third, tilt responses will be organized differently depending on whether your patient is pushed or trips over an obstacle in the environment, whether the application of perturbation is predictable, and whether it is self-induced or elicited.

DYNAMIC POSTUROGRAPHY

Automatic Postural Responses

In the 1970s, Nashner[22,23] reported stereotypical, automatic responses to postural disturbances initiated at the base of support, introducing the measurement of postural reactions on a moving platform as a powerful experimental approach. Since that time, the majority of studies of postural kinematics have concentrated on the electromyographic (EMG) responses from muscles in the lower limb, from which most descriptions about restabilizing actions have been drawn.[22-27] Subjects stand on a platform that could be translated in an anterior and posterior direction, or rotated so that the ankles are moved into plantarflexion or dorsiflexion (Fig. 3–1). The expected response to anterior motion of the platform is backward sway (base of support moved in front of the center of mass), producing a decreased angle at the ankle and a stretch of the ankle muscles on the anterior surface of the body (i.e., tibialis anterior). If the platform moves posteriorly, the subject sways forward (base of support moved behind the center of mass), thereby decreasing the ankle angle and stretching the gastrocnemius and soleus muscles. Rotating the platform into plantar or dorsiflexion would produce equivalent changes at the ankle (see Fig. 3–1), but the center of mass remains in line with the base of support.

Although the monosynaptic stretch reflex does not act functionally to replace the center of mass over the base of support, EMG analysis of the lower limb muscles revealed that the muscles being stretched still tended to respond, at latencies longer than the stretch reflex, to bring the body back over the base of support. These restabilizing ankle muscle responses (at latencies of 90 to 120 msec) were followed within 10 to 20 msec by the muscle in the upper leg on the same side of the body (i.e., soleus followed by the hamstrings; tibialis anterior followed by the quadriceps). Thus, from these early studies, patterns of muscle activation initiated by ankle proprioceptive inputs and arising from distal to proximal lower limb muscles were identified as ascending muscle synergies responsible for restabilization after platform movement.[22,23] Nashner's original conclusion that the body acts as a rigid, inverted pendulum during postural restabilization, reliant primarily on ankle proprioceptive inputs to initiate the restabilizing actions, is now in doubt, however.[22,23] Other findings suggest that the rigid pendulum model is not an adequate model of functional stability,[25,28,29] mostly because the model of the body as an inverted pendulum is based only on EMG measures from the lower limb and is too simple to explain the behaviors of a multisegmental, multisensory system. Even Nashner and his colleagues have begun to revise their original hypothesis and to suggest that posture is a function of the position of all of the different joints[30] and multiple sensory inputs.[27]

Identifying Vestibular Contributions to Automatic Postural Responses

Since the earliest presentation of Nashner's findings, investigators have been attempting to define the contribution of the vestibular system to the automatic postural responses.[7,25-27] Studies in which the labyrinthine receptors were directly stimulated by

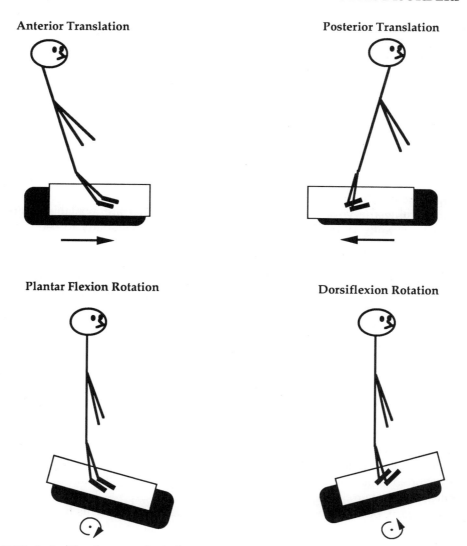

FIGURE 3-1. The four standard directions of posture platform perturbation. Note that in anterior translations and plantar flexion rotations ankle angles increase. In posterior translations and dorsiflexion rotations, ankle angles decrease.

vertically dropping human and animal subjects, thereby producing linear acceleratory stimuli,[31-34] demonstrated that direct labyrinthine stimulation can produce automatic or "triggered" postural reactions in the lower limb. Nashner[24] hypothesized, however, that the vestibular system only contributes to the control of lower limb balance reactions when proprioceptive signals are absent or unreliable. Using a servomechanism, the posture platform was made to match the sway at the hip, thereby maintaining a neutral position at the ankle and, assumably, eliminating any change in the proprioceptive feedback from the ankle during normal quiet standing.[24] In these subjects, automatic postural responses were significantly delayed when the subjects had to rely on vestibular signals in the absence of proprioceptive feedback from the ankles.

Quite possibly the servomechanism did not fully remove the ankle proprioceptor feedback but rather produced distorted or modified signals that altered the automatic postural reactions; or, responses to vestibular inputs during quiet stance may not be transferable to those responses observed during dynamic gait and a loss of balance. In an attempt to resolve the issue of labyrinthine involvement in the generation of postural reactions to support surface displacements, Allum and associates[35] devised a novel experiment. Angular displacement of the ankle was kept equal for both platform translations and rotations, thereby producing equivalent proprioceptive signals from the ankle although the labyrinthine inputs differed. When head acceleration and neck and lower limb muscle EMG responses recorded during both perturbations did not exhibit the same response patterns, the investigators concluded that labyrinthine signals must be directly involved in the generation of lower limb postural reactions.

Altering Sensory Cues

Manipulating the visual and somatosensory inputs that are available during dynamic posturography is another method to isolate a person's ability to use vestibular signals. As mentioned previously, protocols to alter somatosensory inputs include using a servoed platform that matches the normal sway at the ankle during quiet standing or adding a layer of dense foam to the base of support to make somatosensory inputs less effective.[15] Visual conditions have been controlled either by stabilizing or rotating the visual field in an anterior-posterior plane.[16,36,37] When the visual field is rotated in phase with the anterior-posterior sway of the subject, the subject experiences a distortion of visual signals by way of the unexpected and inappropriate visual feedback.

Although normal subjects, elderly individuals, and those with vestibular deficits exhibit an increased tendency to fall under conditions of altered sensory input,[15,16,38,39] concluding that the cause is a vestibulospinal system unable to compensate for the loss of other sensory signals may be premature. Modification of somatosensory and visual inputs is not necessarily equivalent to a loss of those signals, and the central nervous system may well compensate for distorted or minimized inputs by altering the sensorimotor transformation algorithm. For example, the system may select a compensatory strategy that relies on enhancing the gains of somatosensory and visual responsiveness to the distorted inputs rather than shifting responsibility for the response on to the vestibulospinal system.

In summary, postural responses to support surface displacements have been tested by (1) translating a standing subject along the earth's horizontal plane on a moving platform, (2) rotating the foot about the horizontal axis of the ankle into dorsiflexion or plantarflexion, and (3) keeping the platform fixed to the earth horizontal or servoing the angle of the platform to match the angle at the ankle during quiet sway. Experiments using the posture platform have been performed with a wide range of velocities and amplitudes of displacement, thus altering the transmission of forces from the lower limb to the head and making the comparison of vestibular influences on balance difficult across laboratory settings. In fact, Nashner and co-workers[27] have now proposed an approach to studying posture that incorporates the mechanics of body sway with the threshold properties and dynamic characteristics of the labyrinthine receptors. They suggest that knowing the mechanics of the head and motions of the center of mass is necessary to predict the role of canal and otolith feedback in restabilization. Despite this limitation, studies performed on clinical populations continue to employ the posture platform to promote instability as a reliable method for obtaining quantitative measures of postural reactions. Many of the results reported in this chapter have, in fact, depended on the posture platform methodology to examine disturbances in postural control as a result of vestibular dysfunction.

STEPPING TESTS

The Unterberger[40] or stepping test of Fukuda[41] examines the ability of patients to turn about a vertical axis when marching or stepping in place. Marked variability in the amount of rotation produced by even the same subject, however, makes these tests unreliable.[2] Patients with severe disruption of the vestibular system may stagger so uncontrollably that the stepping tests cannot reliably indicate the side of the lesion.[42] A battery of tests developed by Graybiel and Fregly[43] (Ataxia Test Battery) examines subjects standing upright, on one leg, and with feet aligned in tandem position with eyes open or closed, as well as tandem walking in a straight line on the floor or on a narrow rail. This test is useful for patients that have compensated for a labyrinthine deficit because, when a narrowed base of support is required, even those patients score more poorly than normal subjects on measures of deviation from the straight line or of the number of steps made prior to falling from the rail.

POSTURAL REACTIONS IN PERIPHERAL VESTIBULAR DISORDERS

A discussion of etiology and diagnostic testing of vestibular system disease is beyond the scope of this chapter but can be found in other sources.[2,44] The focus here will be on those vestibular disturbances that have been found to produce a postural disturbance and that have been tested for changes in vestibulospinal function. Dysfunction in the vestibulospinal system can be divided into two categories: distortion and deficiency.[45,46] A *deficiency* in the system usually implies that the sensory (i.e., labyrinthine) inputs have been reduced or abolished, resulting mostly in complaints of unsteadiness and instability. *Distortion* means that the signal is present but disturbed and does not correspond with expectations about the sensory feedback. The result would be inappropriate or false motor responses to the existing situation (e.g., vertigo and ataxia). A summary of postural disturbances is presented in Table 3–2 for the disorders discussed in this chapter.

TABLE 3–2 Postural Disturbances Observed
with Vestibular Disorders

Peripheral Vestibular Disorders	
Deficient Inputs	Need more energy to maintain the upright position
	Instability increases in the presence of inappropriate sensory signals
	Amplitudes of EMG and torque are inversely related to severity of deficit
Distorted Inputs	Still able to process vestibular inputs
	Falls increase in the presence of inappropriate sensory signals
Central Vestibular Disorders	
	Impaired perception and location of the gravitational vertical
	Direction-specific ataxia
	Falling tends to occur in the direction of quick phase nystagmus
Aging	
	Longer response latencies and delayed reaction times
	Diminished sensory acuity and impaired signal detection
	Postural response patterns are temporally disordered

Deficient Labyrinthine Inputs

Damage along the eighth nerve or within the vestibular labyrinth produces lost or diminished signals from the peripheral vestibular apparatus.[17] Central disturbances originate at the vestibular nuclei or in the higher central pathways that communicate with the vestibular nuclei. In both cases, patients can experience disequilibrium, imbalance, and ataxia. With unilateral lesions of the peripheral system, the normal symmetry of inputs from the right and left labyrinths become disordered, resulting in a decreased firing rate of the vestibular nuclei on one side. A unilateral lesion affects the system as if the intact side were being stimulated, thus generating an illusion of change in head orientation and movement. The inherent disequilibrium then activates the vestibulospinal system to respond inappropriately, resulting in vertigo, nystagmus, and postural instability.

Another effect of vestibular system stimulation, maintaining tone of the muscles against gravity, appears to be directly correlated with labyrinthine inputs, as the activation of extensor muscles in the extremities of both monkeys[47] and humans[48] with unilateral deficit were found to be enhanced contralateral to the side of the lesion. Postural reactions are more complex than single-pathway vestibular reflexes, however, and cannot be traced and localized as easily as these direct-line responses. For example, when both labyrinths are lesioned, an artificial sense of motion does not occur and neither do the symptoms of nystagmus and vertigo. Yet equilibrium is still disturbed, suggesting that the balance function of the vestibular system is not a simple response to stimulation of the labyrinthine receptors.

INDICATORS OF VESTIBULOSPINAL DYSFUNCTION

Unilateral and Bilateral Labyrinthine Deficit

Variability of the responses measured from the many methods of posturography confirms the complexity of postural responses. After repeated attempts to quantify the results of the Romberg test, the most reliable effort seems to be measuring energy of the power spectral densities of the center of force trajectories when maintaining an upright position.[49] Both in this study and in others using force plates to record sway during quiet stance,[3,14] intersubject variability and overlap between normal and clinical populations reduced the strength of the findings. Results suggest, however, that more energy needs to be expended to maintain an upright position when visual inputs are removed (eyes closed) from patients with a labyrinthine deficit.

In a series of papers presented by Black and Nashner,[38,45,49] postural sway was recorded through a potentiometer placed at the level of the hips. Patients stood on a platform that could be either earth-fixed or moved proportional to body sway (servoed). The visual environment was then manipulated so that patients experienced a visual field that was either (1) earth-fixed, (2) proportional to body sway, or (3) removed by eye closure. Patients with reduced or absent labyrinthine inputs were more unstable than normal controls only when ankle proprioceptive references were proportional to body sway and visual references were either removed or inappropriate (conditions 2 and 3 above). When the only reliable source of feedback was the vestibular inputs, it was believed that patients with vestibular deficiencies would fall because they were dependent on the somatosensory and visual reference to correctly organize their postural responses. From these studies, Black and colleagues[49] suggested that vestibular deficits could be quantified by systematically altering the sensory information provided by the support surface and the visual surround.

Several problems limit our reliance on these results for clinical diagnosis and measurement. First, patients with unilateral or partial bilateral deficits at times were as unstable as patients with total loss of vestibular function,[8] thus rendering this a poor test of graduated function in the vestibular system. Second, the authors tested only well-compensated patients. As will be discussed later, compensation could occur as a central reorganization in the system. Thus, these experiments may not be testing a vestibular deficit but rather a compensatory subsystem that responds inadequately to the presented stimuli. Third, patients with postural instability from other, nonvestibular disorders may have test results similar to those of patients with vestibular deficits (Hain and Herdman, oral communication 1992).

Allum and colleagues[7,9,25,48,50,51] examined both the latencies and amplitudes of muscle EMG responses on a platform that dorsiflexed the ankle. Areas under the EMG bursts in the ankle muscles, soleus and tibialis anterior, and ankle torque recordings of patients with complete bilateral labyrinthine deficit were significantly diminished when compared with normal subjects with eyes both open and closed. Using these data, the presence of a linear correlation between EMG amplitudes and the extent of the peripheral vestibular deficit was explored.[10] The population measured included those with intact labyrinths (normal subjects), acute unilateral labyrinthine deficit patients, chronic unilateral labyrinthine deficit patients, and bilateral labyrinthine deficit patients, thus covering a graduated range of labyrinthine function.

A stepwise discriminant analysis technique performed on the data suggested that muscle response amplitudes in the soleus and tibialis anterior muscles, as well as amplitude of torque exerted on the platform were inversely related to the severity of the labyrinthine deficit. Muscle and torque responses diminished in amplitude as the reception of labyrinthine inputs decreased. Because lower limb EMG activity was still present in the patients with complete loss of labyrinthine inputs, a linear correlation of the amount of EMG activity with extent of peripheral vestibular deficit suggests that lower limb postural reflexes could be triggered by proprioceptive stretch reflexes but that amplitude modulation is under the control of, or requires the presence of, vestibulospinal signals. EMG activity in the neck muscles was not obviously altered in these patients, implying local control of neck muscle responses. Thus the effectiveness of the ankle muscle responses to produce a functional forward torque in patients rotated backward on a platform was diminished, and these patients tended to fall backward.

EMG responses of patients with vestibular deficit during horizontal translations of a platform were also examined.[52] Although latencies of the postural reactions were produced without significant time delays, segmental organization of the postural response did not appear to effectively meet the environmental demands. Determination of this result came from comparing the trajectory of various body segments during postural responses on a wide based platform to those on a narrow beam (see Horak and Schupert[1] for further explanation). Patients with labyrinthine deficit were observed to produce an ankle strategy (greatest motion at the ankle joint) rather than a hip strategy (initial motion at the hip joint) even when the hip strategy was preferable.

There are two explanations for the above observation. First, as suggested by the experimenters, vestibular inputs may be necessary under conditions where changes at the ankle joint are dissociated from changes at the center of mass. Alternatively, there may be either a central or local regulating mechanism that selects the postural strategy on the basis of the state of the system and the available sensory inputs. The second explanation fits the data of Allum and colleagues,[51] who found that angular velocity measures of rotation of the trunk about the hip were not significantly altered in patients with a bilateral peripheral vestibular deficit, and that a hip strategy was a common component in the postural response to platform rotations. These investigators suggest that whichever movement strategy is selected depends on the initial direction of trunk and head acceleration (which is oppositely directed in platform rotations and translations), and is executed as if preprogrammed from the beginning. Although the two laboratories differ in their use of a wide-based versus a narrow-beam base of support, the finding that trunk angular velocities do not correlate with the amplitude of ankle muscle EMG activity[51] seems to overrule the possibility that actions of the trunk are linked to torque forces generated at the ankle.

At this point, studies have not yet been done that overlap methodologic differences and clarify why data from different laboratories present conflicting results about the role of labyrinthine and other inputs during postural instability. In general though, we can conclude that patients with partial or total loss of labyrinthine input exhibit diminished amplitudes of EMG response and thus require greater energy expenditure to maintain balance, particularly when another source of stimulation to the system (e.g., visual inputs) has been removed. These patients also exhibit greater sway in sensory conflict situations, and variability between patients is a common clinical occurrence because of the dynamic central compensatory processes.

Ménière's Syndrome

Ménière's syndrome, or endolymphatic hydrops, is considered to be a vestibular deficiency although it presents as fluctuating vestibular function. Symptoms of acute Ménière's syndrome include hearing loss, tinnitus, and a sensation of fullness or pressure in the ear.[2] Patients with this syndrome exhibit a negative Romberg sign during remission,[53] but symptoms of dizziness and instability can occur for several days following intermittent episodes of vertigo. These episodes appear at irregular intervals for years, and about one third of the patients eventually develop bilateral involvement.[2]

Objective diagnosis of Ménière's syndrome has been dependent on long-term documentation of the fluctuating hearing loss. More recently, quantitative posturography measures have been able to identify consistent changes in the postural response of these patients, even during periods of remission. The movement pattern of the center of gravity was measured during a stepping test after observing that patients deviated toward the affected side even during the remission period.[53] Stepping was performed in the dark with eyes open and closed, and patients were required to perform at a frequency that was both optimal for normal walking and that elicited a smooth rhythmical pattern (i.e., 1.2 Hz). When eyes were closed, the patients exhibited angular deviations of 30 degrees or more toward the affected side after 8 to 12 seconds of stepping. Time to deviation indicated a degrading central motor program that was initiated by visual inputs but which required vestibular inputs (in the absence of vision) to be maintained over time.

Measures of sway during quiet standing have included analyses of the pattern of motion, displacement, and power spectrum of the center of gravity. With all of these measures, position of the center of gravity changed in an irregular fashion and deviated primarily toward the affected side.[54,55] High-frequency components of standing sway were observed during acute phases of Ménière's syndrome but not during remission periods.[55] Patients with Ménière's syndrome who had not developed vestibular hypofunction, as determined from VOR gains, were also tested under conditions of sensory conflict during quiet standing (see earlier description in section on indicators of vestibulospinal dysfunction).[49] These patients responded very much like well-compensated patients with unilateral or bilateral loss of labyrinthine inputs. The group had nearly normal responses on all trials with the platform fixed to earth horizontal. Responses fell outside the normal range when either the platform or the visual field was perceptually stabilized, again suggesting dependence on reliable inputs from the vestibular labyrinths during these test conditions.

Distortion of Labyrinthine Input

To study the effects of distorted labyrinthine inputs on posture, patients with benign paroxysmal positional vertigo (BPPV) have been examined.[49] The key to this syndrome is that brief episodes of vertigo (usually less than 1 minute) are generated with position change. Paroxysmal positional nystagmus can be observed with rapid changes of position. After a period of several attacks, symptoms can become more prolonged and include dizziness and nausea lasting for hours or days.[2] Degeneration of the utricular macula-releasing otoconia that settle on the cupula of the posterior semicircular canal is strongly implicated as the cause of BPPV and could result from a variety of causes (i.e., trauma, infection, ischemia). The intensity of BPPV depends on the velocity of the positional changes, and attacks can be avoided if positions are assumed very slowly.[56]

Because of the positional component of this syndrome, postural changes are easily recorded during quiet standing by having patients alter the position of their head in space. After tilting the head, large amplitudes of anterior-posterior sway and sway ipsilateral to the direction of head tilt were observed.[56] Instability gradually decreased as the vertigo diminished, but with eyes closed the sway could not be compensated by other inputs, and falling occurred.

Unlike patients with a loss of vestibular inputs, patients with distorted inputs from BPPV reacted normally on a moving platform when forced to rely only on their vestibular inputs. More disturbing to this group of patients were inappropriate (perceptually stabilized) visual circumstances whether the platform was earth-fixed or moving proportional to body sway.[8,45,49] Patients with BPPV probably rely primarily on visual information to organize their postural reactions and have suppressed their response to the potentially unreliable vestibular inputs.

Central Vestibular Lesions

One could erroneously assume that function of the vestibular labyrinths is directly representative of the functional integrity of the vestibular system. Although receiving direct inputs from the peripheral labyrinths, the vestibular nuclear complex also receives visual and somatosensory inputs.[17] Convergence of vestibular and somatosensory input onto the vestibulospinal and reticulospinal[57] neurons can take place at the level of the vestibular nuclear complex, at the adjacent reticular formation, and on spinal interneurons[58,59] and motoneurons.[57] Inputs from either of these modalities are not necessarily redundant because each represents different parameters and is effective within a particular frequency domain.[60-62] In fact, the frequency of stimulation is important to control with compensated patients because motor output of the visual system as well as the vestibular system has been found to be frequency dependent.[60,61,63] Thus it is unlikely that normal postural responses are reflective of the isolated labyrinthine and neck reflexes observed in the decerebrate animal.[64-66] Instead, postural reactions probably emerge from a combination of the available sensory signals.

Several clinical findings have been suggested to differentiate between a peripheral and central disturbance in the vestibular system. Gradually increasing disturbances of standing, walking, and falling in the direction of the quick phase of spontaneous nystagmus have been identified as indications of a central vestibular lesion.[67] Balance disorders as a result of abnormalities of the vestibular nuclear complex have been observed[68,69] but are poorly documented. The majority of the literature about central vestibular brain-stem lesions reports only oculomotor abnormalities, but Brandt and colleagues[69] have attempted to relate well-defined central vertigo syndromes to characteristics of postural imbalance. Briefly, these investigators reported five conditions for which postural imbalance has been consistently reported: downbeat nystagmus vertigo syndrome, ocular tilt reaction, Wallenberg's syndrome, paroxysmal and familial ataxia, and brain-stem lesions that mimic labyrinthine dysfunction. One should recognize, however, that structures other than the vestibular system may be damaged and affect balance.

Downbeat nystagmus is specific for a lesion of the paramedian craniocervical junction (30 percent of cases owing to Arnold-Chiari malformation), inducing a direction-specific vestibulospinal ataxia. Static head tilts modulate the intensity of the nystagmus and the postural sway, suggesting involvement of otolith function. The typical postural imbalance in this condition is an anterior-posterior sway with a tendency to fall backward, but many of these patients do not complain of vertigo or balance problems. Brandt and associates[69] suggest that the backward sway is a vestibulospinal compensation to the forward vertigo resulting from the downbeat nystagmus. *Ocular tilt reaction* is actually a triad of responses, including ipsilateral head-trunk tilt, ocular torsion, and ocular deviation. This condition has been observed in patients with brain-stem abscess, multiple sclerosis, and acute Wallenberg's syndrome. Patients seem to have a readjustment in their perception of the vertical that matches tilt deviation of the eye, head, and trunk. *Wallenberg's syndrome* is an infarction of the dorsolateral medulla resulting in ipsilateral dysmetria of the extremities, pain and temperature loss, and a lateropulsion of the eyes and head causing the body to deviate toward the side of the lesion and, consequently, fall. *Paroxysmal and familial ataxia* share the broad-based, unsteady gait that defines ataxia. Finally, pontomedullary lesions near the vestibular nuclei at the entry of the eighth nerve can mimic a peripheral labyrinthine disorder, and *drop attacks* (a sudden, unpredictable forward falling) can occur with basilar insufficiency. Thus, the evidence from clinical reports suggests that a central vestibular dysfunction results in impaired perception and location of the gravitational vertical exhibited throughout the whole-body postural system. With all of these syndromes, however, other motor structures are affected as well and may contribute to the impairment.

POSTURAL DYSFUNCTION WITH PATHOLOGY OF OTHER SENSORY-MOTOR CENTERS

The vestibular nuclear complex communicates with motor as well as sensory centers.[67] In fact, extensive reciprocal connections between the vestibular nuclei and the cerebellum[70] argue for a prominent role of the cerebellum in regulating the output of the vestibulospinal system, and lesions of the cerebellum result in severe postural disturbances. Three kinds of cerebellar ataxia have been identified, suggesting different pathophysiologic mechanisms that are dependent on the site of the lesion.[71] A test of the sway-stabilizing responses on a posture platform of patients with late cortical atrophy of the anterior lobe of the cerebellum revealed that response latencies were within normal limits following dorsiflexion rotations on a platform, but amplitudes and durations of response were two to three times greater than normal,[72] and habituation to the stimulus was absent.[73] A characteristic sway frequency of 3 Hz has been recorded in this population.[74] Intersegmental counterbalancing actions were enhanced in these patients, so that falling was not commonly observed, but the patients tended to exhibit a stiff-legged gait. Thus, in these patients, stabilizing responses occurred, but they lacked the balance between opposing muscle forces and grading of response over time.

The postural system of patients with lesions of the *vestibulocerebellum* (flocculus, nodulus, and uvula) may be so severely impaired that these patients cannot walk. Ataxia of the head and trunk is observed while sitting, standing, and walking. These patients exhibit unusually large sway in all directions with predominantly low frequencies of less than 1 Hz, and visual stabilization appears to be reduced when the Romberg test with eyes open and closed is compared. These patients tend to fall even when sitting down, which may be owing to diminished intersegmental movement for counterbalancing or to truncal ataxia.[71,75] Neocerebellum lesions produce little postural instability or disturbance of stance even with eyes closed. Control of position of the body's center of mass seems to be disturbed, as these patients exhibit ataxia during a limb and trunk pursuit task.[71] Reports of head and trunk deviation to the side of the lesion have also appeared.[75]

With basal ganglia disorders, such as Parkinson's disease, equilibrium reactions are often delayed or absent.[18] An anticipatory postural response in the soleus muscle normally seen in response to a perturbation of the forearm is absent or reduced in these patients,[76] although long latency responses to direct stretch of a muscle have been observed to be enhanced in the Parkinson population in both the upper arm[77] and lower limb.[78] Inferring the contribution of the basal ganglia to postural reactions from this patient population, however, is difficult because the motor impairments could be as much an effect of akinesia, rigidity, or aging as of disruptions in the postural control system.

Lesions in motor cortex have also resulted in disturbances to the automatic postural reactions. Patients with spastic paresis rarely exhibit disturbances of posture during quiet standing as in the Romberg test, but reactions to rapid displacements of the support surface indicate deficits in the dynamic postural reactions.[79] Hemiplegic adults demonstrate delayed onsets, a failure to respond, and disparate responses of agonist and antagonist mucles in the paretic lower limb during postural perturbations on a platform.[80] With augmented feedback, such as a warning tone and knowledge of perturbation direction, however, timing of the postural responses improved.[81] When balancing on a seesaw apparatus, patients with spastic hemiparesis minimized the high-frequency anteroposterior sway on the affected side with a corresponding reduction of the EMG response in tibialis anterior.[82,83] Electrical stimulation of the tibial nerve in patients on the seesaw revealed a delayed and diminished EMG response of tibialis anterior in the affected leg, thereby interfering with the normal compensatory response to displacement of the support surface. Spastic paraparetic patients were observed to produce qualitatively similar results.[82,83]

Children with cerebral palsy were also studied on a posture platform.[84] Their instability seemed to correlate with the clinical diagnosis so that children with spastic hemiplegia exhibited reversals in the expected order of muscular activation, whereas children with ataxia demonstrated normal muscle sequencing yet fell frequently. The timing, direction, and amplitude of their postural reactions were disturbed, particularly when the expected sensory inputs had been altered (see the paradigm described in the section on indicators of vestibulospinal dysfunction). Thus postural abnormalities of children with cerebral palsy were owing either to muscle incoordination or instability as a result of an inability to deal with sensory conflict.

Results of these clinical studies suggest that the long-latency, polysynaptic postural adjustments can be elicited at the spinal level but require modulation by supraspinal structures to develop a sufficient response threshold and gain. Possibly there are an inappropriate number of nerve fibers within the damaged motor pathway to excite the motoneuron pool, or the damaged pathway sends a reduced drive to the interneurons at segmental levels that would normally facilitate the polysynaptic reflex response.[79]

MECHANISMS FOR RECOVERY OF POSTURAL STABILITY

Identification of compensatory mechanisms will improve therapeutic interventions that teach compensation for, or adaptation to, destabilizing conditions. These mechanisms are studied through clinical research, but we must be cautious about conclusions drawn about the function of an anatomic site that are based strictly on the absence of motor control in the presence of specific deficits or damage. We must remember that responses generated in the absence of a sensory or motor signal do not reveal the function of that input. Rather, these responses demonstrate how the system operates in the absence of certain inputs.

Sensory Substitution

Vestibular, visual, and somatosensory signals influence the organization of a normal postural response. When any one of these signals is lost or distorted, a central reweighting occurs so that the remaining sensory inputs are used to elicit postural reactions, albeit in some altered fashion (Table 3–3). Changes in the postural response organization with loss of labyrinthine inputs has been described in detail in earlier sections of this chapter. Two modifications in particular should be noted. First, in the absence of labyrinthine signals, the normal postural reactions to dorsiflexion of the ankle are elicited, but with significantly diminished amplitudes.[7] Thus, the response does not reach an appropriate gain to maintain stability, and restabilizing torques at the ankle are inadequate to prevent falls.

TABLE 3–3 Modifications to Postural Stability Following
Loss of Specific Sensory Inputs

Labyrinthine Deficits
  Stiffening between body segments
  Increased sway at high frequencies
Somatosensory Deficits
  Low-frequency sway during quiet stance
  Delayed restabilization
  Increased lateral sway
Visual Deficits
  Increased sway at low frequencies
  Increased sway at high frequencies when labyrinthine inputs are also absent

Second, peripheral vestibular deficit patients tend to exhibit ankle rather than hip synergies, with the neck stiff so that little free head movement occurs.[52] An analysis of the temporal relationship between angular acceleration of the head and trunk in the flexor and extensor directions demonstrates that patients move the head in the same direction as the body, while normal subjects exhibit a counterbalancing action of the head and body in the sagittal plane.[51] This finding correlates with clinical observations that vestibular deficit patients increase gain of neck muscles to hold the head stiff in relation to the body. A fast Fourier transform performed on the head and trunk angular acceleration recordings revealed a loss of the normal 2- to 3-Hz peak in the power spectrum of patients with bilateral labyrinthine deficit.[7] This frequency has been cited as the operating frequency for the vestibulocollic reflexes in studies of normal subjects attempting to stabilize the head during vertical and horizontal rotations in the seated position[85] and is typical of natural movements during locomotion.[86,87] Stiffening of the muscles may, therefore, be one compensatory strategy that actually works against successful restabilization by interfering with the normal balance of movement-dependent torques at the different body segments, and with the reception of stimuli necessary to produce vestibular adaptation.

Somatosensory inputs provide powerful feedback about motion of the limbs and stabilizes body sway at the lower frequencies (less than 1 Hz). When proprioceptive feedback from the ankle was excluded or suppressed in normal subjects during perturbations on a posture platform,[22,88] a characteristic low-frequency (1-Hz) sway emerged. Postural abnormalities have been observed with impairment of spinal pathways such as occurs with Friedreich's ataxia, a hereditary disorder affecting the spinocerebellar pathways and posterior columns.[89] In the absence of feedback from these pathways to the cerebellum, a significant delay of the restabilizing response of the tibialis anterior muscle following dorsiflexing ankle rotations on a posture platform has been observed.[72] These patients exhibit large lateral sway deviations in the low-frequency range (less than 1 Hz) with eyes closed, as do patients with tabes dorsalis.[88] Patients with sensory polyneuropathy of the lower extremities demonstrate ataxia and instability during quiet stance. Falls tend to occur when the eyes are closed,[89] suggesting that visual inputs are necessary along with vestibular inputs in the absence of lower limb proprioceptor signals. Finally, cervical proprioceptors have been the focus of investigations related to the diagnosis of dizziness and ataxia.[90,91] The neck proprioceptors have intimate connections with the vestibular system and are probably used both as feedforward and feedback to the vestibulocollic reflexes.[92] Cervical ataxia is a controversial diagnosis, however, because there are no hard signs to identify the neck as the source of the dizziness.[91]

Visual signals are used to accurately detect and reduce motion relative to the surround.[93,94] In normal subjects, vision can be influential but does not appear to be an essential input for the recovery of balance. Many studies have shown that simply removing vision will not produce significant changes in the postural response organization, although greater sway amplitudes may appear.[7,36,37] Instead, visual information is thought to be redundant unless both vestibular and somatosensory inputs are lost.[94] To test the importance of visual inputs in the absence of labyrinthine inputs, sway was measured in subjects standing on a stabilometer placed within a laterally tilting room.[16] At low frequencies of sinusoidal tilt (0.0025 to 0.1 Hz), patients with unilateral and bilateral labyrinthine deficits exhibited sway similar to that of normals. At higher frequencies (0.2 Hz), the patients' sway increased beyond normal limits, indicating that patients with vestibular deficit could rely on visual inputs at lower frequencies but suffered for the loss of vestibular signals at higher frequencies.[6,95] Labyrinthine-deficit patients on a stabilometer were better able to stabilize sway when fixating on a stationary light.[96] When an optokinetic stimulus was introduced, the patients became unstable, suggesting that velocity information received through peripheral vision is the cause of the increased sway.

In summary, patients lacking labyrinthine inputs become more dependent on accurate ankle proprioceptive and visual references to correctly organize their postural responses. Inappropriate or distorted signals along either of these sensory pathways will produce increased sway and falls in these patients. Although the sensory signals often provide congruent information, inputs from any of these modalities are not necessarily redundant because each represents different parameters and is affective within a particular frequency domain.[6,60,61] Thus, the falls observed in vestibular-deficit patients, particularly following a platform perturbation or in the absence of other sensory signals, may be owing to uncontrolled or poorly compensated oscillations of intersegmental structures at particular frequencies of sway.

Compensatory Processes

Compensation for vestibular pathology is a gradual process of functional recovery that is probably of central origin.[97,98] Numerous structures have been identified as participating in vestibular compensation, including the vestibular nuclei, spinal cord, visual system, cerebellum, inferior olive, and more.[98] Thus, focusing specifically on a single site for functional recovery of postural control would be difficult. In fact, studies have shown that in both humans and animals, methods of compensation for vestibular dysfunction are not comparable either across subjects or within a subject for different functions.[98,99] The only consistency seems to be that the goal of postural compensation is to reorganize the neural circuitry so that bilateral stimulation of the vestibular system is kept in balance.

Central control over postural responses can be measured in studies examining predictive processes. For example, Guitton and associates[63] assessed the influence of mental set on the relative importance of visual and vestibular cues for head stabilization in humans. Normal subjects and patients with bilateral vestibular deficit were tested on their ability to stabilize their heads voluntarily with visual feedback and in the dark, and while distracted with a mental arithmetic task while being rotated horizontally using a random (white noise) stimulus with a bandwidth of 0 to 1 Hz. Normal subjects stabilized their heads best when voluntarily attempting to keep the head coincident with a stationary visual target. Vestibular-deficit patients had comparable gains with vision present but much lower gains when vision was removed. Thus, vestibular inputs provided a necessary signal for head stability in the dark. The apparent lack of head stabilization when all subjects performed mental arithmetic suggested that the short-latency (approximately 50 msec) head-stabilizing reflexes provided little effective head stabilization in humans at these frequencies of rotation. An analysis of response latencies revealed that long latency or voluntary mechanisms (occurring at greater than 150 msec) were primarily responsible for the observed head stabilization.

Anticipatory presetting of the static and dynamic sensitivity of the postural control system also assists in stabilization of the head at high frequencies.[100,101] Practice or prior experience with a postural task influences EMG output. With practice, decreasing size of the EMG response to a plateau level has commonly been observed during stabilizing reactions,[7,23,50] suggesting central habituation of these responses at the cortical or spinal levels. Selection of postural strategies on a translating platform is influenced by prior experience as well as current feedback information.[102] When the task is well practiced, subjects are able to combine complex movement strategies and respond quickly under a variety of different posture platform paradigms. Even chronic patients with labyrinthine deficits eventually demonstrate normal sway,[14] indicating that a central regulatory mechanism is compensating for the peripheral dysfunction.

AGING AND VESTIBULAR DYSFUNCTION

The gradual loss of labyrinthine acuity with age prompts viewing the elderly population as a model for compensation to vestibular dysfunction. In the elderly, however, sensory loss occurs as a slow process along several feedback pathways, not just the vestibular pathways.[103-108] Their compensatory approach to postural instability may not be the same as in those patients that have experienced an acute but sustained loss of a single input (see Table 3–2). Age-related trends in the VOR and optokinetic reflex have been shown to correlate well with anatomic changes found in the peripheral vestibular system.[104,105] Anatomic studies have revealed a gradually decreasing density of labyrinthine hair-cell receptors beginning at age 30, and a steeper decline in the number of vestibular receptor ganglion cells beginning around 55 to 60 years of age.[106-108] Although caloric measures of the peripheral vestibular system have demonstrated declining function with age,[107] these changes are not present in the central vestibular neurons. Thus, changes in postural function and the increased propensity in falling found in many elderly individuals could be a result of impaired event detection as a result of the diminished sensory feedback rather than of an impaired central vestibular system.

Studies of postural instability and compensation in the elderly demonstrate disruption or deterioration of the mechanisms controlling stability.[109,110] On a posture platform, the stabilizing muscle synergies found to appear in a temporally consistent fashion in young normal subjects exhibit a disorganized order of onset in the elderly.[39,110] Latencies of EMG responses and of reaction times are increased in the elderly population.[109-111] Quiet sway tends to increase, although no correlation has been found between sway and falling.[112,113] A recent study of elderly individuals on a rotating posture platform[114] has explored whether delayed latencies of lower limb muscle responses are responsible for the failure to produce torque outputs necessary to compensate for unexpected falling. Results indicate that a disordered temporal relationship between tibialis anterior and soleus muscles, which are concurrently activated in younger individuals,[7] resulted in decreased stabilizing ankle torques. Weakness of the tibialis anterior muscle has also been described in the elderly,[115] and could be a major contributor to the diminished torque response. Because there is no significant difference in the trunk angular acceleration responses, we can infer that the elderly compensate for diminished ankle torque by increasing hip torque. Thus, impaired balance in the elderly may be produced by altered response synergies that are generated by delayed vestibulospinal and propriospinal reflex responses as a result of increased sensory thresholds and an aging musculoskeletal system.

SUMMARY

We can draw the following conclusions about mechanisms that contribute to postural stability from the existing data. First, central neural processes influence stability in the form of both automatic, long-latency reactions and voluntary movements. Second, the presence or absence of specific sensory inputs (e.g., vestibular or proprioceptive) alters the magnitude or temporal onset of the muscle response pattern, whereas distortion of sensory inputs seems to rearrange the directional organization of the muscle response patterns. Third, learning, attention, and predictive processes influence the performance of postural reactions, as does the motor activity in which the individual is currently engaged when the postural behavior is required. Finally, a particular compensatory strategy adopted by a patient may interfere with, rather than assist, postural stability. Thus, clinicians and researchers should identify the preplanned and automatic components of a postural response to determine how best to influence the postural response organization. Recognizing the multiple factors that contribute to the outcome of a postural response should assist clinicians in determining the approach and effectiveness of their intervention strategies for retraining and restoration of postural function.

REFERENCES

1. Horak, F and Shupert, C: Role of the vestibular system in postural control. In Herdman, S: Vestibular Rehabilitation. Philadelphia, FA Davis, 1993.
2. Baloh, RW and Honrubia, V: Clinical neurophysiology of the vestibular system. FA Davis, Philadelphia, 1979.
3. Norre, ME, Forrez, G, and Beckers, A: Functional recovery of posture in peripheral vestibular disorders. In Amblard, B, Berthoz, A, and Clarac, F (eds): Posture and gait: Development, adaptation and modulation. Elsevier, Amsterdam, 1988, p 291.
4. Romberg, MH: Manual of nervous diseases of man. Sydenham Society, London, 1853, pp 395–401.
5. Wall, C, III and Black, FO: Postural stability and rotational tests: Their effectiveness for screening dizzy patients. Acta Otolaryngol 95:235, 1983.
6. Xerri, C, et al: Synergistic interactions and functional working range of the visual and vestibular systems in postural control: Neuronal correlates. In Pompeiano, O and Allum, JHJ (eds): Vestibulospinal Control of Posture and Movement. Progress in Brain Research. Elsevier, Amsterdam, 1988, p 193.
7. Keshner, EA, Allum, JHJ, and Pfaltz, CR: Postural coactivation and adaptation in the sway stabilizing responses of normals and patients with bilateral peripheral vestibular deficit. Exp Brain Res 69:66, 1987.
8. Black, FO: Vestibulospinal function assessment by moving platform posturography. Am J Otol (suppl) 39, 1985.
9. Allum, JHJ and Keshner, EA: Vestibular and proprioceptive control of sway stabilization. In Bles, W and Brandt, T (eds): Disorders of Posture and Gait. Elsevier, Amsterdam, 1986, pp 19–40.
10. Allum, JHJ, et al: Indicators of the influence a peripheral vestibular deficit has on vestibulo-spinal reflex responses controlling postural stability. Acta Otolaryngol (Stockh) 106:252, 1988.
11. Cohen, H and Keshner, EA: Current concepts of the vestibular system reviewed: II. Visual/vestibular interaction and spatial orientation. Am J Occup Ther 43:331, 1989.
12. Bles, W and de Jong, JMBV: Uni- and bilateral loss of vestibular function. In Bles, W and Brandt, T (eds): Disorders of Posture and Gait. Elsevier, Amsterdam, 1986, pp 127–239.
13. Kapteyn, TS, et al: Standardization in platform stabilometry being a part of posturography. Agressologie 24:321, 1983.
14. Norre, ME and Forrez, G: Posture testing (posturography) in the diagnosis of peripheral vestibular pathology. Arch Otorhinolaryngol 243:186, 1986.
15. Bles, W, et al: The mechansim of physiological height vertigo. II. Posturography. Acta Otolaryngol (Stockh) 89:534, 1980.
16. Bles, W, et al: Compensation for labyrinthine deficits examined by use of a tilting room. Acta Otolaryngol (Stockh) 95:576, 1983.
17. Hain, TC and Hillman, MA: Anatomy and Physiology of the normal vestibular system. In Herdman, S: Vestibular Rehabilitation. FA Davis, 1993.
18. Brock, S and Wechsler, IS: Loss of the righting reflex in man. Arch Neurol Psychiatry 17:12, 1927.
19. Martin, JP: Tilting reactions and disorders of the basal ganglia. Brain 88:855, 1965.
20. McNally, WJ: Labyrinthine reactions and their relation to the clinical tests. Proc Royal Soc Med 30:905, 1937.
21. Weisz, S: Studies in equilibrium reactions. J Nervous Ment Dis 88:150, 1938.
22. Nashner, LM: Adapting reflexes controlling human posture. Exp Brain Res 26:59, 1976.
23. Nashner, LM: Fixed patterns of rapid postural responses among leg muscles during stance. Exp Brain Res 30:13, 1977.
24. Nashner, LM: Vestibular and reflex control of normal standing. In Stein, RB, et al (eds): Control of Posture and Locomotion. Plenum Press, New York, 1973, pp 291–308.

25. Allum, JHJ and Pfaltz, CR: Visual and vestibular contributions to pitch sway stabilization in the ankle muscles of normals and patients with bilateral peripheral vestibular deficits. Exp Brain Res 58:82, 1985.
26. Black, FO, Shupert, CL, and Horak, FB: Abnormal postural control associated with peripheral vestibular disorders. In Pompeiano, O and Allum, JHJ (eds): Vestibulospinal Control of Posture and Movement. Progress in Brain Research. Elsevier, Amsterdam, 1988, p 263.
27. Nashner, LM, et al: Organization of posture controls: An analysis of sensory and mechanical constraints. In Allum, JHJ and Hulliger, M (eds): Afferent Control of Posture and Locomotion. Progress in Brain Research. Elsevier, Amsterdam, 1989, p 411.
28. Keshner, EA, Woollacott, MH, and Debu, B: Neck and trunk muscle responses during postural perturbations in humans. Exp Brain Res 71:455, 1988.
29. Stockwell, CW, Koozekani, SH, and Barin, K: A physical model of human postural dynamics. In Cohen, B (ed): Vestibular and oculomotor physiology. Ann NY Acad Sci 374:722, 1981.
30. Nashner, LM and McCollum, G: The organization of human postural movements: A formal basis and experimental synthesis. Brain Behav 8:135, 1985.
31. Greenwood, R and Hopkins, AL: Muscle responses during sudden falls in man. J Physiol (Lond) 254:507, 1976.
32. Lacour, M and Xerri, C: Compensation of postural reactions to free-fall in the vestibular neurectomized monkey. Exp Brain Res 40:103, 1980.
33. Melvill Jones, G and Watt, DGD: Observations on the control of stepping and hopping movements in man. J Physiol 219:709, 1971.
34. Wicke, RW and Oman, CM: Visual and graviceptive influences on lower leg EMG activity in humans during brief falls. Exp Brain Res 46:324, 1982.
35. Allum, JHJ, Honegger, F, and Pfaltz, CR: The role of stretch and vestibulo-spinal reflexes in the generation of human equilibrating reactions. In Allum, JHJ and Hulliger, M (eds): Afferent Control of Posture and Locomotion. Progress in Brain Research. Elsevier, Amsterdam, 1989, pp 399–410.
36. Nashner, LM and Berthoz, A: Visual contributions to rapid motor responses during postural control. Brain Res 150:403, 1978.
37. Vidal, PP, Berthoz, A, and Millanvoye, M: Difference between eye closure and visual stabilization in the control of posture in man. Aviat Space Environ Med 53:166, 1982.
38. Black, FO, Wall, C, III, and Nashner, LM: Effects of visual and support surface orientation references upon postural control in vestibular deficient subjects. Acta Otolaryngol 95:199, 1983.
39. Woollacott, MH, Shumway-Cook, AT, and Nashner LM: Postural reflexes and aging. In: Mortimer JA (ed): The Aging Motor System. Praeger, New York, 1982, p 98.
40. Unterberger, S: Neue objektive registrierbare vestibulariskorperdrehungen, erhalten durch treten auf der stelle. Der 'Tretversuch'. Arch Ohren Nasen Kehlkopfheilkd 145:478, 1938.
41. Fukuda, T: Statokinetic Reflexes in Equilibrium and Movement. Tokyo University Press, Tokyo, 1983.
42. Bles, W, de Jong, JMBV, and de Wit, G: Somatosensory compensation for loss of labyrinthine function. Acta Otolaryngol (Stockh) 95:576, 1984.
43. Graybiel, A and Fregly, AR: A new quantitative ataxia test battery. Acta Otolaryngol (Stockh) 61:292, 1966.
44. Peitersen, E: Measurement of vestibulospinal responses in man. In Kornhuber, HH (ed): Handbook of sensory physiology, Vol VI (2), Vestibular system. Springer-Verlag, Berlin, 1974, p 267.
45. Black, FO and Nashner, LM: Vestibulo-spinal control differs in patients with reduced versus distorted vestibular function. Acta Otolaryngol (Stockh) 406:110, 1984.
46. Norre, ME: Posture in otoneurology. Acta Oto-Rhino-Laryngol Belgica 44:55, 1990.
47. Dow, RS: The effects of bilateral and unilateral labyrinthectomy in monkey, baboon, and chimpanzee. Am J Physiol 121:392, 1938.
48. Allum, JHJ and Pfaltz, CR: Postural control in man following acute unilateral peripheral vestibular deficit. In Igarashi, M and Black, FO (eds): Vestibular and visual control of posture and locomotor equilibrium. Karger, Basel, 1985, p 315.
49. Black, FO, Wall, C, III, and O'Leary, DP: Computerized screening of the human vestibulospinal system. Ann Otol Rhinol Laryngol 87:853, 1978.
50. Keshner, EA and Allum, JHJ: Plasticity in pitch sway stabilization: Normal habituation and compensation for peripheral vestibular deficits. In Bles, W and Brandt, T (eds): Disorders of Posture and Gait. Elsevier, Amsterdam, 1986, p 289.
51. Allum, JHJ, et al: Organization of leg-trunk-head coordination in normals and patients with peripheral vestibular deficits. In Pompeiano, O and Allum, JHJ (eds): Vestibulospinal Control of Posture and Movement. Progress in Brain Research. Elsevier, Amsterdam, 1988, p 277.
52. Horak, FB, Nashner, LM, and Diener, HC: Postural strategies associated with somatosensory and vestibular loss. Exp Brain Res 82:167, 1991.
53. Okubo, J, et al: Posture and gait in Ménière's disease. In Bles, W and Brandt, T (eds): Disorders of Posture and Gait. Elsevier, Amsterdam, 1986, p 113.
54. Dichgans, J, et al: Postural sway in normals and atactic patients: Analysis of the stabilizing and destabilizing effects of vision. Agressologie 17C:15, 1976.
55. Kapteyn, TS and De Wit, G: Posturography as an auxiliary in vestibular investigation. Acta Otolaryngol 73:104, 1972.

56. Buchele, W and Brandt, T: Benign paroxysmal positional vertigo and posture. In Bles, W and Brandt, T (eds): Disorders of Posture and Gait. Elsevier, Amsterdam, 1986, p 101.
57. Brink, EE, Hirai, N, and Wilson, VJ: Influence of neck afferents on vestibulospinal neurons. Exp Brain Res 38:285, 1980.
58. Peterson, BW: The reticulospinal system and its role in the control of movement. In Barnes, CD (ed): Brainstem control of spinal cord function. Academic Press, New York, 1984, pp 27–86.
59. Wilson, VJ, Ezure, K, and Timerick, SJB: Tonic neck reflex of the decerebrate cat: Response of spinal interneurons to natural stimulation of neck and vestibular receptors. J Neurophysiol 51:567, 1984.
60. Bilotto, G, et al: Dynamic properties of vestibular reflexes in the decerebrate cat. Exp Brain Res 47:343, 1982.
61. Peterson, BW, et al: The cervicocollic reflex: Its dynamic properties and interaction with vestibular reflexes. J Neurophysiol 54:90, 1985.
62. Keshner, EA and Peterson, BW: Motor control strategies underlying head stabilization and voluntary head movements in humans and cats. In Pompeiano, O and Allum, JHJ (eds): Vestibulospinal control of posture and movement. Progress in Brain Research. Elsevier, Amsterdam, 1988, p 329.
63. Guitton, D, et al: Visual, vestibular and voluntary contributions to human head stabilization. Exp Brain Res 64:59, 1986.
64. Roberts, TDM: Reflex balance. Nature 244:156, 1973.
65. Suzuki, J and Cohen, B: Head, eye, body and limb movements from semicircular canal nerves. Exp Neurol 10:393, 1964.
66. Magnus, R: Physiology of posture. Lancet 2:531, 585, 1926.
67. Uemura, T, et al: Neuro-otological Examination. University Park Press, Baltimore, 1977.
68. Rudge, P: Clinical Neurootology. Churchill Livingstone, London, 1983.
69. Brandt, T, Dieterich, M, and Buchele, W: Postural abnormalities in central vestibular brain stem lesions. In Bles, W and Brandt, T (eds): Disorders of Posture and Gait. Elsevier, Amsterdam, 1986, p 141.
70. Shimazu, H and Smith, CM: Cerebellar and labyrinthine influences on single vestibular neurons identified by natural stimuli. J Neurophysiol 34:493, 1971.
71. Mauritz, KH, Dichgans, J, and Hufschmidt, A: Quantitative analysis of stance in late cortical cerebellar atrophy of the anterior lobe and other forms of cerebellar ataxia. Brain 102:461, 1979.
72. Diener, HC, et al: Characteristic alterations of long-loop "reflexes" in patients with Friedreich's disease and late atrophy of the cerebellar anterior lobe. J Neurol Neurosurg Psychiatry 47:679, 1984.
73. Nashner, LM and Grimm, RJ: Analysis of multiloop dyscontrols in standing cerebellar patients. In Desmedt, JE (ed): Cerebellar Motor Control in Man: Long Loop Mechanisms. Karger, Basel, 1978, p 300.
74. Dichgans, J and Mauritz, KH: Patterns and mechanisms of postural instability in patients with cerebellar lesions. In Desmedt, JE (ed): Motor control mechanisms in health and disease. Raven Press, New York, 1983, p 633.
75. Dichgans, J and Diener, HC: Different forms of postural ataxia in patients with cerebellar diseases. In Bles, W and Brandt, T (eds): Disorders of Posture and Gait. Elsevier, Amsterdam, 1986, p 207.
76. Traub, MM, Rothwell, JC, and Marsden, CD: Anticipatory postural reflexes in Parkinson's disease and other akinetic-rigid syndromes and cerebellar ataxia. Brain 103:393, 1980.
77. Berardelli, A, Sabra, AF, and Hallett, M: Physiological mechanisms of rigidity in Parkinson's disease. J Neurol Neurosurg Psychiatry 46:45, 1983.
78. Allum, JHJ, et al: Disturbance of posture in patients with Parkinson's disease. In Amblard, B, Berthoz, A, and Clarac, F (eds): Posture and Gait: Development, Adaptation and Modulation. Elsevier, Amsterdam, 1988, p 245.
79. Benecke, R and Conrad, B: Disturbance of posture and gait in spastic syndromes. In Bles, W and Brandt, T (eds): Disorders of Posture and Gait. Elsevier, Amsterdam, 1986, p 231.
80. DiFabio, RP and Badke, MB: Influence of cerebrovascular accident on elongated and passively shortened muscle responses after forward sway. Phys Ther 68:1215, 1988.
81. Badke, MB, Duncan, PW, and Di Fabio, RP: Influence of prior knowledge on automatic and voluntary postural adjustments in healthy and hemiplegic subjects. Phys Ther 67:1495, 1987.
82. Dietz, V, Mauritz, KH, and Dichgans, J: Body oscillations in balancing due to segmental stretch reflex activity. Exp Brain Res 40:89, 1980.
83. Dietz, V and Berger, W: Interlimb coordination of posture in patients with spastic paresis. Brain 107:965, 1984.
84. Nashner, LM, Shumway-Cook, A, and Marin, O: Stance posture control in select groups of children with cerebral palsy: Deficits in sensory organization and muscular coordination. Exp Brain Res 49:393, 1983.
85. Keshner, EA and Peterson, BW: Mechanisms of human head stabilization during random sinusoidal rotations. Soc Neurosci Abstr 14:1235, 1988.
86. Keshner, EA and Peterson, BW: Frequency and velocity characteristics of head, neck, and trunk during normal locomotion. Soc Neurosci Abstr 15:1200, 1989.
87. Gresty, M: Stability of the head: Studies in normal subjects and in patients with labyrinthine disease, head tremor, and dystonia. Movement Disorders 2:165, 1987.
88. Mauritz, KH and Dietz, V: Characteristics of postural instability induced by ischaemic blocking of leg afferents. Exp Brain Res 38:117, 1980.

89. Kotaka, S, Croll, GA, and Bles, W: Somatosensory ataxia. In Bles, W and Brandt, T (eds): Disorders of Posture and Gait. Elsevier, Amsterdam, 1986, pp 178–183.
90. Cohen, LA: Role of eye and neck proprioceptive mechanisms in body orientation and motor coordination. J Neurophysiol 24:1, 1961.
91. de Jong, JMBV and Bles, W: Cervical dizziness and ataxia. In Bles, W and Brandt, T (eds): Disorders of Posture and Gait. Elsevier, Amsterdam, 1986, p 185.
92. Wilson, VJ and Melvill Jones, G: Mammalian vestibular physiology. Plenum Press, New York, 1979.
93. Gantchev, GN, Draganova, N, and Dunev, S: Influence of the stabilogram and statokinesigram visual feedback upon the body oscillations. In Igarashi, M and Black, FO (eds): Vestibular and visual control of posture and locomotor equilibrium. Karger, Basel, 1985, p 135.
94. Paulus, W, Straube, A, and Brandt, T: Visual postural performance after loss of somatosensory and vestibular function. J Neurol Neurosurg Psychiatry 50:1542, 1987.
95. Waespe, W and Henn, V: Neuronal activity in the vestibular nuclei of the alert monkey during vestibular and optokinetic stimulation. Exp Brain Res 27:523, 1977.
96. Kotaka, S, Okubo, J, and Watanabe, I: The influence of eye movements and tactile information on postural sway in patients with peripheral vestibular lesions. Auris-Nasus-Larynx, Tokyo, 13 (Suppl II):S153, 1986.
97. Pfaltz, CR: Vestibular habituation and central compensation. Advances in Oto-Rhino-Laryngology 22:136, 1977.
98. Igarashi, M: Vestibular compensation. Acta Otolaryngol (Stockh) (suppl) 406:78, 1984.
99. Hart, CW, McKinley, PA, and Peterson, BW: Compensation following acute unilateral total loss of peripheral vestibular function. In Graham, MD and Kemink, JL (eds): The vestibular system. Neurophysiologic and clinical research. Raven Press, New York, 1987, p 187.
100. Viviani, P and Berthoz, A: Dynamics of the head-neck system in response to small perturbations: Analysis and modelling in the frequency domain. Biol Cybernet 19:19, 1985.
101. Jeannerod, M: The contribution of open-loop and closed-loop control modes in prehension movements. In Kornblum, S and Requin, J (eds): Preparatory States and Processes. Lawrence Erlbaum Assoc, Hillsdale, NJ, 1984, p 323.
102. Horak, FB and Nashner, LM: Central programming of postural movements: Adaptation to altered support-surface configurations. J Neurophysiol 55:1369, 1986.
103. Skinner, HB, Barrack, RL, and Cook, SD: Age-related declines in proprioception. Clin Orthop 184:208, 1984.
104. Peterka, RJ, Black, FO, and Schoenhoff, MB: Age-related changes in human vestiublo-ocular reflexes: Sinusoidal rotation and caloric tests. J Vestib Res 1:49, 1990.
105. Peterka, RJ and Black, FO: Age-related changes in human vestiublo-ocular reflexes: Pseudorandom rotation tests. J Vestib Res 1:61, 1990.
106. Bergstrom, B: Morphology of the vestibular nerve. II. The number of myelinated vestibular nerve fibers in man at various ages. Acta Otolaryngol 76:173, 1973.
107. Richter, E: Quantitative study of human Scarpa's ganglion and vestibular sensory epithelia. Acta Otolaryngol 90:199, 1980.
108. Rosenhall, U: Degenerative patterns in the aging human vestibular neuro-epithelia. Acta Otolaryngol 76:208, 1973.
109. Studenski, S, et al: The role of instability in falls among older persons. In Duncan, PW (ed): Balance. American Physical Therapy Association, 1990, p 57.
110. Woollacott, MH: Gait and postural control in the aging adult. In Bles, W and Brandt, T (eds): Disorders of Posture and Gait. Elsevier, New York, 1986, p 325.
111. Stelmach, GE, et al: Age-related decline in postural control mechanisms. Int J Aging Hum Develop 29:205, 1989.
112. Hasselkus, BR and Shambes, GM: Aging and postural sway in women. J Gerontol 30:661, 1975.
113. Overstall, PW, et al: Falls in the elderly related to postural imbalance. Br Med J 1:261, 1977.
114. Keshner, EA, Allum, JHJ, and Honegger F: Predictors of less stable postural responses to support surface relations in healthy human elderly. J Vest Res, in press.
115. Whipple, RH, Wolfson, LI, and Amerman, PM: The relationship of knee and ankle weakness to falls in nursing home residents: An isokinetic study. J Am Geriatr Soc 35:13, 1987.

CHAPTER 4

Vestibular Adaptation

David S. Zee, MD

A robust and versatile capability for adaptive control of vestibular motor behavior is essential if an organism is to maintain optimal visual function and stable balance throughout life. Changes associated with normal development and aging, as well as with disease and trauma, demand mechanisms both to detect errors in performance and to correct them. An understanding of such mechanisms is crucial in the design and in the evaluation of the programs of physical therapy that are used to rehabilitate patients with vestibular disorders.[1] The purpose of this chapter is to review new information about adaptive mechanisms that bears on the management of patients with disorders of their vestibular systems. By necessity, we emphasize studies of the vestibulo-ocular reflex (VOR or head-eye loop), because most is known about its adaptive control. When possible, however, we also refer to vestibulospinal (VSR or head-body loop); vestibulo-collic (VCR or head-neck loop); and cervico-ocular (COR or neck-eye loop) reflexes.

RECALIBRATION, SUBSTITUTION, AND ALTERNATIVE STRATEGIES

Adaptive control of vestibular reflexes must be looked at in the larger context of overall compensation for vestibular deficits.* Restoring adequate motor behavior by simply readjusting the input-output relationships (e.g., gain, timing, or direction) of the VOR or VSR may be impossible, especially when deficits are large. Other mechanisms of compensation must then be invoked (Table 4-1). Examples include substitution of another sensory input to drive the same motor response (e.g., substitution of the COR for the VOR); substitution of an alternative motor response in lieu of the usual compensa-

---

*We will not make a rigid distinction here between the terms adaptation and compensation, although, in general, the former is used in a more restricted sense to imply adjustment in the basic VOR and VSR, while the latter is used in a larger sense to include the entire repertoire of ways, including substitution, prediction, and other cognitive strategies by which patients recover from, and learn to live with, vestibular disorders.

TABLE 4-1 Compensatory Mechanisms

Adaptation:
  Changing the gain of the vestibular system
Substitution:
  Of other sensory inputs mechanisms (e.g., COR)
  Of alternative motor responses (e.g., saccades)
  Of strategies based on prediction/anticipation

tory motor response (e.g., use of saccades instead of slow phases to help stabilize gaze during head rotation); and the use of strategies based on prediction or anticipation of intended motor behavior (e.g., when there is a complete vestibular loss, subjects learn to prevent gaze overshoot by preprogramming compensatory slow phases in anticipation of a combined eye-head movement toward a new target).

Furthermore, there is considerable variability among subjects about which particular mechanisms are primarily used for compensation. This heterogeneity dictates a need for quantitative testing of vestibular function and eye-head coordination in patients before and during rehabilitation. Any plan of therapy must focus on what is likely to work best and what is working best. The promotion of different goals may require a different therapeutic emphasis, and different therapeutic programs may potentially work at cross purposes. Therefore, planning the program of therapy based on what is most likely to succeed in the context of the type and the degree of deficit and the patient's inherent potential for compensation is essential. To illustrate these points, we first discuss two archetypal paradigms requiring vestibular compensation: unilateral and bilateral loss of labyrinthine function.

UNILATERAL LOSS OF LABYRINTHINE FUNCTION

Perhaps the most common vestibular disturbance that brings a patient to a physician is diminished or absent function in one labyrinth. Unilateral labyrinthectomy (UL) has been used as an experimental model to study motor learning and compensation for more than a hundred years. Yet, until recently, little has been known about the error signals that drive the compensatory process, the precise mechanisms that underlie recovery from both the static and the dynamic disturbances that are created by the loss of labyrinthine input from one side, and the additional strategies that are available to assist in the overall goal of gaze and postural stability during movement.

The Deficit to Be Corrected after Unilateral Labyrinthectomy

Using the VOR as an example, UL creates two general types of deficits for which a correction is required: static imbalance, related to the differences in the levels of tonic discharge within the vestibular nuclei; and dynamic disturbances, related to the loss of one half of the afferent input that normally contributes, in a push-pull fashion, to the generation of compensatory responses during head movement. Spontaneous nystagmus with the head still is an example of the static type of disturbance. Decreased amplitude (gain) and asymmetry of eye rotation during head rotation are examples of the dynamic type of disturbance.

The Error Signals That Drive VOR Adaptation

What might be the error signals that drive VOR adaptation? Image motion or "slip" on the retina, when associated with head movements, is the obvious candidate, as the *raison d'etre* of the VOR is to keep images stable on the retina during head movements. We investigated the role of vision, and especially of visual information mediated by geniculostriate pathways, on both the acquisition and the maintenance of adaptation to UL in monkeys.[2]

We recorded VOR function in three groups of animals. One group had undergone bilateral occipital lobectomy many months before the labyrinthectomy. These "cortically blind" animals were allowed normal light exposure after UL. The other animals had undergone no prior lesions and were divided into two groups: those that were kept in complete darkness for 4 days following UL and those that were allowed normal exposure to light after the UL.

Restoration of Static VOR Balance after UL

The results from this experiment were clear-cut. Restoration of static balance, as reflected in the disappearance of spontaneous nystagmus, proceeded independently of whether or not the animals had undergone a prior occipital lobectomy or whether or not they were kept in the dark after UL. Furthermore, a bilateral occipital lobectomy performed nearly a year after the labyrinthectomy, when compensation to UL had taken place, did not result in the reappearance of spontaneous nystagmus. Thus, both the acquisition and the maintenance of static balance after UL are independent of visual inputs.*

Restoration of Dynamic VOR Function after UL

On the other hand, the restoration of dynamic performance after UL depended critically on visual experience. There was no increase in the amplitude (gain) of the VOR until exposure to light. Similar results occur in monkeys after unilateral plugging of a lateral semicircular canal, which causes a nearly 50 percent decrease in VOR gain.[4] Presumably, it is not light per se but rather the presence of motion of images on the retina during head movements that is the critical stimulus for recalibration of dynamic VOR responses.

Furthermore, the compensatory changes in the gain of the VOR that occurred after UL were lost, over the course of several weeks, following a bilateral occipital lobectomy. The occipital lobectomy itself was unlikely to have been responsible for the decrease in the gain of the VOR, since there are only small alterations in the gain and in the symmetry of the VOR produced by occipital lobectomy in animals that have not undergone any prior vestibular lesions.

Taken together, these findings suggest that adaptation of VOR gain is a dynamic process that requires visual experience for its acquisition and is dependent on the

---

*Another example of restoration of static imbalance after UL is the elimination of cyclotorsion (occular counterroll) that follows UL. It is not known if this readjustment also requires visual inputs.[3]

posterior cerebral hemispheres for its maintenance. Presumably, the contribution of the occipital lobes is that they transmit information about image slip on the retina during head movements to the more caudal structures that, in turn, use this error information to readjust the dynamic performance of the VOR.

Restoration of Spontaneous Activity in the Deafferented Nuclei

One might ask why visual experience is necessary for recalibration of dynamic VOR function but not for restoration of static balance. Without motion of images on the retina during head movements, adaptive mechanisms do not have a reliable error signal that they can use to recalibrate the dynamic VOR. With respect to static imbalance, however, deafferentation of the vestibular nucleus might initiate alterations in the intrinsic properties of the vestibular neurons themselves, or lead to denervation hypersensitivity to remaining sensory inputs, or stimulate sprouting of extralabyrinthine afferents.[5] Each process might lead to an increase in the level of the spontaneous activity of neurons on the lesioned side. Recall that restoring vestibulospinal balance also depends on rebalancing of the vestibular nuclei, and that many neurons within the vestibular nuclei have axons that bifurcate and project both rostrally, to the ocular motor nuclei, and caudally, to the spinal cord. Vestibulospinal compensation would not be expected to rely solely on visual inputs for providing the necessary error signals for central readjustment of balance. Proprioceptive and somatosensory cues are probably more important and could provide the requisite error signals leading to the static rebalancing of the vestibular nuclei that would affect both vestibulo-ocular and vestibulospinal responses.

A Critical Period for VOR Adaptation?

Another finding, potentially of important clinical relevance, emerged from our study. Monkeys that had been kept in the dark for 4 days after UL and then allowed normal visual experience, generally showed a recovery of dynamic VOR performance at about the same rate, and to the same level, as did monkeys allowed visual experience immediately following UL. There was, however, one important exception. For high-velocity rotations directed to the lesioned side, recovery was markedly delayed in the monkeys initially deprived of vision, although the final level reached was close to that of monkeys that had not been deprived of vision immediately after UL.

This finding suggests that there may be a *critical period* during which, if error signals are not provided to the adaptive mechanism, and recalibration does not get under way, the rate of recovery, and perhaps the ultimate degree, may decrease. Restoration of postural control after unilateral labyrinthectomy also appears to be subject to a critical period (reviewed in Lacour and co-workers[6]). If cats are immobilized for a period of days after a unilateral labyrinthectomy, their recovery of locomotor function, even after normal activity is reinstituted, is delayed and limited. Another example of the influence on vestibular adaptation of a restriction of sensory inputs has been demonstrated in guinea pigs.[7] If their head is restrained after UL, the rate of compensation of lateral head deviation (the static vestibulocollic reflex) is altered.

The obvious implication of these findings is that when patients incur enduring vestibular damage, they should be encouraged to move about in the light and to try to engage their VOR and VSR as much as possible. In this way, they will generate and experience the sensorimotor mismatches that make the central nervous system (CNS) aware of a need for adaptive readjustment of its motor reflexes. As a further caveat, heavy sedation, immobilization, and restriction of activity of patients with a recent loss of vestibular function should be discouraged. Such practices may potentially retard or even limit the ultimate degree of compensation after a vestibular lesion.

In the same vein, physical exercise promotes recovery of balance function in monkeys that have undergone either unilateral or bilateral experimental vestibular ablations.[8] Although carefully controlled studies of the effects of different types of activity on vestibular compensation have not yet been performed in human beings, physical therapy will most likely also promote recovery in patients.

Substitution of Saccades for Inadequate Compensatory Slow Phases

Apart from readjustment of VOR gain, other mechanisms may also be invoked to help stabilize the position of the eyes during head motion after UL. Patients may learn to generate catchup saccades (elicited automatically, even in complete darkness) in the same direction as their inadequate compensatory slow phases.[9] This substitution strategy may be necessary because there appear to be inherent limitations, both with respect to maximum velocity and to maximum acceleration, in the ability of subjects with just one labyrinth to generate slow phases of the correct magnitude when the head is rotated toward the side of the lesion (Ewald's second law).[10]

Recovery Nystagmus and Related Phenomena

A practical clinical implication of these ideas about recovery from unilateral labyrinthine lesions relates to the phenomenon of "recovery nystagmus."[11] As indicated earlier, the static imbalance created by unilateral peripheral lesions leads to a spontaneous nystagmus that is compensated by rebalancing the level of activity between the vestibular nuclei. If peripheral function should suddenly recover, central adaptation would become inappropriate, and a nystagmus would appear with slow phases directed away from the paretic side. Recovery nystagmus may confuse the clinician or therapist, who may think that the reappearance of symptoms and of a spontaneous nystagmus are owing to a loss of function on the previously healthy side rather than to a recovery of function on the previously diseased side. In either case, a spontaneous nystagmus ensues that must be eliminated, adaptively, by a further readjustment of levels of activity within the vestibular nuclei. Such a sequence of events may be a relatively common occurrence after vestibular lesions.[12]

A similar mechanism may account for some instances in which nystagmus is provoked by hyperventilation.[11] In these cases, the induced alkalosis alters the amount of calcium available for generating action potentials along the vestibular nerve, and so may lead to a restoration of function on partially demyelinated fibers (e.g., owing to multiple sclerosis, chronic microvascular compression, petrous bone tumors [e.g., cholesteatoma] or cerebellopontine angle tumors [e.g., acoustic neuroma]). Hyperventilation, however, may also produce nystagmus in patients with a perilymphatic fistula by altering intracranial pressure that is then transmitted to the labyrinth.

There may even be a *dynamic equivalent of recovery nystagmus*. After sustained head shaking, patients who have a unilateral peripheral vestibular loss often develop a transient eye nystagmus with slow phases directed toward the impaired ear—so-called head-shaking nystagmus.[13] The initial phase of head-shaking nystagmus may be followed by a reversal phase in which nystagmus is directed oppositely to the initial phase. The primary phase of head-shaking nystagmus is related to a dynamic asymmetry in the VOR such that excitation (rotation toward the intact side) elicits a larger response than inhibition (rotation toward the impaired side). Head-shaking nystagmus is another manifestation of Ewald's second law. The secondary phase is often attributed to short-term (with a time constant of about 1 minute) vestibular adaptation, probably reflecting adaptive processes in both the peripheral nerve and in central structures.

If recovery occurs peripherally, however, any prior central VOR gain adaptation (which would increase the dynamic response during rotation toward the impaired side) could lead to a head-shaking–induced nystagmus with the slow phases of the primary phase directed *away* from the impaired ear. Thus, one can appreciate the pivotal role that adaptation plays in determining the particular pattern and direction of any spontaneous or induced nystagmus that may appear during the process of recovery.

BILATERAL LOSS OF LABYRINTHINE FUNCTION

An even more challenging problem for the CNS is to compensate for a *complete* bilateral loss (BL) of labyrinthine function. In the case of a truly complete loss, there is no labyrinthine-driven VOR to recalibrate so that alternative mechanisms—sensory substitution, motor substitution, predictive and anticipatory strategies—must be invoked.

Complete Versus Partial Vestibular Loss

Whether or not labyrinthine function is completely absent helps to determine what type of program of physical therapy should be prescribed. Because the response of the VOR to high frequencies of head rotation is usually spared until the labyrinthine loss is complete, caloric responses (which primarily simulate a low-frequency rotational stimulus) may be absent even when the patient has a relatively functional VOR. Recall that the response to the high-frequency components of head rotation requires the fast-acting labyrinthine-driven VOR; visual stabilizing reflexes are adequate to ensure stabilization for the low-frequency components of head rotation. Accordingly, the results of a rotational test are necessary to determine the degree of preservation of labyrinthine function, because such information may help the therapist choose whether to prescribe a program of rehabilitation that stresses recalibration of a deficient but present VOR or a program that emphasizes sensory substitution and alternative strategies.

Experimental Results in Nonhuman Primates

Dichgans and co-workers[14] first described compensatory mechanisms of eye-head coordination in monkeys that had undergone bilateral labyrinthine destruction. They identified three major adaptive strategies used to improve gaze stability during head movements: (1) potentiation of the COR (neck-eye loop), as reflected in slow-phase eye movements elicited in response to body-on-head (head stable in space) rotation; (2) preprogramming of compensatory slow phases in anticipation of intended head motion;

and (3) a decrease in the saccadic amplitude-retinal error relationship, selectively during combined eye-head movements, to prevent gaze overshoot. With respect to the last phenomenon, saccades made with head movements would normally cause gaze to overshoot the target if there were no functioning VOR to compensate for the contribution of the movement of the head to the change in gaze. Dichgans and co-workers[14] showed that saccades were programmed to be smaller when an accompanying head movement was also anticipated. When the head was persistently immobilized, however, saccades were programmed to be of their usual size.

Additional Strategies in Human Patients with Bilateral Loss

The compensatory mechanisms described by Dichgans and associates[14] in monkeys without labyrinthine function have also been identified in human beings who have a complete BL of labyrinthine function. The degree to which one or another mechanism is adopted, however, varies from patient to patient. In addition, several additional strategies have been identified in humans that are also quite idiosyncratic from patient to patient (Table 4–2).[15-18] These strategies include (1) *substitution of small saccades* in the direction opposite to head rotation, to augment inadequate compensatory slow phases; (2) *enhanced visual following reflexes; (3) use of predictive strategies* to improve gaze stability during tracking of targets jumping periodically, or during self-paced tracking between two stationary targets; and (4) use of an *effort of spatial localization*, as judged by a much better compensatory response to head rotation when the patient imagines the location of stationary targets, as opposed to the response while performing mental arithmetic. As a corollary to these last two mechanisms, responses during active (self-generated) head rotations occur at a shorter latency, and usually with a larger gain, than those during passive head rotations. Even somatosensory cues from the feet can be used to augment inadequate compensatory slow phases of the eyes—producing so-called stepping-around nystagmus.[19] Finally, perceptual mechanisms—suppression of oscillopsia (illusory movement of the environment) despite persistent retinal image motion—may also be part of the "compensatory" response to vestibular loss.[17,20]

Another example of potentiation of a reflex that is normally vestigial in human beings can be shown in the ocular motor response to static lateral tilt of the head. This presumably otolith-mediated reflex is comprised of a static torsion of the eyes, opposite to the direction of lateral head tilt—so-called ocular counterrolling. In labyrinthine defective human beings, but not in normal subjects, ocular counterrolling can be produced by lateral tilt of the *trunk* with respect to the (stationary, upright) head.[21] This response probably reflects a potentiation of a static COR in lieu of the missing otolith signals. Patients with BL also show an increased sensitivity to visually induced tilt. With

TABLE 4–2 Compensatory Mechanisms Following
Bilateral Vestibular Deficits

Potentiation of COR
Substitution of saccades for slow phases
Central preprogramming of compensatory slow phases
Decreased saccade amplitude during combined eye-head gaze changes
Enhanced visual following
Effort of spatial localization
Suppression of perception of oscillopsia

the loss of the inertial frame of reference, normally provided by the dominating labyrinthine inputs, visual inputs become more potent stimuli to vestibular reflexes.

A new reliance on visual inputs is a necessary and useful adaptation to labyrinthine loss, although it may become a liability if visual inputs should become incongruent with the actual motion or position of the head. For example, when one is reading a newspaper in a moving elevator or escalator, visual inputs (from the motion of the image of the newspaper on the retina) provide misleading information about the position or the movement of the head, and if relied on (as BL patients may), would lead to an inappropriate (or lack of) compensatory response and possibly a fall.

STUDIES OF VOR ADAPTATION IN NORMAL SUBJECTS

Adaptive control of the VOR has been investigated in normal subjects by artificially creating motion of images on the retina, using optical or other means, during head rotation. For example, in the pioneering experiments of Melvill Jones and colleagues[22,23] subjects wore right-left reversing prisms, which required, and led to, a reversal in the direction of the slow phase of nystagmus with respect to the direction of head motion. Likewise, magnifying and minifying spectacle lenses (used to correct for far-sightedness, and near-sightedness, respectively) require and produce an adaptive increase and decrease, respectively, in VOR gain.[24] A practical consequence of this phenomenon is that normal subjects wearing a spectacle correction undergo an adaptive change in VOR gain to meet the needs of the new visual circumstances created by their optical correction.* Such gain changes must be considered in evaluating the results of vestibular function tests in individuals who habitually wear spectacles.[25] Furthermore, if a patient does show a change in VOR gain in response to wearing spectacles, one can infer that the patient has at least some capability to undergo adaptive VOR recalibration.

VOR adaptation can also be studied by prolonged rotation of subjects while artificially manipulating the visual surround. One can use an optokinetic drum that surrounds the subject and rotate it in phase — in the same direction as chair rotation — to produce a decrease in VOR gain, or out of phase — opposite the direction of chair rotation — to produce an increase in VOR gain. If the amplitude of drum rotation is exactly equal to that of the chair, then the required VOR gain would be 0.0 for in-phase viewing (so-called $\times 0$ viewing) and 2.0 for out-of-phase viewing (so called $\times 2$ viewing). The usual duration for VOR training in these types of paradigms is 1 or 2 hours, although VOR adaptation can probably be detected within minutes of the onset of the change in the relationship between the visual and vestibular stimuli.[26,27]

Imagination and Effort of Spatial Localization in Vestibular Adaptation

Finally, we note that one's *imagination* can be a potent substitute for the real stimulus to VOR adaptation — motion of images on the retina during head rotation. Melvill Jones and colleagues[22] have shown that the VOR of normal subjects can be

---

*Note that wearing contact lenses does not require an adaptive change in VOR gain because contacts rotate with the eye and are therefore unassociated with a rotational magnification effect.

adaptively modified (as measured in darkness and tested under the same mental set) with just a few hours of imagining a visual stimulus moving in such a way that it would normally create slip of images on the retina if it were actually visible. Thus, what are usually called psychologic factors — motivation, attention, effort, interest — may actually play a more specific role in promoting adaptive recovery. The habit of professional athletes — downhill skiers or ice skaters, for example — of going through their routines in their minds as they prepare for the actual event, is probably an example of using this "cognitive" capability to create an internal model of the external environment (and the sensory consequences of moving within it) in which to rehearse their motor performance.

Similar types of paradigms, in which the motion of the visual surround is artificially manipulated with respect to the motion of the head, have been used to induce an alteration in the phase (timing) but without a change in the amplitude of the VOR;[28] and a change in the direction of the VOR, so-called cross-axis plasticity.[29,30] In the latter paradigm, the visual surround is rotated in a direction orthogonal to the direction of rotation of the head. A clinical consequence of a disturbance of cross-axis VOR plasticity is the occurrence of "perverted" nystagmus; nystagmus in which the slow phases are in the wrong direction relative to that of the stimulus. A strong vertical nystagmus induced during caloric stimulation is such an example and usually occurs with central vestibular lesions.

These short-term rotation experiments probably test only one particular type of vestibular adaptation, since the learned response is not sustained in the absence of continued stimulation. There is also a long-term adaptive process, taking days rather than hours, which gradually supervenes and leads to a more enduring, resilient adaptive change. Thus, one must be cautious when extrapolating the results from these short-term experiments to the long-term problems of patients adapting to chronic vestibular deficits.

Adaptive capabilities have been investigated in elderly subjects,[31] by measuring changes in VOR gain after wearing of ×2 (magnifying) lenses for 8 hours. At higher frequencies (above about 0.75 Hz), the ability to increase VOR gain adaptively is significantly diminished in older individuals. Because the labyrinthine-induced VOR is most needed to compensate for the high-frequency components of head rotation, a loss of adaptive capability in elderly patients could account for the more devastating and persistent symptoms after a vestibular loss.

Context Specificity

One recent finding, which may have important clinical implications, is the demonstration that VOR gain adaptation is context-specific. Baker and co-workers[32] showed that cats can be trained to adaptively change the gain of their canal-induced (rotational) VOR in one way, when the head is oriented with respect to gravity in one particular position (e.g., right ear down), and in another way, when the head is oriented in the opposite position with respect to gravity (e.g., left ear down). Thus, even though the pattern of canal activation is the same, the pattern of static otolith inputs determines or gates different central responses to an identical input from the semicircular canals.

We have recently shown that VOR adaptation in humans also depends on the static orientation of the head in which the training of the canal-induced VOR took place.[33] Shelhamer and associates[34] have also shown that adaptation of the gain of the VOR can be made to depend on the position of the eye in the orbit in which the training took place. In their paradigm, the *horizontal* VOR gain was trained to depend on the *vertical* position of the eye in the orbit. Such a capability would be particularly useful for individuals who wear a bifocal spectacle correction. When viewing through the lower part of the lenses, which has the stronger prescription needed to overcome the effects of presbyopia, subjects require a higher VOR gain during head rotation than when viewing through the top part of the spectacles. Potentially, then, simply putting one's glasses on (or perhaps just the frames, or putting on the glasses in complete darkness) might be enough of a cue to generate a different vestibular response. Just such an effect of spectacles has been shown for another type of ocular motor adaptation in which the eyes are required to rotate disconjugately.[35]

Thus, context specificity of vestibular learning, which potentially can be derived from a variety of cues—both vestibular and nonvestibular—must be considered in the design of programs of physical therapy. Will the particular training paradigm that is being used to promote vestibular compensation "transfer" to the more natural circumstances in which the patient usually becomes symptomatic?

Neurophysiologic Substrate of VOR Adaptation

Where might be the structures within the CNS that elaborate the various types of vestibular plasticity that we have discussed? First, we should remember that one must distinguish between static and dynamic VOR adaptation (Table 4–3). The cerebellum, and especially the flocculus, seem to play an important role in the acquisition of adaptive changes in VOR gain.[36,37] Furthermore, potentiation of the COR as an adaptive strategy during head rotation is lost in patients with bilateral vestibular loss who also have cerebellar atrophy, implying a role for the cerebellum in this aspect of vestibular adaptation as well.[38] The exact sites of these types of vestibular learning are still unsettled; evidence for both a cerebellar cortex and a brain-stem (vestibular nuclei) locus exists.[39,40] Long-term, more hard-wired changes in the VOR may take place in the vestibular nuclei themselves.

Finally, there is some evidence that the vestibular commissure may mediate signals important for dynamic VOR adaptation. Following interruption of the vestibular commissure, cats lose their ability to undergo plastic *gain changes* in a short-term VOR adaptation paradigm.[41] However, the same may not be true in the monkey.[42]

In contrast to VOR gain adaptation, section of the vestibular commissure does not appear to interfere with rebalancing of the vestibular nuclei for restoration of static VOR function after a unilateral labyrinthine loss.[43] Likewise, the mechanism of restoration of balance between the vestibular nuclei—for example, to remove spontaneous nystagmus—does not appear to depend on the flocculus.[44] The deep cerebellar nuclei,

TABLE 4–3 Potential Neuroanatomic Substrates
of VOR Adaptation

Static disturbance	Dynamic disturbance
Deep cerebellar nuclei	Flocculus
Inferior olive	Inferior olive
	Vestibular commissure

however, may be important for static adaptation, and it is likely that the inferior olive is important for both dynamic and static VOR adaptation.[45]

Still unclear are the substrates for the variety of strategies and cognitive influences (e.g., context and imagination, and effort of spatial localization) that are incorporated as part of the compensatory response to vestibular damage. A possible anatomic substrate for such higher-level influences may reside in the reciprocal connections between the vestibular nuclei and the cerebral cortex.[46]

SUMMARY

We have emphasized here that a consideration and a knowledge of the adaptive capabilities of the brain are essential to the diagnosis and management of patients with vestibular disorders. The proper interpretation of the symptoms and the signs shown by patients with vestibular dysfunction, the design of an optimal plan of physical therapy to promote recovery from vestibular dysfunction, and an objective analysis of any salutary effects of physical therapy, cannot be accomplished without paying constant attention to the actions of the variety of compensatory mechanisms that are used to cope with abnormal vestibular function. Furthermore, we have reemphasized that compensation is far more than a simple readjustment of low-level, largely subconscious reflexes. The role of anticipation and prediction, altered motor strategies, sensory substitution, and cognitive factors related to mental set, psychologic effort, imagination, and context are all important in the adaptive process. We are only now beginning to identify the wide repertoire of compensatory mechanisms available to us. The challenge now is for us to learn to marshall these adaptive mechanisms to best promote recovery in our patients.

ACKNOWLEDGMENTS

This research was supported by NIH Grant DC00979.

REFERENCES

1. Zee, DS: The management of patients with vestibular disorders. In Barber, HO and Sharpe, JA (eds): Vestibular Disorders. Year Book Medical Publishers, Chicago, 1988, p 254.
2. Fetter, M, Zee, DS, and Proctor, LR: Effect of lack of vision and occipital lobectomy upon recovery from unilateral labyrinthectomy in rhesus monkey. J Neurophysiol 59:394, 1988.
3. Curthoys, IS, Dai, MJ, and Halmagyi, GM: Human ocular torsional position before and after unilateral vestibular neurectomy. Exp Brain Res 85:218, 1991.
4. Paige, GD: Vestibuloocular reflex and its interactions with visual following mechanisms in the squirrel monkey: II. Response characteristics and plasticity following unilateral inactivation of horizontal canal. J Neurophysiol 49:152, 1983.
5. Smith, PF and Curthoys, IS: Mechanisms of recovery following unilateral labyrinthectomy: A review. Brain Res Rev 14:155, 1989.
6. Lacour, M, et al: Vestibular Compensation: Facts, Theories and Clinical Perspectives. Elsevier, Amsterdam, 1989.
7. Jensen, DW: Reflex control of acute postural asymmetry and compensatory symmetry after a unilateral vestibular lesion. Neuroscience 4:1059, 1979.
8. Igarashi, M: Physical exercise and acceleration of vestibular compensation. In Lacour, M, et al (eds): Vestibular Compensation: Facts, Theories and Clinical Perspectives. Elsevier, Amsterdam, 1989, p 131.
9. Segal, BN and Katsarkas, A: Long-term deficits of goal-directed vestibulo-ocular function following total unilateral loss of peripheral vestibular function. Acta Otolaryngol (Stockh) 106:102, 1988.
10. Halmagyi, GM, et al: The human horizontal vestibulo-ocular reflex in response to high-acceleration stimulation before and after unilateral vestibular neurectomy. Exp Brain Res 81:479, 1990.

11. Leigh, RJ and Zee, DS: The Neurology of Eye Movements, ed 2. FA Davis, Philadelphia, 1991.
12. Lockemann, U and Westhofen, M: On the course of early vestibular compensation after acute labyrinthine lesions. Laryngo-Rhino-Otol 70:326, 1991.
13. Hain TC, Fetter, M, and Zee, DS: Head-shaking nystagmus in patients with unilateral peripheral vestibular lesions. Am J Otolaryngol 8:36, 1987.
14. Dichgans J, et al: Mechanisms underlying recovery of eye-head coordination following bilateral labyrinthectomy in monkeys. Exp Brain Res 18:548, 1973.
15. Kasai, T and Zee, DS: Eye-head coordination in labyrinthine-defective human beings. Brain Res 144:123, 1978.
16. Takahashi, M, et al: Recovery of gaze disturbance in bilateral labyrinthine loss. ORL 51:305, 1989.
17. Gresty, MA, Hess, K, and Leech, J: Disorders of the vestibulo-ocular reflex producing oscillopsia and mechanisms compensating for loss of labyrinthine function. Brain 100:693, 1977.
18. Huygen, PLM, et al: Compensation of total loss of vestibulo-ocular reflex by enhanced optokinetic response. Acta Otolaryngol (Stockh) (suppl) 468:359, 1989.
19. Bles, W, de Jong, JMBV, and de Wit, G: Somatosensory compensation for loss of labyrinthine function. Acta Otolaryngol (Stockh) 97:213, 1984.
20. Bronstein, AM and Hood, JD: Oscillopsia of peripheral vestibular origin. Central and cervical compensatory mechanisms. Acta Otolaryngol (Stockh) 104:307, 1987.
21. Bles, W and De Graaf, B: Ocular rotation and perception of the horizontal under static tilt conditions in patients with labyrinthine function. Acta Otolaryngol (Stockh) 111:456, 1991.
22. Melvill Jones, G, Berthoz, A, and Segal, B: Adaptive modification of the vestibulo-ocular reflex by mental effort in darkness. Exp Brain Res 56:149, 1984.
23. Gonshor, A and Melvill Jones G: Extreme vestibulo-ocular adaptation induced by prolonged optical reversal of vision. J Physiol 256:381, 1976.
24. Demer, JL, et al: Vestibulo-ocular reflex during magnified vision: Adaptation to reduced visual-vestibular conflict. Aviat Space Environ Med 58 (suppl):A175, 1987.
25. Cannon, SC, et al: The effect of the rotational magnification of corrective spectacles on the quantitative evaluation of the VOR. Acta Otolaryngol (Stockh) 100:81, 1985.
26. Collewijn, H, Martins, AJ, and Steinman, RM: Compensatory eye movements during active and passive head movements: Fast adaptation to changes in visual magnification. J Physiol (Lond) 340:359, 1983.
27. Melvill Jones, G, Guitton, D, and Berthoz, A: Changing patterns of eye-head coordination during 6 h of optically reversed vision. Exp Brain Res 69:531, 1988.
28. Peterson, W and Houk, JC: A model of cerebellar-brainstem interaction in the adaptive control of vestibuloocular reflex. Acta Otolaryngol (Stockh) (suppl) 481:428, 1991.
29. Schultheis, LW and Robinson, DA: Directional plasticity of the vestibulo-ocular reflex in the cat. Ann NY Acad Sci 374:504, 1981.
30. Khater, TT, Baker JF, and Peterson, BW: Dynamics of adaptive change in human vestibulo-ocular reflex direction. J Vest Res 1:23, 1990.
31. Paige, GD: The aging vestibulo-ocular reflex (VOR) and adaptive plasticity. Acta Otolaryngol (Stockh) 481:297, 1991.
32. Baker, JF, et al: Simultaneous opposing adaptive changes in cat vestibulo-ocular reflex direction for two body orientations. Exp Brain Res 69:220, 1987.
33. Tiliket, C, et al: Adaptation of the vestibulo-ocular reflex with the head in different orientations and positions relative to the axis of body rotation. J Vest Res 3:181, 1993.
34. Shelhamer, M, Robinson, DA, and Tan, HS: Context specific adaptation of the gain of the vestibulo-ocular reflex in humans. J Vest Res 2:89, 1992.
35. Oohira, A, Zee, DS, and Guyton, DL: Disconjugate adaptation to long-standing, large-amplitude spectacle-corrected anisometropia. Invest Ophthal Vis Sci 32:1693, 1991.
36. Ito, M and Nagao, S: Comparative aspects of horizontal ocular reflexes and their cerebellar adaptive control in vertebrates. Comp Biochem Physiol 98C:221, 1991.
37. Lisberger, SG, Miles, FA, and Zee, DS: Signals used to computer errors in the monkey vestibulo-ocular reflex: Possible role of the flocculus. J Neurophysiol 52:140, 1984.
38. Bronstein, AM, Mossman, S, and Luxon, LM: The neck-eye reflex in patients with reduced vestibular and optokinetic function. Brain 114:1, 1991.
39. Ito, M: Long-term depression. Ann Rev Neurosci 12:85, 1989.
40. Lisberger, SG: The neural basis for learning of simple motor skills. Science 242:728, 1988.
41. Cheron, G: Effect of incisions in the brainstem commisural network on the short-term vestibulo-ocular adaptation of the cat. J Vest Res 1:223, 1990.
42. Katz, E, et al: Effects of midline medullary lesions on velocity storage and the vestibulo-ocular reflex. Exp Brain Res 87:505, 1991.
43. Smith, PF, Darlington, CL, and Curthoys, IS: Vestibular compensation without brainstem commissures in the guinea pig. Neurosci Lett 65:209, 1986.
44. Haddad, GM, Friendlich, AF, and Robinson, DA: Compensation of nystagmus after VIIIth nerve lesions in vestibulo-cerebellectomized cats. Brain Res 135:192, 1977.
45. Llinas, R, et al: Inferior olive: Its role in motor learning. Science 190:1230, 1975.
46. Ventre, J and Faugier-Grimaud, S: Projections of the temporo-parietal cortex on vestibular complex in the macaque monkey (Macaca fascicularis). Exp Brain Res 72:653, 1988.

CHAPTER 5

Vestibular System Disorders

M. Fetter, MD

Peripheral vestibular dysfunction, which involves the vestibular end organs and/or the vestibular nerve, can produce a variety of signs and symptoms. A thorough evaluation by a physician is needed to identify the specific pathology behind the patient's complaints of vertigo or disequilibrium. In many cases, a firm diagnosis cannot be reached. Determining whether vestibular rehabilitation is appropriate and, if it is, which approach should be used is in part based on the patient's diagnosis. This chapter describes the clinical presentation of the more common peripheral vestibular disorders. The results of diagnostic tests, and the medical, surgical, and rehabilitative management of each of these disorders is presented as an overview only, because this material is covered in detail in other chapters.

BENIGN PAROXYSMAL POSITIONAL VERTIGO

Benign paroxysmal positional vertigo (BPPV) is the most common cause of vertigo. Typically, a patient with BPPV will complain of brief episodes of vertigo precipitated by rapid change of head posture. Sometimes symptoms are brought about by assuming very specific head positions. Most commonly these head positions involve rapid extension of the neck, often with the head turned to one side (like looking up to a high shelf or backing a car out of a garage) or lateral head tilts toward the affected ear. The symptoms are often encountered while rolling from side to side in bed. Patients can usually identify the offending head position, which they often studiously avoid. Many patients also complain of mild postural instability between attacks. The vertigo will last only 1 to 2 minutes and will go away even if the precipitating position is maintained. Hearing loss, aural fullness, and tinnitus are not seen in this condition, which most commonly occurs spontaneously in the elderly population but can be seen in any age group after even mild head trauma. Women are more commonly affected than men. Bilateral involvement can be found in 10 percent of the spontaneous cases and 20 percent of the traumatic cases. Spontaneous remissions are common, but recurrences can occur, and the condition may trouble the patient intermittently for years.

Evaluation should include a careful neurotologic examination, the most important part being the history. A key diagnostic maneuver is the Dix-Hallpike positioning test[1] while observing the eyes with a pair of Frenzel lenses or in combination with electronystagmography (ENG) monitoring. A typical response is induced by rapid position changes from the sitting to the head-hanging right or left position. Vertigo and nystagmus begin with a latency of 1 or more seconds after the head is tilted toward the affected ear and increase in severity within about 10 seconds to a maximum accompanied by a sensation of discomfort and apprehension that will sometimes cause the patient to cry out and attempt to sit up. The symptoms reduce gradually after 10 to 40 seconds and ultimately abate, even if the precipitating head position is maintained. The nystagmus is usually slightly disconjunctive, being more torsional in the lower eye (on the side of the dependent ear) and more vertical in the upper eye. The nystagmus is mixed upbeat and torsional. The nystagmus changes with the direction of gaze: becoming more torsional on looking toward the dependent ear and becoming more vertical on looking toward the higher ear. A small horizontal component, greater in the lower eye, with fast phases toward the dependent ear, may also be evident. The pattern of nystagmus corresponds closely to the results of experimental stimulation of the posterior semicircular canal of the dependent ear. Sometimes, a low-amplitude, secondary nystagmus, directed in the opposite direction, may occur. If the patient then quickly sits up, a similar but usually milder recurrence of these symptoms occurs, the nystagmus being directed opposite to the initial nystagmus. Repeating this procedure several times will decrease the symptoms. This adaptation of the response is of diagnostic value because a clinical picture similar to that of BPPV can be created by cerebellar tumors. In the latter, however, there is no habituation of the response with repetitive testing. Further diagnostic criteria pointing toward a central positional nystagmus is that the condition does not subside with maintenance of the head in the precipitating position; the nystagmus may change direction when different head positions are assumed; or it may occur as downbeat nystagmus only in the head-hanging position. BPPV must be differentiated from positional nystagmus in *Ménière's disease, perilymph fistulas,* and *alcohol intoxication.*

A few patients do not display the typical torsional upbeat nystagmus but, for example, show a strong horizontal nystagmus (with the fast phases in the opposite direction to that usually observed) which, nevertheless, follows a similar pattern of buildup and decline but often over a longer period. This horizontal nystagmus may indicate a lateral canal variant of BPPV.

The classic explanation of the underlying pathophysiology (cupulolithiasis) was first described by Schuknecht[2] in 1969. His study of the temporal bones of two patients afflicted with this disorder showed deposition of otoconial material in the cupula of the posterior semicircular canal. Further support of this etiology is the relief of symptoms obtained by sectioning the posterior ampullary nerve in those patients with persistent problems after conservative treatment. Whether the otoliths actually adhere to the cupula and intermittently weigh it down, retard its return to the resting position after a head rotation, or obstruct the flow of endolymph, the net result is to produce false signals from the affected posterior semicircular canal. There has been some controversy as to whether this pathologic finding is indeed the cause of symptoms in these patients.

If symptoms persist longer than expected, then further investigation such as an MRI (magnetic resonance imaging) scan should be done to assess for unusual causes of positional vertigo such as acoustic neuroma or tumors of the fourth ventricle.

BPPV is usually a self-limiting disorder and will commonly resolve spontaneously within 6 to 12 months. Simple vestibular exercises or maneuvers aimed at dispersing the otolithic debris from the cupula can speed recovery; antivertiginous drugs are not helpful. One approach is to instruct the patient to assume repeatedly the positions that bring on the symptoms.[3] The period of recovery varies from immediate after one positioning maneuver (physical displacement) to usually 6 weeks to 6 months. More recently, two single-treatment approaches have been shown to be effective in treating patients with BPPV[4-6] (see also Chapter 16). In a few patients, usually the more elderly, the symptoms persist despite compliance with vestibular exercises. For more severe symptoms unresponsive to exercises, three surgical options are available for relief. The first is transmeatal posterior ampullary nerve section (also known as singular neurectomy). The other two options are complete vestibular nerve section and occlusion of the posterior semicircular canal.

VESTIBULAR NEURITIS (NEURONITIS)/LABYRINTHITIS

Acute unilateral (idiopathic) vestibular paralysis, also known as vestibular neuritis, is the second most common cause of vertigo. The term "vestibular neuronitis" should be replaced by "vestibular neuritis" because the neuron itself cannot become inflamed.

The most common form of vestibular neuritis is due to viral infection. Although in most cases a definitive cause is never proved, evidence to support a viral cause comes from histopathologic changes of branches of the vestibular nerve in patients who have suffered such an illness[7] and the sometimes epidemic occurrence of the condition. Onset is often preceded by the presence of a viral infection of the upper respiratory or gastrointestinal tracts. The associated viral infection may be coincident with the vestibular neuritis or may have preceded it by as much as two weeks. The chief symptom is the acute onset of prolonged severe rotational vertigo that is exacerbated by movement of the head, associated with spontaneous horizontal-rotatory nystagmus beating toward the good ear, postural imbalance, and nausea. Hearing loss is not usually present, but when it is, then mumps, measles, and infectious mononucleosis, among other infections, have been incriminated. The latter condition should also alert the physician to consider other diagnoses (i.e., ischemia of labyrinth artery, Ménière's disease, acoustic neuroma, herpes zoster, Lyme disease, or neurosyphilis).

The condition mainly affects those aged between 30 and 60 years, with a peak for women in the fourth decade and men in the sixth decade.

If examined early, the patient may manifest an irritative nystagmus from the acute phases of the inflammation. Usually the patient is examined after these initial findings have given way to a more paralytic, or hypofunctional, pattern. Caloric testing invariably shows ipsilateral hyporesponsiveness or nonresponsiveness (horizontal canal paresis). The symptoms usually abate after a period of 48 to 72 hours, and gradual return to normal balance occurs over approximately 6 weeks. Rapid head movements, however, can still cause slight oscillopsia of the visual scene and impaired balance for a second. Recovery is produced by the combination of central compensation of the vestibular tone imbalance, aided by physical exercise, and peripheral restoration of labyrinthine function. The latter is found in about two thirds of the patients.

The differential diagnosis should initially include other causes of vertigo, and careful history taking, physical examination, and an audiogram are required. Physical examination should include neurologic examination with attention to cranial nerve findings and cerebellar testing. Careful otoscopy is performed to rule out the presence of a potential otologic infectious process as the source of a toxic serous labyrinthitis. Fever in the presence of chronic ear disease and labyrinthitis suggests suppuration and meningitis. Commonly, a toxic labyrinthitis is the result of a well-defined event such as surgery or trauma.

The initial treatment of the condition is accomplished with the use of vestibular suppressants such as the antihistamine dimenhydrinate or the anticholinergic scopolamine. In addition, bed rest is very helpful early on in the course of the disease. After the most severe vertigo and nausea have passed (after 24 to 72 hours), then ambulation may resume with assistance; independent ambulation may be achieved over the next few days. At the same time, the administration of vestibular suppressants should be greatly diminished or, even better, stopped completely because they prolong the time required to achieve central compensation. To further speed up the process of recuperation, vestibular exercises challenge the compensatory mechanisms of the central nervous system (CNS), stimulating adaptation. These exercises are designed to improve both gaze stability and postural stability (see Chapter 14). The symptomatology is usually self-limited to a course of approximately 6 weeks.

Animal experiments have shown that alcohol, phenobarbital, chlorpromazine, diazepam, and ACTH antagonists retard compensation; caffeine, amphetamines, and ACTH accelerate compensation. The use of drugs for acceleration of compensation in patients has still to be proven.[8]

MÉNIÈRE'S DISEASE, MÉNIÈRE'S SYNDROME, AND ENDOLYMPHATIC HYDROPS

Ménière's disease is a disorder of inner-ear function that can cause devastating hearing and vestibular symptoms. The typical attack is experienced as an initial sensation of fullness of the ear, a reduction in hearing, and tinnitus, followed by rotational vertigo, postural imbalance, nystagmus, and nausea and vomiting after a few minutes. This severe disequilibrium (vertigo) will persist anywhere from approximately 30 minutes to 24 hours. Gradually, the severe symptoms will abate, and the patient is generally ambulatory within 72 hours. Some sensation of postural unsteadiness will persist for days or weeks, and then normal balance will return. During this recuperation time, hearing gradually returns. Hearing may return to the preattack baseline or there may be residual permanent sensorineural hearing loss, most commonly in the lower frequencies. The rare transient improvement of hearing during the attack is known as the *Lermoyez phenomenon*. Tinnitus will also usually diminish as the hearing returns. As the disease progresses, hearing fails to return after the attack, and after many years, the symptoms of vertigo may gradually diminish in frequency and severity. Some patients may suddenly fall without warning; these events, which may occur in later stages of the disease, are referred to as Tumarkin's otolithic crises and should be differentiated from other forms of drop attack.

The typical form of Ménière's disease is sometimes not complete and is called *vestibular Ménière's disease*, if only vestibular symptoms and aural pressure are present, or *cochlear Ménière's disease*, if only cochlear symptoms and aural pressure are encountered. The distinction between Ménière's disease (or "idiopathic," that is, as yet unknown, origin) from *Ménière's syndrome* (of known origin) is not very helpful because the current understanding of the pathogenesis of Ménière's disease is still imprecise. The newer nomenclature, therefore, uses the term "Ménière's disease" for all cases demonstrating the characteristic symptom complex.[9]

The disease is about equally distributed between the sexes and usually has its onset in the fourth to sixth decade of life. However, there are reports of children as young as 6 years of age with classical Ménière's disease.[10] About 15 percent of the patients have blood relatives with the same disease, suggesting genetic factors. The incidence of bilaterality of involvement ranges between 33 and 50 percent.[11]

A phenomenon fundamental to the development of Ménière's disease is *endolymphatic hydrops*. Whether endolymphatic hydrops itself is the cause of the symptoms characteristic of Ménière's disease or whether it is a pathologic change seen in the disease is still unclear. The development of hydrops is generally a function of malabsorption of endolymph in the endolymphatic duct and sac. Malabsorption may itself be a result of disturbed function of components comprising the endolymphatic duct and sac, mechanical obstruction of these structures, or altered anatomy in the temporal bone. Endolymph is produced primarily by the stria vascularis and flows both longitudinally (along the axis of the endolymphatic duct toward the endolymphatic sac) and radially (across the membrane of the endolymphatic space into the perilymph system). Ménière's disease is generally a consequence of altered longitudinal flow usually evolving over a course of many years. Experimental obstruction of the endolymphatic duct will routinely result in endolymphatic hydrops in many animal models.[12] Lesions in the temporal bone that have been associated with the development of hydrops include fractures of the temporal bone, perisaccular fibrosis, atrophy of the sac, narrowing of the lumen in the endolymphatic duct, otitis media, otosclerotic foci enveloping the vestibular aqueduct, lack of vascularity surrounding the endolymphatic sac, syphilitic osteitis of the otic capsule, and leukemic infiltrations, to name just a few. Anatomically, ears affected by Ménière's disease are likely to demonstrate hypodevelopment of the endolymphatic duct and sac, the periaqueductal cells, and the mastoid air cells. Therefore, one can postulate a cause-and-effect relationship between constricted anatomy in the temporal bone and malabsorption of endolymph.

Any explanation of the clinical symptoms of Ménière's disease should account for all of the symptoms, including rapid or prolonged attacks of vertigo, disequilibrium, positional vertigo during and between attacks, fluctuating progressive sensorineural hearing loss, tinnitus, aural pressure, inability to tolerate loudness, and diplacusis. These symptoms probably result from both chemical and physical mechanisms. Physical factors can tamponade the cochlear duct, contributing to fluctuating progressive sensorineural hearing loss and other cochlear symptoms, whereas distension of the otolithic organs can physically affect the crista ampullaris, resulting in vestibular symptoms. The prolonged nystagmus and vertigo are commonly believed to be caused by periodic membrane ruptures with subsequent transient potassium palsy of vestibular nerve fibers.

Useful diagnostic tests include the audiogram and electronystagmography. Typically, the audiogram displays a unilateral sensorineural hearing loss involving the lower frequencies of the involved ear. Fluctuation in discrimination scores is often seen, with a long-term trend toward poor scores. ENG may demonstrate a unilateral vestibular weakness on caloric testing, again involving the ear symptomatic for pressure, hearing loss, and tinnitus. Electrocochleography is useful in cases that are unclear. The finding of enlarged summating potentials in the suspected ear is diagnostic of endolymphatic hydrops.

A brain stem–evoked acoustic response (BEAR) must be done in those cases with findings of retrocochlear pathology on routine audiometry to screen for cochlear nerve or brain-stem pathology. If the BEAR is found to be positive, then MRI scanning with the use of intravenous gadolinium should be done to assess for CNS pathology or eighth nerve schwannoma.

Treatment in the remission phase aims to reduce the frequency of the attacks and to preserve hearing without distressing tinnitus. Dietetic programs, including restriction of salt, water, alcohol, nicotine, and caffeine, are as valueless in treating the disease as are physical exercise or avoidance of exposure to low temperatures. Stellate ganglion blocks, diuretics, vasoactive agents, tranquilizers, neuroleptics, and lithium have been employed under the mistaken assumption that diminishing endolymphatic hydrops is possible by changing inner-ear blood flow, osmotic diuresis, or central sedation. There has never been prospective proof of the efficiency of these therapies. The histamine derivative betahistine has been advocated as the drug of first choice. Findings from a 1-year prospective double-blind study showed that this treatment is preferable to leaving the disease untreated.[13] The action is attributed to improvement of microcirculation of the stria vascularis, but betahistine also has inhibitory effects on polysynaptic vestibular neurons. Adjunctive medications in the form of vestibular suppressants other than betahistine are to be used primarily during the acute episodes of vertigo and should be discouraged as a chronic daily medication.

In addition to pharmacologic therapies, many patients with Ménière's disease require psychologic support to help cope with the frustrations and changes brought about by their medical condition.

Those patients in whom the vertigo becomes disabling by virtue of increased severity or frequency of attacks, despite maximal medical therapy, would then be considered candidates for surgical intervention. Only about 1 to 5 percent of patients ultimately require surgical treatment, because the success of regular endolymphatic sac shunt operations has been shown to be a placebo effect.[14]

Sacculotomy has been proposed by a variety of authors as a method of relieving the pressure buildup in the endolymphatic chamber. Long-term success rates for this procedure are not yet available, but significant hearing loss is observed in 50 percent of patients undergoing cochleosacculotomy. Advantages are ease of performance, utility in elderly patients as a first procedure under local anesthesia, and little risk other than hearing loss.

Intratympanic treatment with ototoxic antibiotics such as gentamicin sulfate, 8 to 24 mg instilled daily via a plastic tube inserted behind the annulus via the transmeatal approach, is obviously able to damage selectively the secretory epithelium (and thereby to improve endolymphatic hydrops) before significantly affecting vestibular and cochlear function.[15] Instillation (up to 10 days) should be stopped when daily audiograms or a check of spontaneous nystagmus indicate end-organ dysfunction.

The current treatment most successful is the vestibular nerve section. This procedure is indicated in individuals with serviceable hearing in whom maximal medical therapy has been unsuccessful in controlling vertigo. Success rates in the range of 90 to 95 percent have been reported by numerous authors. The newer technique of focused ultrasound seems to have an advantage over open surgery in that partial ablation of vestibular function (with preservation of hearing) can be performed without invading the labyrinth.

Surgical fistulization in various parts of the membranous labyrinth has been used in patients with Ménière's disease. Cochlear endolymphatic shunt operation is the current solution, and Schuknecht and Bartley[16] report that 72 percent of the cases were relieved of vertigo, but hearing was worse in 45 percent of the cases.

In patients with hearing loss, destructive procedures are also possible like transmeatal, transmastoid, or translabyrinthine labyrinthectomy. The success rate is 95 percent. An extension of this surgery is the translabyrinthine vestibular nerve section, shown to eliminate vertigo in 98 percent of cases. However, particularly in elderly patients, ablative surgical procedures may cause long-lasting postural imbalance because of the reduced ability of central mechanisms to compensate for the postoperative vestibular tone imbalance.

Vestibular exercises are not appropriate in patients with Ménière's disease unless there is permanent loss of vestibular function. Vestibular exercises are designed to induce long-term changes in the remaining vestibular system or to foster the substitution of other strategies to compensate for the loss of vestibular function. In Ménière's disease, the vestibular dysfunction is episodic and between episodes, the system usually returns to normal function. Some patients developed a loss of vestibular function at the end stages of the disease, and for those patients, vestibular rehabilitation may be appropriate. Vestibular exercises are also beneficial in those patients who have surgical destruction of the inner ear.

PERILYMPHATIC FISTULA

Perilymphatic fistula is a disruption of the limiting membranes of the labyrinth, creating a fistula between the perilymph and middle ear. Most commonly, these fistulas occur through the round and oval windows of the middle ear. Classically, a history of (often minor) head trauma, barotrauma, mastoid or stapes surgery, penetrating injury to the tympanic membrane, or vigorous straining precedes the onset of sudden vertigo, hearing loss, and loud tinnitus. The patients often report a "pop" in the ear during the precipitating event. Later on, patients with fistula may complain of imbalance, positional vertigo, and nystagmus as well as hearing loss. Tullio phenomenon — vestibular symptoms that include vertigo, oscillopsia, nystagmus, ocular tilt reaction, and postural imbalance induced by auditory stimuli — is usually due to perilymph fistula, but sublaxation of the stapes foot plate and other ear pathology may be responsible. The symptoms will often subside while at rest only to resume with activity. Sneezing, straining, nose blowing, and other such maneuvers can elicit the symptoms after the initial event. Perilymph fistulas probably account for a considerable proportion of those patients presenting with vertigo of unknown cause. Diagnosing perilymph fistula is difficult because of the great variability of signs and symptoms and the lack of a pathognomonic test. In the acute phase, medical treatment is universally recommended because these fistulas usually heal spontaneously, and the results of surgical interventions are not encouraging.[17]

Physical examination, particularly otoscopy, is important. In the cases of head trauma and barotrauma, hemotympanum is often seen as an early finding. In cases of penetrating injury to the ear, a tympanic membrane perforation makes the likelihood of ossicular discontinuity with fistula very high. A useful clinical test consists of applying manual pressure over the tragus or applying pressure to the tympanic membrane with the pneumatic otoscope; a positive test is indicated by the evocation or exacerbation of vertigo (Hennebert's sign) or the elicitation of nystagmus. Audiometric findings usually demonstrate a mixed or sensorineural hearing loss, depending on the mechanism of injury. This loss may be quite severe and usually involves the high frequencies more than the low frequencies. ENG with caloric testing may be normal or show a unilateral weakness in the affected ear. The specificity of the clinical fistula tests can be augmented by recording eye movements or measuring body sway as pressure on the tympanic membrane is increased. Despite refinements, these tests remain unreliable in detecting all fistulas. The diagnosis remains, essentially, a historical one, and in those patients with a suggestive history and symptoms, treatment is indicated. Often the only manner in which the diagnosis is made definitively is at the time of surgical exploration by tympanoscopy as the patient performs Valsalva maneuvers.

Medical treatment consists of absolute bed rest, with the head elevated, for 1 to 3 weeks. Mild sedation with tranquilizers; avoidance of straining, sneezing, coughing, or head-hanging positions; and the use of stool softeners is important for reduction of further explosive and implosive forces that may activate perilymph leakage.[18]

When symptoms persist for more than 4 weeks, or if hearing loss worsens, exploratory tympanotomy is indicated. Considerable controversy persists surrounding the frequency with which perilymph fistulas are found at surgery. Surgical management consists of middle ear exploration and packing of the oval and round window areas with fat, Gelfoam, and areolar and/or fibrous tissue. These areas are packed whether or not a clear-cut fistula is demonstrated. Reported success rates for this treatment vary between 50 and 70 percent and likely reflect some element of variable patient selection.

BILATERAL VESTIBULAR DISORDERS

Bilateral vestibulopathy may occur secondary to meningitis, labyrinthine infection, otosclerosis, Paget's disease, polyneuropathy, bilateral tumors (acoustic neuromas in neurofibromatosis), endolymphatic hydrops, bilateral sequential vestibular neuritis, cerebral hemosiderosis, ototoxic drugs, inner-ear autoimmune disease, or congenital malformations.

Autoimmune conditions affecting the inner-ear are rare but distinct clinical entities,[19] characterized by a progressive, bilateral sensorineural hearing loss often accompanied by a bilateral loss of vestibular function. Other autoimmune-mediated disease is often present in the afflicted patients; examples include rheumatoid arthritis, psoriasis, ulcerative colitis, and Cogans's syndrome (iritis accompanied by vertigo and sensorineural hearing loss). The history is the most useful diagnostic tool. Support for the diagnosis can be obtained by blood testing for complete blood count, erythrocyte sedimentation rate, rheumatoid factor, and antinuclear antibodies. Western blot precipitation studies to look for anticochlear antibodies can be done in some research centers and may be the future definitive test of choice in these cases.

Little is known about how autoimmune disorders cause otologic symptoms. As with other autoimmune conditions, the otologic symptoms may occur as a direct assault by the immune system in the form of humoral and cellular immunity directed at the inner-ear. Another mechanism of injury may be related to the deposition of antibody-antigen complex in capillaries or basement membranes of inner-ear structures. Further immunologic studies of temporal bones harvested from deceased patients who had clinical evidence of autoimmune inner-ear involvement may shed some light on the underlying process.

Because autoimmune vestibulopathy usually affects both ears, therapy is almost exclusively medical. Vestibular suppressants are most useful in controlling the more severe exacerbations of vertigo. The use of corticosteroids and some cytotoxic agents (cytoxan, methotrexate) has been shown to provide relief in some patients. There is some newer evidence to suggest that serum plasmapheresis may play a more prominent role in controlling this disease in the future. The natural history of the disease leads to eventual bilateral vestibular ablation. This end result is almost inevitable unless the underlying process can be arrested with treatment or arrests spontaneously.

The most common *toxic* cause of acute vertigo is ethyl alcohol. We know that positional changes exacerbate the vertigo of a hangover. The reason may be that alcohol diffuses into the cupula and endolymph at different rates and so creates a density gradient, making the cupula sensitive to gravity.[20] Other agents that may produce vertigo include organic compounds of heavy metals and aminoglycosides. The aminoglycosides are notorious for causing irreversible failure of vestibular function without vertiginous warning or hearing loss. Thus, monitoring of vestibular function may be necessary during such therapy.

Independent of vestibulopathies produced by ototoxins, single cases of "progressive vestibular degeneration" of unknown origin have been described, with the following factors in common: repeated episodes of dizziness relatively early in life, bilateral loss of vestibular function with retention of hearing, and freedom from other neurologic disturbances.[21]

Alport's (inherited sensorineural deafness associated with interstitial nephritis); Usher's (inherited sensorineural deafness associated with retinitis pigmentosa); and Waardenburg's syndromes (inherited deafness associated with facial dysplasia) usually cause bilateral labyrinthine deficiency if they affect the vestibular system. Congenital vestibular loss is secondary to either abnormal genetic or intrauterine factors including infection (most commonly rubella and cytomegalovirus); intoxication (thalidomide); or anoxia.

Controlled physical exercises can improve the condition in patients with permanent bilateral vestibulopathy by recruiting nonvestibular sensory capacities such as the cervico-ocular reflex and proprioceptive and visual control of stance and gait (see Chapter 15).

SUMMARY

This chapter describes the clinical presentation of the more common peripheral vestibular disorders and the differential diagnosis to central origins of vertigo. Although

TABLE 5–1 Summary of Vestibular System Disorders

	BPPV	Vestibular Neuritis	Ménière's Disease	Fistula	Bilateral Vestibular Disorder
Vertigo	+	+	+	+	−
Type	Rotational	Rotational	Rotational	Rotational/ linear	−
Nystagmus	+	+	+	+	−
Duration	½–2 min	48–72 hr	30 min–24 hr	Seconds	Permanent
Nausea	−/(+)	+	+	−	−
Postural ataxia	−/(+)	+	+	+	++
Specific symptoms	Onset latency, adaptation	Acute onset	Fullness of ear, hearing loss, tinnitus	Loud tinnitus, Tullio sign, Hennebert sign	−
Precipitating action	positioning, turning in bed	−	−	Head trauma, ear surgery, sneezing, straining, nose blowing	−

the symptomatology of a certain peripheral vestibular disorder might be rather specific, as in acute unilateral vestibular loss, the cause can be rather different, ranging from infection to ischemia to traumatic lesions. A thorough evaluation, therefore, should, in addition to the specific otoneurologic investigation, always include a detailed history and a general physical examination. For a quick review, Table 5–1 summarizes the hallmarks of the peripheral vestibular disorders treated in this chapter.

REFERENCES

1. Dix, R and Hallpike, CS: The pathology, symptomatology and diagnosis of certain common disorders of the vestibular system. Ann Otol Rhinol Laryngol 6:987, 1952.
2. Schuknecht, HF: Cupulolithiasis. Arch Otolaryngol 90:765, 1969.
3. Brandt, T and Daroff, RB: Physical therapy for benign paroxysmal positional vertigo. Arch Otolaryngol 106:484, 1980.
4. Semont A, Freyss, G, and Vitte, E: Curing the BPPV with a liberatory maneuver. Adv Oto-Rhino-Laryngol 42:290, 1988.
5. Epley, JM: The canalith repositioning procedure: For treatment of benign paroxysmal positional vertigo. Otolaryngol Head Neck Surg 107:399, 1992.
6. Herdman, SJ, et al: Single treatment approaches to benign paroxysmal positional vertigo. Arch Otolaryngol Head Neck Surg 119:450–454, 1993.
7. Schuknecht, HF and Kitamura, K: Vestibular neuritis. Ann Otol Rhinol Laryngol 90 (suppl 79): 1, 1981.
8. Zee, DS: Perspectives on the pharmacotherapy of vertigo. Arch Otolaryngol 111:609, 1985.
9. Paparella, MM and Kimberley, BP: Pathogenesis of Ménière's disease. J Vest Res 1:3, 1990.
10. Paparella, MM and Meyerhoff, W: Ménière's disease in children. Laryngoscope 88:1504, 1978.
11. Balkany, T, Sires, B, and Arenberg, I: Bilateral aspects of Ménière's disease: An underestimated clinical entity. Otolaryngol Clin North Am 13:603, 1980.
12. Kimura, R: Animal models of endolymphatic hydrops. Am J Otol 3:447, 1982.
13. Meyer, ED: Zur Behandlung des Morbus Ménière mit Betahistindimesilat—Doppelblindstudie gegen Plazebo. Laryngol Rhinol Otol 64:269, 1985.
14. Thomson, J, et al.: Placebo effect in surgery for Ménière's disease. Arch Otolaryngol 107:271, 1981.
15. Lange, G: Die intratympanale Behandlung des Morbus Ménière mit ototoxischen Antibiotika. Laryng Rhinol 56:409, 1977.
16. Schuknecht, HF and Bartley, M: Cochlear endolymphatic shunt for Ménière's disease. Ann J Otol (suppl) 20:2, 1985.
17. Singleton, GT, et al: Perilymph Fistulas. Diagnostic criteria and therapy. Ann Otol Rhinol Laryngol 87:1, 1978.
18. Brandt, T: Episodic vertigo. In Rakel, RE (ed): Conn's Current Therapy. WB Saunders, Philadelphia, 1986, p 723.
19. Hughes, GB, et al: Clinical diagnosis of immune inner ear disease. Laryngoscope 98:251, 1988.
20. Brandt, T: Positional and positioning vertigo and nystagmus. J Neurol Sci 95:3, 1990.
21. Baloh, RW, Jacobson, K, and Honrubia, V: Idiopathic bilateral vestibulopathy. Neurology 39:272, 1989.

CHAPTER 6

Clinical Changes In Vestibular Function over Time after Lesions: The Consequences of Unilateral Vestibular Deafferentation

G. Michael Halmagyi, MD
Ian S. Curthoys, PhD

For more than a century, we have known that acute total deafferentation or destruction of a previously intact labyrinth—unilateral vestibular deafferentation (UVD)—invariably causes a profound and stereotyped disruption of equilibrium in species as diverse as amphibians, birds, rodents, monkeys and humans. The paradox is that although the deafferentation is permanent, the disruption it causes is only temporary. The process of spontaneous recovery from the neurologic effects of acute UVD is termed "vestibular compensation" (for a recent review see Smith and Curthoys[1]).

Acute total UVD is a common clinical event that occurs spontaneously as a result of diseases, such as acute vestibular neuritis, or deliberately as a result of surgical treatment such as vestibular neurectomy. This chapter describes the pattern of onset and resolution and the pathophysiologic basis of the UVD syndrome in humans.

CONSEQUENCES OF UNILATERAL VESTIBULAR DEAFFERENTATION IN HUMANS

Immediately after UVD humans invariably experience intense disequilibrium. This disequilibrium has sensory and motor components with profound disturbances of position and motion perception and of posture and movement control. The sensory and the motor components of the UVD syndrome can be categorized as *static* or *dynamic*. Static components are those present at rest, whereas dynamic components are those evident only during movement—that is, during stimulation of the sole remaining labyrinth by angular or linear acceleration.

The UVD syndrome is totally stereotyped in pattern and duration in each species. Certain components are invariably present, and each of these component changes in time with a characteristic temporal profile. This rule is normally so reliable that if certain components of the UVD syndrome are missing, or if their temporal profile fails to change as described, then we can assume that there has either been an error of observation or that another process has intervened. To measure precisely the pattern and resolution of the UVD syndrome in humans, the same patients should be studied before and after surgical deafferentation of one intact labyrinth. Although such cases and the facilities for studying them are few, some long-term quantitative data on the precise sensory and motor consequences of UVD in humans have recently become available.[2-4] Following UVD, there are abnormalities of perception of both linear and angular acceleration. The abnormalities of motion perception present at rest are called the *static sensory components* of the UVD syndrome; the abnormalities of motion perception during motion are called the *dynamic sensory components* of the UVD syndrome. Some of these abnormalities of motion perception are temporary, whereas others appear to be permanent.

Static Sensory Components of the UVD Syndrome

Immediately after recovering from the anesthesia for the UVD, patients will experience two different false spatial sensations (i.e., illusions). Both occur at rest, and both resolve within 1 to 2 days. One is an illusion of angular motion in yaw and the other is an illusion of linear tilt in roll.

ANGULAR MOTION ILLUSION

This is a false sense of angular motion (i.e., rotation) either of self or of the world, that is, vertigo. With the eyes closed, the illusion is of self-motion with the body turning about its long or yaw axis toward the UVD side. With the eyes open, the illusion is of world motion, now in the opposite direction.

LINEAR TILT ILLUSION

This is a false sense of body roll-tilt about the naso-occipital or roll axis again toward the UVD side.

Both these illusions are probably due to the asymmetry in resting neural activity between the two vestibular nuclei (see Section IV). This asymmetry occurs as a result of the sudden profound decrease in resting activity in the deafferented vestibular nucleus. These illusions occur because whenever the level of neural activity in one vestibular nucleus exceeds the level of activity in the other, this will be interpreted by the brain as rotation toward the side generating the higher level of activity. The higher level of neural activity in the medial vestibular nucleus on the intact side, as compared to the level of activity on the deafferented side, is interpreted by the brain as rotation toward the intact side. Similarly, the relatively higher level of resting neural activity in the lateral vestibular nucleus of the intact side is interpreted by the brain as roll-tilt toward the intact side.

Dynamic Sensory Components of the UVD Syndrome

Deficits in the perception of angular and acceleration stimulation have been found after UVD. Although both these deficits improve with time after UVD, in some patients some deficit appears to be permanent.

ANGULAR ACCELERATION PERCEPTION

To evaluate the precision of yaw angular acceleration perception, subjects seated in a rotating chair were asked in a recent study to counterrotate themselves following a passive rotation in the dark.[5] Metcalfe and Gresty[5] showed that normal subjects passively rotated in a chair by 30 to 180 degrees at 80 deg/sec can, when given control over chair rotation, return the chair precisely back to its starting position. Some chronic UVD patients consistently underresponded to rotations toward the UVD side, whereas they were able to respond correctly to rotations toward the intact side. Other UVD patients were able to respond correctly to rotations to either side. These results were taken to indicate that perception of rotation toward the lesioned side is impaired following UVD and that this impairment compensates with time in some patients.

LINEAR ACCELERATION (ROLL-TILT) PERCEPTION

Normal Roll-Tilt Perception

A normal subject on earth is continuously stimulated by the linear acceleration of gravity. If the subject is upright, then the direction of the gravitational vector corresponds to longitudinal axis of the body. If tilted in the coronal (i.e., roll) plane, about the naso-occipital axis, then the angle between the subject's head long axis and the gravitational linear acceleration vector, the roll-tilt angle, increases and the subject is said to be experiencing roll-tilt stimulation. Roll-tilt stimulation activates otolithic receptors in the utricle and the saccule of each labyrinth.

Another method of producing roll-tilt stimulation is centrifugation. If a subject, seated upright on a centrifuge with the interaural axis parallel to the centrifuge arm, is rotated at constant angular velocity (linear but no angular acceleration), he or she will experience a centrifugal linear acceleration. (For convenience, we refer to centrifugal rather than to centripetal accelerations as the otolithic receptor hair cells are bent in the direction of the centrifugal acceleration and not in the direction of the centripetal acceleration). The centrifugal linear acceleration and the gravitational linear acceleration will sum to produce a resultant gravitoinertial force. Because this resultant force is in the coronal plane and is directed away from the body long axis, it is called a *roll-tilt stimulus*. If the subject is now centrifuged in total darkness to exclude visual cues to verticality, he or she will experience an irresistible sensation of being tilted in the roll plane.[2]

Roll-tilt perception is the conscious sensation of body tilt produced by roll-tilt stimulation. If during centrifugation the subject views a luminous, rotatable bar attached to the centrifuge chair and aligned with his or her interaural axis, the bar will appear to the subject to have tilted (i.e., rolled) with his or her body, away from the preceived gravitational horizontal, by approximately the same amount as the body. This tilt of the subjective visual horizontal with respect to the perceived gravitational horizontal during centrifugation is called the *oculogravic illusion*. A subject's ability to sense the direction of the resultant gravitoinertial vector during centrifugation can be accurately measured by requiring the subject to indicate the perceived direction of the gravitational horizontal with respect to the interaural axis.

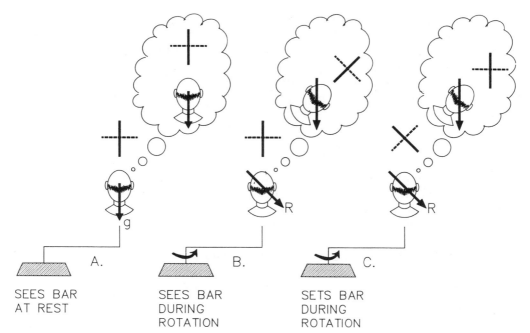

SEES BAR
AT REST

SEES BAR
DURING
ROTATION

SETS BAR
DURING
ROTATION

FIGURE 6–1. Measurement of linear acceleration perception using the oculogravic illusion. (*A*) With the centrifuge at rest in an otherwise darkened room, a normal subject (shown from behind), seated with his interaural axis parallel to the long axis of the centrifuge arm and with his left ear toward the axis of rotation, views a dimly illuminated, gravitationally horizontal, rotatable bar shown here with interrupted lines. At rest, he correctly perceives the bar as aligned not only with the gravitational horizontal, but also with his interaural axis. (*B*) When the centrifuge with its 1-m arm turns at a constant velocity of 180 deg/sec the gravito-inertial resultant force will be directed 45 degrees from the gravitational vector, toward the subject's right labyrinth. In the otherwise darkened room, the subject can now only assume that the resultant force is the gravitational force and therefore perceives that his own body long axis has rotated 45 degrees to his right; that is, he will sense a 45-degree roll-tilt to his right. The illuminated bar is, however, still physically aligned with his own interaural axis and not with the resultant force, so that he perceives the bar as also having rolled with him, 45 degrees to the right. (*C*) When required to set the bar to the perceived gravitational horizontal, the subject does so by rotating the bar 45 degrees to his left (i.e., counterclockwise) and so accurately aligns the bar normal to the resultant force. (From Dai et al,[2] p 316, with permission.)

Consider a subject sitting upright on a centrifuge, 1 m from the rotation axis, with the left ear directed toward the rotation axis (Fig. 6–1). The centrifuge rotates at a constant 30 rpm (equals 180 deg/sec or π radians/sec) in darkness. In the absence of vision, the main source of the subject's sensation of verticality will be otolithic. Because gravitational acceleration and linear acceleration are identical physical forces, the subject now cannot but regard the gravitoinertial resultant as his or her subjective gravitational vertical. Because the resultant is now directed from the subject's left to right, the only perception that will accord with the subject's sensations is that he or she has been tilted onto the right side.

The angle of resultant linear acceleration is simple to calculate, in this case, 45 degrees. In response to this stimulus, a normal subject will sense the direction of this resultant vector accurately and will therefore perceive that his or her body has been tilted 45 degrees to the right. If the subject now views a dimly illuminated, rotatable light bar that is attached to the centrifuge chair and is aligned parallel to the interaural axis (and therefore also normal to the gravitational vertical), the subject will see that the bar has tilted with him or her to the right, also by 45 degrees. The subject can now indicate the precise angle of perceived body tilt by rotating the bar to the left until it is set to the perceived gravitational horizontal (i.e., normal to the resultant vector). Normal subjects centrifuged in darkness can indicate their perception of roll-tilt accurately; they can set a light bar to within 5 degrees of the gravitational horizontal on 95 percent of attempts. These observations show that roll-tilt perception can be accurately measured by nulling the oculogravic illusion, and they raise the possibility of using roll-tilt perception to measure otolith function clinically.

Unilateral Vestibular Deafferentation and Roll-Tilt Perception

Because roll-tilt perception largely depends on otolithic sensation and because normal subjects have accurate roll-tilt perception, testing otolith function clinically by means of the oculogravic illusion is now possible.

In a study of 30 patients before and after UVD,[2] we found that 1 week after operation all 30 patients showed a loss of sensitivity to linear accelerations that were medially directed with respect to the single functioning utricle (Fig. 6–2). This loss of sensitivity became increasingly evident with increasing roll-tilt stimulus angles. Further-

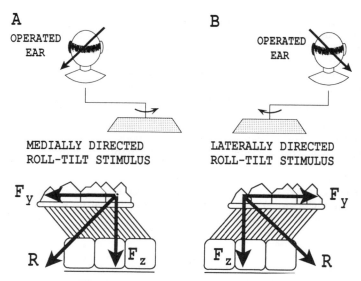

FIGURE 6–2. Medial versus lateral roll-tilt stimulation following unilateral vestibular deafferentation. Schematic representation of roll-tilt stimulation of the remaining intact right labyrinth of a patient who has had a left vestibular deafferentation. The patient, viewed from behind, sits across the centrifuge arm so that his interaural axis is co-linear with the centrifugal linear acceleration. If his intact right labyrinth is positioned away toward the rotation axis (A), then its otoconial membrane will be displaced medially, toward the center of the head, and he is said to be subject to a *medially directed roll-tilt stimulus*. If his intact right labyrinth is positioned away from the rotation axis (B), its otoconial membrane will be displaced laterally, away from the center of the head, and he is said to be subject to a *laterally directed roll-tilt stimulus*. The direction of the centrifugal acceleration indicates the direction of bending of the hair cells. The resultant (R) has two components: Fy, the roll-shear component, which acts in the interaural axis, across the mean utricular plane, and Fz, the component due to gravitational acceleration, which acts as a compressive force in the body longitudinal axis. Fz is constant at 1g during centrifugation. (From Dai et al,[2] p 316, with permission.)

more, even when tested 6 months after operation, these UVD patients still showed a significant loss of sensitivity to linear accelerations that were medially directed with respect to the single functioning utricle (Fig. 6–3).

These results indicate that total UVD causes a deficit in roll-tilt perception of linear accelerations directed toward the lesioned side and that although this deficit compensates over time, this compensation is incomplete, and a small but detectable deficit in roll-tilt perception toward the lesioned side is a permanent legacy of UVD.

The clinical significance of these results is that oculogravic tests of roll-tilt perception could prove a useful means of detecting severe unilateral loss of otolith function and could provide a way of monitoring a sensory component of vestibular compensation.

Static Motor Components of the UVD Syndrome

The *static motor components* of the UVD syndrome all reflect a motor offset or bias toward the deafferented side.

SPONTANEOUS NYSTAGMUS

A spontaneous horizontal nystagmus is invariably present immediately after UVD. The slow phases are always directed toward the lesioned side and are coupled to quick phases directed toward the intact side. The essential characteristics of UVD nystagmus are the same as that of any other peripheral vestibular nystagmus. The nystagmus is largely horizontal, unidirectional, and suppressed by visual fixation. Visual fixation suppression can be so effective that the nystagmus will only be apparent when visual fixation is completely excluded, emphasizing the need to check for nystagmus in the absence of visual fixation in all patients with suspected UVD (Fig. 6–4). Clinically, it is possible to exclude visual fixation by using Frenzel glasses or by using an ophthalmoscope to view the fundus of one eye while the other eye is covered.[5] The *presence* of nystagmus in the absence of visual fixation, combined with the *absence* of nystagmus in the presence of visual fixation is virtually pathognomonic of a peripheral vestibular lesion, opposite the side toward which the quick phases are directed.

Typically, the patient will have primary position (i.e., second-degree) nystagmus even with visual fixation for the first day after UVD, and then first-degree gaze-evoked nystagmus until the end of the first week. Even after a month there will still be a low-velocity (2 to 3 deg/sec) first-degree gaze-evoked nystagmus, present only in the absence of visual fixation. This nystagmus appears to be a permanent legacy of UVD.

Recent studies suggest that the spontaneous nystagmus is due to loss of resting activity in type I secondary horizontal semicircular canal (HSCC) neurons in the medial vestibular nucleus on the same side as the lesion (called here "ipsilesional"). The intensity of the spontaneous nystagmus could be an accurate index of the relative resting rates of ipsilesional and contralesional type I HSCC canal neurons (see Section IV).

Because the two vertical semicircular canals on one side are also deafferented by UVD, it is surprising that the torsional vector of UVD nystagmus is so much less apparent than the horizontal vector. In fact, a prominent torsional vector usually indicates that the lesion is in the vestibular nucleus rather than in the labyrinth or vestibular nerve. There appears to be no entirely satisfactory explanation for these observations, probably because so few objective measurements of the torsional nystagmus component following UVD have been made.

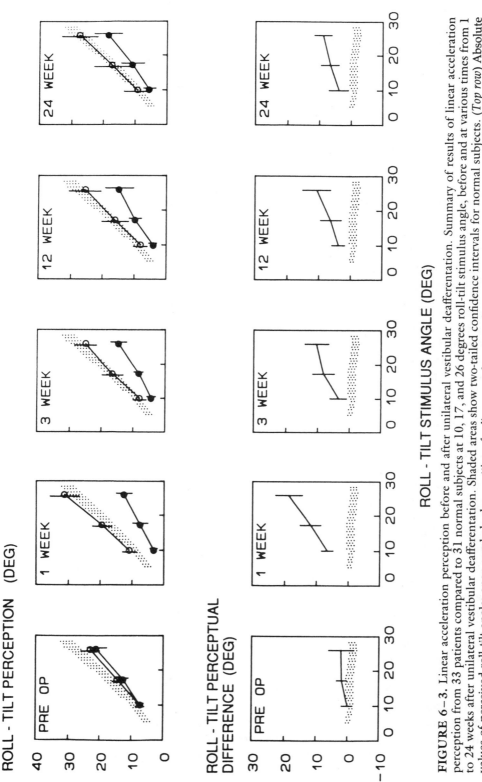

ROLL - TILT PERCEPTION (DEG)

ROLL - TILT PERCEPTUAL DIFFERENCE (DEG)

ROLL - TILT STIMULUS ANGLE (DEG)

FIGURE 6-3. Linear acceleration perception before and after unilateral vestibular deafferentation. Summary of results of linear acceleration perception from 33 patients compared to 31 normal subjects at 10, 17, and 26 degrees roll-tilt stimulus angle, before and at various times from 1 to 24 weeks after unilateral vestibular deafferentation. Shaded areas show two-tailed confidence intervals for normal subjects. (*Top row*) Absolute values of perceived roll-tilt angle: open symbols show settings for linear accelerations directed toward the intact labyrinth (i.e., laterally directed roll-tilt stimulation); filled symbols show settings for linear accelerations directed toward the operated labyrinth (i.e., medially directed roll-tilt stimulation). The large interaural difference present 1 week after operation as decreased by 3 weeks but is still abnormal at all stimulus levels even 24 weeks after operation. (*Bottom row*) Interaural differences in roll-tilt perception remain abnormally high, perhaps indefinitely, after unilateral vestibular deafferentation. (From Dai et al,[2] p 323, with permission.)

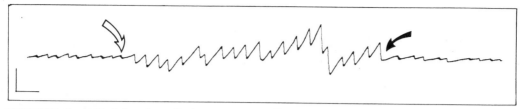

FIGURE 6–4. Peripheral vestibular nystagmus. Oculographic recording shows a left-beating primary-position nystagmus that is obvious only when visual fixation is removed (*open arrow*) and is quickly suppressed again when visual fixation is permitted (*filled arrow*). Peripheral vestibular nystagmus can be detected clinically by viewing the fundus of one eye while occluding the other. The patient had a right vestibular neurectomy the previous day. Upward deflections indicate rightward eye movements, downward deflections indicate leftward eye movements. Bars = 10 degrees and 1 sec.

OCULAR TILT REACTION

The ocular tilt reaction (OTR) is a postural synkinesis consisting of head tilt, conjugate eye torsion, and skew deviation, all in the same direction. Following UVD, there is a tonic ipsilesional OTR so that there is maintained head tilt, ocular torsion, and hypotropia all directed toward the UVD side.[7] Although head tilt and skew deviation are usually subtle, conjugate ipsilesional ocular torsion appears to be invariably present.[4] The direction of the torsion is always ipsilesional: the 12 o'clock meridians of the eyes are rotated toward the side of the UVD. The magnitude of the ocular torsion can be measured by ocular fundus photography (Fig. 6–5). One week after UVD, there is up to 15 degrees of ocular torsion; 1 month after UVD the ocular torsion has diminished to about half the one-week value. A slight but statistically significant ocular torsion (2 to 3 degrees) also appears to be a permanent legacy of UVD.

This change in ocular torsional position can be readily detected in perceptual tests that show a bias in settings of the subjective visual vertical or horizontal toward the UVD side. A normal subject sitting upright in an otherwise *totally* darkened room can accurately align a dimly illuminated bar to within 2 degrees of the gravitational vertical or horizontal.[2] Dai and associates[2] studied 30 patients before and after UVD and showed that whereas their preoperative settings were reasonably accurate, 1 week after operation they invariably set the bar so that it was tilted toward the side of the UVD, in some cases by up to 15 degrees. These patients reported that while seated upright they perceived themselves to be upright, although no nonvisual measures of perceived body position were made. The setting of the bar returned toward the horizontal with time but was still tilted by a mean of 4 degrees 6 months or more after UVD. In all cases, the magnitude of the tilting of the visual horizontal was closely correlated with the magnitude of the ocular torsion. An ipsilesional tilting of the visual horizontal appears to be a permanent legacy of UVD.

The clinical significance of these findings is that careful standardized measurement of the visual horizontal, using a dim light bar in an otherwise totally darkened room gives valuable diagnostic information. A significant tilting of the visual horizontal indicates vestibular, probably otolithic, hypofunction on the side to which the patient tilts the bar. Although tilting of the visual horizontal is probably due to ocular torsion, the mechanism of the ocular torsion itself is speculative. This mechanism could be similar to that of spontaneous nystagmus that occurs after UVD and reflects decreased resting activity in secondary vestibular neurons in the ipsilesional vestibular nucleus due to loss of input from primary vestibular neurons.

BEFORE RIGHT VESTIBULAR NEURECTOMY

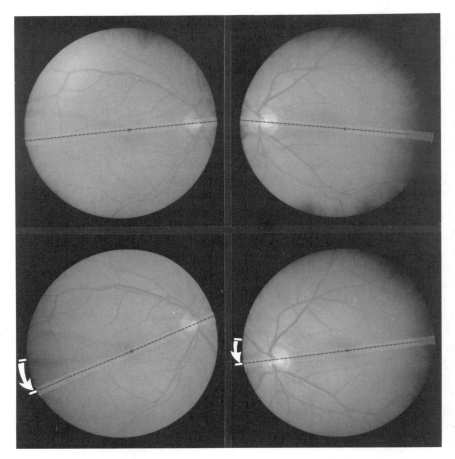

AFTER RIGHT VESTIBULAR NEURECTOMY

FIGURE 6–5. Fundus photographs of the left and right eye of a patient before (*top row*) and 1 week after (*bottom row*) right vestibular neurectomy. After operation, there is tonic rightward torsion of the 12 o'clock meridian of each eye toward the patient's right side. The change in torsion angle measures 18 degrees in the right eye and 16 degrees in the left eye. When the patient was asked to set a luminous bar to the perceived visual horizontal in an otherwise darkened room, he set the bar tilted toward his right side by 14.2 when viewing with the right eye and 15.1 degrees when viewing with the left. (From Curthoys et al,[4] p 221, with permission.)

LATEROPULSION

Following UVD, an *offset* or *lateropulsion* of limb and body posture toward the operated side is invariably evident in the absence of visual fixation. Many clinical tests can be used to demonstrate this, including the Bárány past pointing test, the Fukuda vertical writing test, or the Unterberger stepping test. Although these are all positive in the first postoperative week, they have all returned to normal after about 1 month.

POSTURAL DYSEQUILIBRIUM

Despite this apparent return to normal posture on clinical tests, posturographic tests often show a permanent deficit in postural equilibrium following UVD.[8] This deficit becomes evident if the movements of either the platform alone, or of the platform and the visual surround together, are referenced to the body sway. The relationship of these posturographic abnormalities to the other tests of vestibular function and to the overall clinical state after UVD is not yet clear. There are many unanswered questions. For example, is a permanent posturographic deficit after UVD simply the result of the UVD? Or does this deficit imply a subclinical abnormality in the remaining labyrinth that was not detected before deafferentation? What is the relationship between an abnormal posturogram and symptomatic chronic vestibular insufficiency? These questions have an impact on both the physical and surgical treatment of vestibular disorders, and further studies are needed to answer them.

Dynamic Motor Components of the UVD Syndrome

HORIZONTAL VESTIBULO-OCULAR REFLEXES

The changes that occur in the horizontal vestibulo-ocular reflex (HVOR) after UVD have been investigated in many species, including monkeys and humans. The results obtained depend on the stimulus used. In response to low-frequency (<1 Hz) low-acceleration (100 deg/sec^2) symmetrical (i.e., sinusoidal) head rotations, immediately after UVD there is a severe and asymmetrical HVOR deficit. The deficit persists, for about a month in humans, and then improves so that by 1 year after UVD the HVOR (in response to this type of stimulus) is normal or near normal.[9,10] This improvement in the low-frequency, low-acceleration HVOR is commonly used as an index of vestibular compensation.

If high-acceleration stimulation is used, a different result is obtained. In monkeys, immediately after operation there is a profound deficit of both the ipsilesional and contralesional HVOR, but some recovery is already apparent even by the second postoperative day. The vestibulo-ocular reflex deficit is most apparent with the fastest head movements. Fetter and Zee[11] have shown using a constant 125 deg/sec^2, angular acceleration stimulation for 2 to 3 seconds that 3 months after operation the ipsilesional HVOR still only has a mean gain that is 60 percent of normal and the contralesional HVOR a gain that is 80 percent of normal.[11] Using head impulses with acceleration up to 3000 deg/sec^2, we have shown that the ipsilesional HVOR gain years after operation is on average still only 25 percent of normal[3] (Figs. 6–6, 6–7). From this finding, one can presume that the high-acceleration response of the HVOR is never restored to normal after UVD. It appears that dynamic equilibrium, just like static equilibrium, is permanently impaired by UVD.

Two signs of HVOR asymmetry can be detected clinically: head-shaking nystagmus[10] and the head-impulse sign.[13] Head-shaking nystagmus is horizontal nystagmus with quick phases directed toward the normal ear that appears for 3 to 10 seconds after 20 seconds or so of active horizontal head shaking. Like any other type of peripheral vestibular nystagmus, head-shaking nystagmus is absent in the presence of visual fixation and present only in the absence of visual fixation. Head-shaking nystagmus is most readily observed using Frenzel glasses. Head-shaking nystagmus is a direct result of the inherent right-left behavioral asymmetry of each horizontal semicircular canal (Ewald's second law), signaling to a brain-stem neural network that normally perserverates the peripheral vestibular input (velocity storage). Head-shaking nystagmus requires a properly functioning neural integrator and can be absent after UVD.[14]

The head-impulse sign consists of compensatory saccades toward the intact ear during rapid passive head impulses toward the affected ear. The sign is always positive

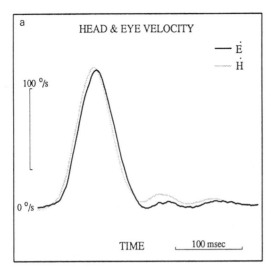 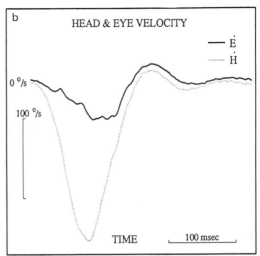

FIGURE 6–6. Single head impulses from a patient 3 years after unilateral vestibular neurectomy. Head velocity is shown in interrupted lines, eye velocity in continuous lines. (*a*) Eye velocity more or less mirrors head velocity in response to the ampullopetal excitation produced by head rotation toward the intact side. (*b*) In contrast, eye velocity lags head velocity from the onset of head rotation in response to ampullofugal disfacilitation produced by head rotation toward the deafferented side. (From Halmagyi, et al,[50] p 412, with permission.)

in patients with severe unilateral loss of HSCC function. The head-impulse test also depends on Ewald's second law and the ability of rapid head impulses to drive the afferents of the single remaining HSCC to silence.

VERTICAL VESTIBULO-OCULAR REFLEXES

Normal subjects have a symmetric near-unity gain *vertical vestibulo-ocular reflex* (VVOR) in response to 0.4 to 1.6 Hz active sinusoidal head oscillation both in the upright and in the onside positions.[15] In response to passive low-acceleration onside pitch stimulation in UVD patients, no long-term VVOR deficit was found.[16] The reason for this negative finding could have been that the acceleration used was too low to demonstrate the inherent on-off direction nonlinearity of the vertical semicircular canal (VSCC).

In response to high-acceleration passive head impulses in the upright position, normal subjects have a symmetrical VVOR with near-unity gain. Following UVD, there is a consistent bidirectional VVOR deficit, indicating that a single labyrinth is not adequate to produce a normal VVOR.[17] Moreover, the VVOR deficit is asymmetrical: it is more marked for upward head impulses that excite the sole functioning posterior SCC and disfacilitate the sole functioning anterior SCC, than for downward impulses that excite the sole functioning anterior SCC and disinhibit the sole functioning posterior SCC.[17] There could be many reasons for this asymmetry. Perhaps the simplest explanation is in terms of the planar orientation of the VSCCs with respect to the sagittal plane. In humans, the plane of the anterior canal makes an angle of about 41 degrees with the sagittal plane, whereas the plane of the posterior canal makes an angle of about 55 degrees.[18] The projection of these mean VSCC planes to the sagittal plane yields a posterior to anterior canal ratio of (0.74), a value close to the upward/downward VVOR gain asymmetry (0.72). The reason that the VVOR asymmetry after UVD is not as

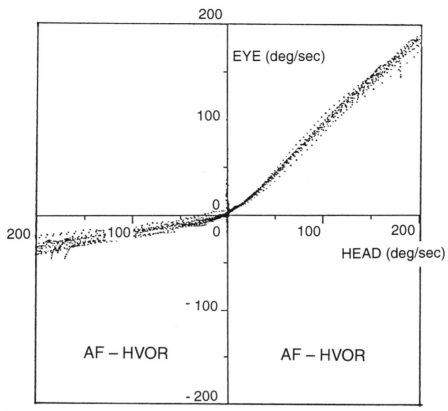

FIGURE 6–7. Horizontal eye velocity plotted as a function of horizontal head velocity for 20 horizontal head impulses in a patient who had undergone a left vestibular neurectomy 3 years previously. There is a profound HVOR deficit in response to head impulses directed toward the deafferented side — the ampullofugal (AF) HVOR. In contrast, the HVOR in response to head impulses directed toward the intact side is normal — the ampullopetal (AP) HVOR. (From Halmagyi, et al,[50] p 413, with permission.)

marked as the HVOR asymmetry[3] could be that there are still two SCCs driving the VVOR as opposed to the one SCC driving the HVOR.

Summary of Changes in Vestibular Function with Time after Lesions

1. *Angular rotation illusion:* Maximum during first few hours, completely resolved by third day.
2. *Roll-tilt illusion:* Maximum during first few hours, completely resolved by third day.
3. *Angular acceleration perception deficit:* Maximum during first week; in some cases, completely resolved at 1 year, but in other cases, deficit still present. Data incomplete.
4. *Linear acceleration perception deficit:* Maximum during the first week; largely but incompletely resolved within 1 year.

5. *Spontaneous nystagmus:*   Maximum during the first 2 days; improved at 1 week; largely but incompletely resolved within 1 year.
6. *Ocular torsion:*   Maximum during the first week; largely but incompletely resolved within 1 year.
7. *Lateropulsion:*   Maximum during the first 3 days; improved by 1 week; completely resolved within 1 year.
8. *Postural disequilibrium:*   Maximum during first week; incompletely resolved within 1 year.
9. *Horizontal vestibulo-ocular reflex deficit:*   Maximum during the first week; partial recovery at 1 month, near-complete recovery within 1 year in response to low-acceleration stimulation; no significant recovery at all in response to high-acceleration stimulation.
10. *Vertical vestibulo-ocular reflex deficit:*   Persistent deficit at 1 year in response to high-acceleration stimulation; data incomplete.

INFLUENCES ON THE RESTORATION OF STATIC AND DYNAMIC EQUILIBRIUM

There is little reliable quantitative information on the effects of any physical or chemical interventions on the rate or extent of vestibular compensation in humans. The data that are available come from studies on cats, monkeys, and guinea pigs, and are incomplete, inconclusive, or contradictory (for a recent review see Smith and Curthoys[1]). One reason for these contradictions could be that the large number of different inputs to the vestibular nuclei could all directly or indirectly affect the activity of vestibular nucleus neurons. In general, the restoration of static equilibrium—that is, static compensation—is remarkably robust: very little appears to hasten or hinder it. In contrast, the restoration of dynamic equilibrium—dynamic compensation—appears to depend at least in part in intact visual, vestibular, and proprioceptive sensory inputs, and is often incomplete.

Visual Inputs

Visual deprivation has no effect on the resolution of spontaneous nystagmus[19,20] but may impede the recovery of roll head tilt,[21,22] which is part of the ocular tilt reaction, and the HVOR in response to low-frequency, low-acceleration stimulation.[20,23] Although bilateral occipital lobectomy has no effect on the resolution of spontaneous nystagmus, it does impede the recovery of the HVOR to low-acceleration stimulation.[20] Visual inputs do augment the diminished muscle responses to linear acceleration[24] and the deficient righting reflexes[25] that occur after UVD. Visual motion deprivation delays recovery of locomotor equilibrium.[26]

Vestibular Inputs

There are only scant data on the effects on vestibular stimulation or vestibular deprivation on static or dynamic compensation. In frogs, otolithic stimulation hastens, whereas otolithic deprivation delays static compensation of head tilt.[27] In cats, low-frequency combined visuo-vestibular stimulation helps reverse the symmetrical deficit in HVOR gain that occurs in response to low-frequency stimulation following UVD[28] but has no effect on the asymmetry of the HVOR. There are no data on the effects of vestibular deprivation on vestibular compensation in mammals.

Proprioceptive Inputs

Cervical proprioceptive input could be important in static compensation as head restraint retards resolution of head tilt and spontaneous nystagmus.[29] Somatosensory proprioceptive deprivation appears to retard static compensation,[24] whereas somatosensory proprioceptive stimulation appears to facilitate the restoration of dynamic postural equilibrium.[30] Acute spinal lesions can produce a temporary decompensation of static postural symptoms.[31]

Drugs

The restoration of near-normal levels of spontaneous activity in the neurons of the ipsilesional vestibular nucleus in the absence of reinnervation could have a neurochemical basis. Investigations so far have not revealed any changes in glutamate, dopamine, norepinephrine, acetylcholine, histamine, or serotonin receptors that could account for the restoration of spontaneous activity (for a recent review see Smith and Darlington[32]). In several species, treatment with an ACTH fragment accelerates static compensation.[33,34] In cats, amphetamine and trimethobenzamide could facilitate both static and dynamic compensation.[35]

Lesions

Data on the effects of lesions of the cerebellum or its connections on vestibular compensation are contradictory. Whereas some cerebellar lesion studies[36] show a marked delay in the resolution of spontaneous nystagmus, others[37] show no effect. Although bilateral occipital lobectomy has no effect on the resolution of spontaneous nystagmus, it does impede the recovery of the HVOR to low-acceleration stimulation.[20] Lesions of the brain stem[38] or transcerebellar vestibular commissures[39] do not impede static compensation, at least in mammals. This finding suggests that input from the contralesional (intact) vestibular nucleus is not essential for static compensation. Sections of the brain-stem commissures might, however, abolish the HVOR.[40]

In patients with fluctuating vestibulopathies, such as Ménière's disease, the attacks of vertigo are brief compared to the time required for compensation. In humans, compensation takes 3 to 5 days to get under way and 1 month or more to achieve a functionally useful level. Vestibular compensation cannot help the patient with recurrent or paroxysmal vertigo as the process is too slow. Compensation does, however, help the patient to recover after a permanent UVD.

Chronic Vestibular Insufficiency Following Unilateral Vestibular Deafferentation

Chronic vestibular insufficiency (CVI) is a clinical syndrome consisting of gait ataxia and oscillopsia (see Chapter 13). The gait ataxia is always most evident when visual and proprioceptive inputs are disrupted, for example, when the patient tries to walk on uneven ground in the dark. The oscillopsia is only evident during head movement, for example, when the patient walks or runs, or when he or she looks rapidly from side-to-side while driving or crossing a road.[41] CVI can be due to central or peripheral vestibular lesions and invariably occurs in patients who have severe bilateral loss of vestibular function as evidenced by absent HVOR responses to rapid accelerations and to 0°C caloric stimulation. A common cause of severe bilateral loss of vestibular function is aminoglycoside ototoxicity. Although the CVI can be asymptomatic in some patients with severe bilateral vestibular loss during the activities of daily living, the symptoms and abnormalities can always be demonstrated under certain provocative conditions such as rapid head movements and eye closure while standing on a soft surface.

We have found that certain UVD patients also experience symptomatic CVI. Considering that recent data show permanent and in some cases severe deficits of horizontal and vertical VOR and of postural equilibrium following UVD this finding is not entirely surprising.[3,8,17] What is surprising is that most UVD patients do not experience symptoms of CVI, even though their VOR and posturographic results are apparently indistinguishable from the results of those patients who do. From the therapeutic viewpoint, one should determine what differences there are between those patients who do and those who do not experience symptoms of CVI following UVD. Do the symptomatic UVD patients have a subtle defect in the contralesional sole functioning labyrinth, or do they have some defect in the compensation process? This question merits further investigation.

NEURAL ACTIVITY IN THE VESTIBULAR NUCLEI DURING VESTIBULAR COMPENSATION

To appreciate the mechanisms of the UVD syndrome and vestibular compensations, we should examine the changes in neural activity underlying these changes in behavior (for recent reviews see Goldberg and Fernandez[42] and Smith and Curthoys[1]).

Normal Medial Vestibular Nucleus Activity

Two types of HSCC–driven neurons have been found in the medial vestibular nuclei of monkeys, cats, and guinea pigs. Both types of vestibular nucleus neurons, just like primary vestibular neurons, discharge spontaneously, that is, at rest, at rates sometimes in excess of 80 impulses/sec. The discharge rate of type I neurons increases when the head acceleration is ipsilateral and decreases when the head acceleration is contralateral. The reverse applies to type II neurons that increase their discharge rate in response to contralateral head accelerations and decrease their discharge rate in response to ipsilateral head accelerations (Fig. 6–8). The reason why type I and type II neurons respond differently is that whereas type I neurons are excited by ipsilateral HSCC, primary afferent neurons are inhibited by ipsilateral type II neurons; type II neurons themselves are excited by contralateral type I neurons via commissural pathways. Motor and sensory equilibrium requires equal resting activity in the two medial vestibular nuclei. Type I neurons drive the HVOR by excitatory projections to abducens motoneurons and interneurons in the contralateral abducens nucleus.

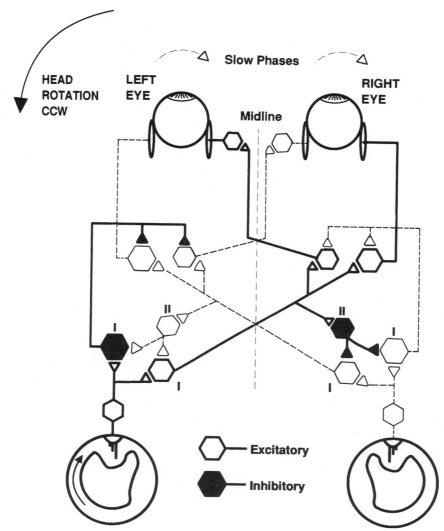

FIGURE 6-8. Schematic simplified representation of the responses in some of the identified connections of the normal HVOR pathways, in response to a counterclockwise (i.e., leftward) head acceleration. Neurons from the left HSCC are shown by solid lines; neurons from the right HSCC are shown by dotted lines. Primary HSCC neurons, excitatory type I medial vestibular nucleus neurons, abducens motoneurons, abducens interneurons, and medial rectus motoneurons are shown by open hexagonal symbols. Inhibitory type II medial vestibular nucleus neurons are shown by filled hexagonal symbols.

Ipsilesional Medial Vestibular Nucleus Activity

Immediately after UVD, there are changes in the activity of both type I and type II neurons in the medial vestibular nucleus on the operated side.[43-46] The resting activity of type I neurons is decreased, whereas the resting activity of type II neurons is increased. The decrease in resting activity of type I neurons reflects the loss of excitatory drive by HSCC primary afferent neurons. The increase in resting activity of type II neurons could reflect increased excitatory drive by contralesional type I neurons that have become disinhibited by the decrease in the activity of contralesional type II neurons, which are themselves normally excited by ipsilesional type I neurons (see Fig. 6–8). As well as showing a reduced resting discharge rate, immediately after UVD, ipsilesional type I neurons show a decrease in sensitivity to angular acceleration. The sensitivity of type II neurons to angular acceleration remains unchanged. In the days and weeks that follow, a remarkable series of changes occur in the resting activity of ipsilesional medial vestibular nucleus neurons. The resting discharge rates of both type I and type II neurons are restored to normal rates even though the medial vestibular nucleus no longer receives any afferent drive from its labyrinth. Data so far, mainly from the guinea pig and the gerbil, have shown a limited restoration of sensitivity of type I neurons to angular accelerations. This restoration of resting activity in type I neurons could also underlie the recovery of humans from the disabling consequences of UVD and the restoration of normal static equilibrium.

Contralesional Medial Vestibular Nucleus Activity

Immediately after unilateral deafferentation, there is an increase in the resting activity of contralesional type I neurons without much change in their sensitivity.[44–47] There is also a decrease in the sensitivity of contralesional type II neurons without much change in resting activity. This increase in resting activity of type I neurons is due to decreased inhibition by type II neurons that are themselves normally excited by ipsilesional type I neurons, now silenced. In the following days and weeks, the resting activity of contralesional type I neurons is restored to normal and the resting activity of contralesional type II neurons increases to above normal. These changes in the resting activity of contralesional medial vestibular nucleus neurons occur despite the fact that the ipsilesional vestibular nucleus remains isolated from its labyrinth. However, the remarkable restoration of resting activity in ipsilesional type I neurons described above can account for the changes in activity of contralateral medial vestibular nucleus neurons. The restoration of contralesional type I resting activity to normal is presumably the result of the increased inhibition by contralesional type II neurons, now excited by the restored resting activity of ipsilesional type I neurons. Together with the decrease of contralesional type I resting activity to normal, there is a late decrease in contralesional type I sensitivity, whereas contralesional type II sensitivity remains low.

Normal Lateral Vestibular Nucleus Activity

Primary otolithic neurons project to secondary vestibular neurons mainly in the lateral (and descending) vestibular nuclei. The predominant response of lateral vestibular nucleus neurons is an increase in firing rate from the resting level in response to ipsilateral tilts (i.e., laterally directed linear accelerations), the alpha response. The commissural connections between secondary otolithic neurons are poorly understood. Unlike the commissural connections of the HSCC, secondary neurons in the medial vestibular nucleus that are direct and functionally inhibitory, the commissural connections between the secondary otolithic neurons in the lateral vestibular nucleus apparently are indirect and functionally excitatory. There are also interconnections between the lateral and the medial vestibular nuclei, and some medial vestibular nucleus neurons respond to both semicircular canal and to otolithic stimulation. The changes that occur in the lateral vestibular nucleus after UVD vary between the rostroventral and dorsocaudal areas of the nucleus, which project to the cervicothoracic and lumbosacral segments of the spinal cord, respectively.

Ipsilesional Lateral Vestibular Nucleus Activity

There is a decrease in the proportion of roll-tilt responsive neurons in the rostroventral area, but not in the dorsocaudal area, as well as an overall decrease in the average resting activity of neurons.[48] In contrast, there are increases in the number of position-sensitive neurons, in the tilt sensitivity of dorsocaudal neurons, and in the number of beta responses (increase firing with medially directed linear acceleration). With compensation, there is little recovery in the resting activity of either alpha or beta neurons. The proportion of neurons in the rostroventral areas responsive to roll-tilt increases to normal while the sensitivity remains normal. The sensitivity of dorsocaudal neurons decreases to normal. The proportion of position-sensitive neurons and beta responses does not change.

Contralesional Lateral Vestibular Nucleus Activity

The proportion of roll-tilt–sensitive neurons is normal. The overall resting activity is slightly reduced. As in the ipsilesional lateral vestibular nucleus, there is an increase in position-sensitive neurons and in beta responses and a decrease in the roll-tilt sensitivity of neurons in the rostroventral areas. There are scant data on the changes with compensation, but there appear to be few differences in the contralesional neuronal activity in normal and in uncompensated cats.[49]

SUMMARY

This chapter describes the neurophysiologic changes that occur following unilateral vestibular deficits. Both the static and dynamic components of vestibular function follow a characteristic temporal pattern of change that is reflected in the clinical changes in vestibulo-ocular and vestibulospinal responses. For example, spontaneous nystagmus and the ocular tilt reaction reflect the effects of UVD on the static component of vestibular function and head-shaking–induced nystagmus and the inability to maintain visual fixation during rapid head thrusts reflect the disruption of the dynamic component. Visual, vestibular, and somatosensory inputs have varying effects on the recovery of the static and dynamic vestibular responses.

ACKNOWLEDGMENTS

This work was supported by the Australian National Health and Medical Research Council and by the RPA Hospital Neurology Department Trustees.

REFERENCES

1. Smith, PF and Curthoys, IS: Mechanisms of recovery following unilateral labyrinthectomy: A review. Brain Res Rev 14:155, 1989.
2. Dai, MJ, Curthoys, IS, and Halmagyi, GM: Perception of linear acceleration before and after unilateral vestibular neurectomy. Exp Brain Res 77:315, 1989.
3. Halmagyi, GM, et al: The human horizontal vestibulo-ocular reflex in response to high-acceleration stimulation before and after unilateral vestibular neurectomy. Exp Brain Res 81:471, 1990.
4. Curthoys, IS, Dai, MJ, and Halmagyi, GM: Ocular torsional position before and after unilateral vestibular neurectomy. Exp Brain Res 85:218, 1991.
5. Metcalf, ET and Gresty, M: Self-controlled reorienting movements in response to rotational displacements in normal subjects with labyrinthine disease. Ann NY Acad Sci May: 22695, 1992.
6. Zee, DS: Ophthalmoscopy in the examination of patients with vestibular disorders. Ann Neurol 3:373, 1978.
7. Halmagyi, GM, Gresty, MA, and Gibson WPR: Ocular tilt reaction due to peripheral vestibular lesion. Ann Neurol 6:80, 1979.
8. Black, FO, et al: Effects of unilateral loss of vestibular function on the vestibulo-ocular reflex and postural control. Ann Otol Rhinol Laryngol 98:884, 1989.
9. Jenkins, HA: Long-term adaptive changes of the vestibulo-ocular reflex in patients following acoustic neuroma surgery. Laryngoscope 95:1224, 1985.
10. Paige, GD: Nonlinearity and asymmetry in the human vestibulo-ocular reflex. Acta Otolaryngol 108:1, 1989.
11. Fetter, M and Zee, DS: Recovery from unilateral labyrinthectomy in rhesus monkey. J Neurophysiol 59:370, 1988.
12. Hain, TC, Fetter, M, and Zee, DS: Head-shaking nystagmus in patients with unilateral peripheral vestibular lesions. Am J Otolaryngol 8:36, 1987.
13. Halmagyi, GM and Curthoys, I: A clinical sign of canal paresis. Arch Neurol 45:737, 1988.
14. Fetter M, et al: Head-shaking nystagmus during vestibular compensation in humans and rhesus monkeys. Acta Otolaryngol 110:175, 1990.
15. Baloh, RW and Demer, J: Gravity and the vertical vestibulo-ocular reflex. Exp Brain Res 83:427, 1991.
16. Allum, JHJ, Yamane, M, and Pfaltz, CR: Long-term modifications of vertical and horizontal vestibulo-ocular reflex dynamics in man. Acta Otolaryngol 105:328, 1988.
17. Halmagyi, GM, et al: The human vertical vestibulo-ocular reflex in response to high-acceleration stimulation after unilateral vestibular neurectomy. Ann NY Acad Sci May: 22732, 1992.
18. Blanks, RHI, Curthoys, IS, and Markham, CH: Planar relationships of the semicircular canals in man. Acta Otolaryngol 80:185, 1975.
19. Maoli, C, Precht, W, and Ried, S: Short and long-term modifications of vestibulo-ocular response dynamics following unilateral vestibular nerve lesions in the cat. Exp Brain Res 50:259, 1983.
20. Fetter, M, Zee, DS, and Proctor, LR: Effect of lack of vision and of occipital lobectomy upon recovery from unilateral labyrinthectomy in rhesus monkey. J Neurophysiol 59:394, 1988.
21. Putkonen, PT, Courjon, JH, and Jeannerod, M: Compensation of postural effects of hemilabyrinthectomy in the cat. A sensory substitution process? Exp Brain Res 28:249, 1977.
22. Smith, PF, Darlington, CL, and Curthoys, IS: The effect of visual deprivation on vestibular compensation in the guinea pig. Brain Res 364:195, 1986.
23. Courjon, JH, et al: The role of vision in compensation of the vestibulo-ocular reflex in the cat. Exp Brain Res 28:235, 1977.
24. Lacour, M and Xerri, C: Vestibular compensation: New perspectives. In Flohr, H and Precht, W (eds): Lesion-Induced Neuronal Plasticity in Sensorimotor Systems. Springer-Verlag, Berlin 1981, p 240.
25. Igarashi, M and Guitirrez, O: Analysis of righting reflex in cats with unilateral and bilateral labyrinthectomy. Otorhinolaryngology 445:279, 1983.
26. Xerri, C and Zennou, Y: Sensory, functional and behavioural substitution processes in vestibular compensation. In Lacour, M, et al (eds): Vestibular compensation: Facts, Theories and Clinical Perspectives. Elsevier, Paris, 1989, p 35.
27. Flohr, H, et al: Concepts of vestibular compensation. In Flohr, H and Precht, W (eds): Lesion-induced Neuronal Plasticity in Sensorimotor Systems. Springer-Verlag, Berlin 1981, p 153.
28. Maoli, C and Precht, W: On the role of vestibulo-ocular reflex plasticity in recovery after unilateral peripheral vestibular lesions. Exp Brain Res 59:267, 1985.
29. Pettorossi, VE and Petrosini, L: Tonic cervical influences on eye nystagmus following labyrinthectomy: Immediate and plastic effects. Brain Res 324:11, 1984.
30. Igarashi M: Physical exercise and the acceleration of vestibular compensation. In Lacour, M, et al (eds): Vestibular Compensation: Facts, Theories and Clinical Perspectives. Elsevier, Paris, 1989, p 131.
31. Jensen, DW: Vestibular compensation: Tonic spinal influence upon spontaneous descending vestibular nuclear activity. Neuroscience 4:75, 1979.
32. Smith, PF and Darlington, CL: Neurochemical mechanisms of recovery from peripheral vestibular lesions (vestibular compensation). Brain Res Rev 16:117, 1991.

33. Flohr, H and Luneburg, U: Influence of melanocortin fragments on vestibular compensation. In Lacour, M, et al: Vestibular compensation: Facts, Theories and Clinical Perspectives. Elsevier, Paris, 1989, p 161.
34. Gilchrist, DP, Smith PF, and Darlington, CL: ACTH(4-10) accelerates ocular motor recovery in the guinea pig following vestibular deafferentation. Neurosci Lett 118:14, 1990.
35. Peppard, SB: Effect of drug therapy on compensation from vestibular injury. Laryngoscope 96:878, 1986.
36. Courjon, JH, et al: The role of the flocculus in vestibular compensation after hemilabyrinthectomy. Brain Res 239:251, 1982.
37. Haddad, GM, Friendlich, AR, and Robinson, DA: Compensation of nystagmus after VIIIth nerve lesions in the vestibulo-cerebellectomized cat. Brain Res 135:192, 1977.
38. Smith, PF, Darlington, CL, and Curthoys, IS: Vestibular compensation without brainstem commissures in the guinea pig. Neurosci Lett 65:209, 1986.
39. Newlands, SD and Perachio, AA: Effects of commisurotomy on vestibular compensation in the gerbil. Soc Neurosci Abstr 12:254, 1986.
40. Precht, W, Shimazu, H, and Markham CH: A mechanism of central compensation of vestibular function following hemilabyrinthectomy. J Neurophysiol 26:996, 1966.
41. Halmagyi, GM and Henderson, CJ: Visual symptoms of vestibular disease. Austr N Zeal J Ophthalmol 16:177, 1988.
42. Goldberg, JM and Fernandez, C: The vestibular system. In Handbook of Physiology. The Nervous System. Sensory Processes, Sec 1, Vol 3, Chap 21, Physiological Society, Bethesda, MD, 1981, pp 977–1022.
43. Smith, PF and Curthoys, IS: Neuronal activity in the ipsilateral medial vestibular nucleus of the guinea pig following unilateral labyrinthectomy. Brain Res 444:308, 1988.
44. Newlands, SD and Perachio, AA: Compensation of horizontal canal-related activity in the medial vestibular nucleus following unilateral labyrinth ablation in the decerebrate gerbil. I. Type I neurons. Exp Brain Res 82:359, 1990.
45. Newlands, SD and Perachio, AA: Compensation of horizontal canal-related activity in the medial vestibular nucleus following unilateral labyrinth ablation in the decerebrate gerbil. II. Type II neurons. Exp Brain Res 82:373, 1991.
46. Smith, PF and Curthoys, IS: Comments to SD Newlands and AA Perachio: Neuronal activity in the medial vestibular nucleus following unilateral labyrinthectomy. Exp Brain Res 86:679, 1991.
47. Smith, PF and Curthoys, IS: Neuronal activity in the contralateral medial vestibular nucleus of the guinea pig following unilateral labyrinthectomy. Brain Res 444:295, 1988.
48. Xerri, C, et al: Compensation of central vestibular deficits. I. Reponse characteristics of lateral vestibular neurons to roll tilt after ipsilateral labyrinth deafferentation. J Neurophysiol 50:428, 1983.
49. Lacour, M, et al: Central compensation of vestibular deficits. III. Response characteristics of lateral vestibular nucleus neurons to roll tilt after contralateral labyrinthine deafferentation. J Neurophysiol 54:988, 1985.
50. Halmagyi, GM, et al: Unilateral vestibular neurectomy in man causes a severe permanent horizontal vestibulo-ocular reflex deficit in response to high-acceleration ampullofugal stimulation. Acta Otolaryngol S481:411, 1991.

SECTION II

Medical Assessment

CHAPTER 7

Quantitative Vestibular Function Tests and the Clinical Examination

Vicente Honrubia, MD, DMSc

The maintenance of equilibrium and posture and the awareness of spatial orientation in everyday life are complex functions depending on multiple organs and neural centers in addition to the peripheral labyrinth. Visual and proprioceptive reflexes must be integrated with vestibular reflexes. Consequently, the evaluation of the "vestibular system" requires the study of the function of all these systems, not only that of the vestibular organs. The physician must investigate through medical history, physical evaluation, and signs and symptoms every aspect relevant to this contemporary view of vestibular function.

The most common symptom of vestibular dysfunction is *dizziness*, and the most common signs are spontaneous nystagmus and abnormal voluntary eye movements. Dizziness or some form of disequilibrium or disorientation can be produced by lesions in sites other than the vestibular system. Clinical evaluation of the patient remains the most important aspect of the vestibular diagnosis. The history provides many clues to the cause of symptoms, and the physical examination provides objective data about the operation of various components of the vestibular system. Careful evaluation of information obtained by the physician is necessary to complement the objective and quantitative laboratory evaluation of data on eye movements and other reflexes. This integration makes it possible in many instances to determine if the site of the lesion is the inner ear, vestibular centers, or pathways in the central nervous system (CNS).

Radical improvement in the management of patients has occurred during the past 10 years, with the creation of technology that has led to new tests for differential diagnosis and the evaluation of treatment of vestibular patients. The vestibular tests used most often are those to evaluate maintenance of gaze, as this is one of the primary functions of the vestibular system. Eye movements produced for this purpose are the result of three basic systems with different dynamics and neuroanatomic pathways: the

113

saccadic system, the smooth-pursuit and optokinetic systems, and the vestibulo-ocular system. Tests for evaluation of these types of eye movement have become important parts of the modern neurotologic examination. Besides their intrinsic value, they represent a powerful method of evaluating the state of large parts of the CNS.

CLINICAL EVALUATION OF PATIENTS WITH VESTIBULAR PROBLEMS

The neurotologic evaluation consists of a detailed history to ascertain the character of dizziness, physical examination of the ear, evaluation of the function of vestibulo-visuo-ocular and equilibrium reflexes and hearing, and overall neurologic assessment. This section emphasizes the more "vestibular" aspects of the examination during the first interaction between patient and clinician and describes the most important details of the history of dizziness and the clinical evaluation of vestibular-dependent and visual-dependent eye movements.

Dizziness

The individual's description of dizziness can be of help in determining which part of the systems involved in orientation is responsible for the symptoms. *Vertigo* is an illusion of movement that is specific for vestibular system disease, and rotation is the most commonly described experience. The illusion of linear displacement or rocking is less frequently noted and suggests otolithic organ involvement. Other terms used by persons to describe dizziness are less specific: giddiness, one's head is swimming, lightheadedness, floating, or a feeling of drunkenness. These sensations can be associated with disorders of other systems.

Intensity, duration, and frequency of attacks, precipitating or relieving factors, and characteristics of associated symptoms (tinnitus, hearing loss, ear pain, and infections) are all important elements in elucidating the underlying cause of dizziness.

Vertigo always indicates an imbalance within the vestibular system, although the symptom per se does not indicate where in the system the imbalance originates: the inner ear, deep paravertebral stretch receptors of the neck, vestibular centers, the cerebellum, or upper cerebral pathways and cortex. The distinction between peripheral and central causes of vertigo can be suspected on the basis of history. Peripheral vertigo is often severe and associated with other physiologic changes, such as hearing loss, and with autonomic symptoms, such as nausea. Vertigo of central origin is more moderate and more persistent.

Peripheral vestibular vertigo invariably occurs in episodes, usually abrupt in onset, and decreasing in intensity as the precipitating factor disappears. Continuous vertigo and/or dizziness without fluctuation for long periods is not typical of vestibular disorders of peripheral origin. Typically, the duration of attacks associated with peripheral disorders varies from seconds, as in benign postural vertigo, to minutes, even hours, as in Ménière's disease or during a vascular compromise of the inner ear. In these cases, the episode is followed by lightheadedness, fatigue, and generalized weakness that subside during the day. If the vestibular damage is severe, recovery may take several days to 1 week. Even at such times, differentiating spontaneous episodes of vertigo, as may occur in Ménière's disease, from the rather brief episodes of disorientation associated with quick head movements owing to deficient function of the damaged vestibular receptors is important. Peripherally induced vertigo, even in the case of severe damage, gradually resolves as central compensation occurs, although the duration of symptoms depends on the extent of damage.

Diagnosis of the cause of vertigo can be suspected from events just prior to or at the time of the episode. Fluctuating hearing loss, earache, and appearance of or an increase in tinnitus are typical of Ménière's disease. Positional vertigo may be precipitated by turning over in bed, sitting up from a prone position, extending the neck to look upward, or bending over and straightening up. Patients with perilymph fistula develop brief episodes of vertigo precipitated by changes in middle-ear pressure, such as when coughing, sneezing, or engaging in vigorous physical activities. Occasionally, loud noises can produce vertigo when a fistula is present or when there is inner-ear pathology (syphilis and advanced Ménière's disease). The medical history may also point out a contributing factor in the use of drugs such as alcohol, tranquilizers, anticonvulsants, or barbiturates. A compromised cardiovascular, metabolic, or immunologic condition, impaired vision, or generalized neuropathies may be associated with dizziness. The occurrence of headaches at the time of vertigo may suggest a history of migraines in other members of the family, and, if headaches are associated with ataxia, one should inquire whether other family members experience the same symptoms. Episodes of vertigo can occur from decreased cerebral blood flow, as occurs during changes in position of the body and head in hypotensive conditions and cardiac insufficiency, or spontaneously during transient ischemic episodes in basilar vertebral insufficiency. The latter should be differentiated from Tumarkin episodes occurring in patients with Ménière's disease. Patients with handicapped brain blood flow experience generalized weakness; particularly of the lower extremities, brief disorientation; and finally, near or complete loss of consciousness; whereas patients undergoing Tumarkin crises feel irresistibly catapulted to the ground without loss of consciousness. Both conditions can occur in elderly patients with Ménière's disease. Dizziness in a continuous static fashion without episodic vertigo has a central origin and should lead to inquiry about other CNS symptoms or signs (e.g., cranial nerve function evaluation).

Finally, the association of dizziness or vertigo with psychologic conditions such as panic attacks, agoraphobia, anxiety, or hyperventilation should be considered. Anxiety is also an important component of the status of the patient at the time of clinical examination and should be differentiated from other conditions in which it is the primary cause of dizziness.

Nystagmus

Nystagmus can be defined as nonvoluntary rhythmic oscillation of the eyes. It usually has clearly defined fast and slow components beating in opposite directions. Figure 7–1 shows diagrammatically the various components of typical horizontal nystagmus. By convention, the direction of the fast component defines the direction of nystagmus.

CLASSIFICATION OF NYSTAGMUS

Physiologic nystagmus can be induced with natural or experimental stimuli in normal subjects; *pathologic nystagmus* can appear with or without external stimulation in patients

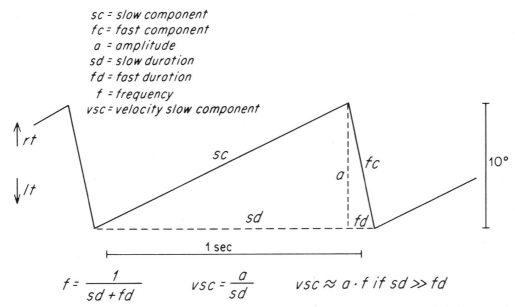

sc = slow component
fc = fast component
a = amplitude
sd = slow duration
fd = fast duration
f = frequency
vsc = velocity slow component

$$f = \frac{1}{sd + fd} \qquad vsc = \frac{a}{sd} \qquad vsc \approx a \cdot f \text{ if } sd \gg fd$$

FIGURE 7–1. A theoretic beat of nystagmus, indicating major components and their approximated values. (From Baloh and Honrubia,[41] p 132, with permission.)

with vestibular disorders. Physiologic nystagmus is produced by vestibular (caloric, rotatory, or linear acceleration) or visual (optokinetic) stimulation, or with extreme lateral gaze (endpoint nystagmus). The characteristics (direction, intensity, shape) of pathologic nystagmus and the method used to induce it often offer clues to the involved pathology. Pathologic nystagmus can be spontaneous (present with head erect and gaze centered); positional (induced by change in head position); or gaze-evoked (induced by change in eye position). Pathologic nystagmus can be affected by interference with fixation (darkness, use of special lenses) and gaze position (e.g., congenital) (see Table 7–1). The cause of spontaneous nystagmus can be lesions of the peripheral or central vestibular system as well as lesions of other CNS pathways involved in the control of eye movements, or it can be visuo-ocular in origin (congenital). The combined effects on nystagmus of vision (or its absence), position of the head, and direction of gaze are helpful in elucidating its origin.[1]

Methods of Examination of Pathologic Nystagmus

The search for pathologic nystagmus can be accomplished during clinical examination of the patient and should always be part of the laboratory evaluation of vestibular function.

TABLE 7–1 Types of Nystagmus

Physiologic	Pathologic
Rotational-induced	Spontaneous
Caloric-induced	Gaze-evoked
Optokinetic	Positional
End point	Congenital

The clinical examination search for pathologic nystagmus should include a systematic study of the eyes during changes in (1) fixation, (2) eye position, and (3) head position. In addition, a "fistula" test should be conducted to determine the possibility of inducing nystagmus associated with slow pressure variation in the external ear canal. The control of fixation during physical examination is accomplished with Frenzel glasses, which consist of +30 lenses mounted in a frame. A battery-power internal light or an external flashlight held by the examiner enables observation of the patient's eyes. Examination with Frenzel glasses in a darkened room is easier to accomplish and, in addition, prevents the patient from fixating (at least partially) through the lenses on lighted objects.

The effect of change in eye position is evaluated by having the patient fixate on a target 30 degrees to the right, left, up, and down from center. Because horizontal eye deviation beyond 40 degrees may result in low-amplitude, high-frequency torsional nystagmus in normal subjects (so-called end-point nystagmus), extreme eye positions should be avoided. Each eye position is held for at least 20 seconds and should be repeated at least once. First-degree nystagmus refers to nystagmus that is present only on gaze in the direction of the fast component; second-degree nystagmus is present in the midposition and on gaze in the direction of the fast component; and third-degree nystagmus is present even on gaze away from the fast component. These terms, however, are not applicable to all varieties of nystagmus and, therefore, can lead to confusion. A simple description can be summarized with a box diagram as illustrated in Figure 7–2. The size, shape, and direction of the arrows provide information about the amplitude and direction of the fast component of nystagmus in the five primary eye positions.

The effect of head position is evaluated with two types of positional testing—slow and rapid. First, the patient slowly moves into supine, right lateral, and left lateral positions. The nystagmus is observed for 20 to 60 seconds as the patient looks straight ahead. Rapid positional changes are used to induce paroxysmal positional nystagmus, which, owing to the moving maneuver, cannot be confused with the physiologic nystagmus. Both tests can be conducted with fixation and, using Frenzel glasses, without fixation.

The *fistula test* is easily performed during otoscopic examination with the aid of a

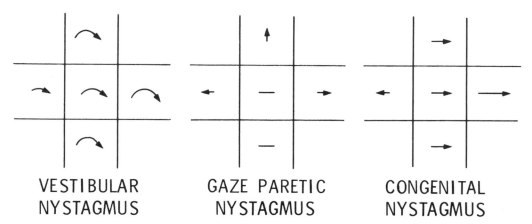

VESTIBULAR   GAZE PARETIC   CONGENITAL
NYSTAGMUS   NYSTAGMUS   NYSTAGMUS

FIGURE 7–2. Method for describing the effect of eye position on nystagmus amplitude and direction. Arrows indicate direction of nystagmus (direction of fast component) and its relative magnitude in each of five primary eye positions. (From Baloh and Honrubia, [119] p 109, with permission.)

pneumatic otoscope. After a speculum is selected that tightly fits the canal, pressure is applied (approximately 200 to 300 ml H_2O) while the tympanic membrane and the skin of the auditory meatus are observed in order to verify the effect of successive periodic pressure variations of about 2- to 3-second cycles. In our clinic, a Siegle speculum is mounted on the regular otoscope by means of an adapter. Tympanic membrane motion and change in skin color owing to interference with blood flow in the dermis of the external canal are good indications of the use of adequate pressure. An assistant should observe the eyes, which are behind Frenzel glasses, to prevent fixation, and the patient should be asked to describe any unusual sensations, mainly the illusion of motion, during the test. The resulting eye movement is not necessarily a burst of nystagmus but can be a back-and-forth motion related to the pressure variation in either the horizontal or vertical plane. A positive test should be repeated with electronystagmography recordings at a later time.

Method of Recording Nystagmus and Other Types of Eye Movement

In addition to observation, the recording and quantitative measurement of nystagmus form the ideal basis of many vestibular tests and provide objective documentation of vestibular function. The search for nystagmus in the laboratory is made with the aid of electro-oculography, which is the simplest and most readily available method for recording many eye movements.[2,3] With this technique, a voltage surrounding the orbit is measured, whose magnitude is proportional to the amplitude of eye movement. When used for evaluating vestibular function, the technique has also been termed *electronystagmography* (ENG).[4,5] ENG provides a permanent record for comparison with eye movement and nystagmus findings from other patients. Because of the transient nature of many types of nystagmus, a permanent record is invaluable.

RECORDING PATHOLOGIC NYSTAGMUS

A systematic search for pathologic nystagmus should be conducted during the ENG examination. Recording with eyes closed or with eyes open in darkness is more effective than the use of Frenzel glasses for identifying spontaneous and positional nystagmus of peripheral origin. Even with the use of Frenzel glasses to prevent fixation, patients can inhibit spontaneous nystagmus by converging on the light inside the lenses or on other unexpected references. Approximately 20 percent of normal subjects have spontaneous nystagmus, and as many as 75 percent have positional nystagmus when tested with eyes closed or with eyes open in darkness.[6,7] Apparently, in many otherwise normal individuals, the vestibular system alone is unable to stabilize the position of the eyes when visual signals are removed. In our clinic, an average slow component velocity of spontaneous or positional nystagmus exceeding 4 deg/sec is considered a sign of vestibular impairment.[6,8]

Principle of Electronystagmography

The principle of ENG is illustrated in Figure 7-3. A potential difference exists between the cornea and the retina, oriented in the direction of the long axis of the eye. In relation to an indifferent remotely located electrode, an electrode placed in the vicinity of the eye becomes more positive when the eye rotates toward it and less positive when the

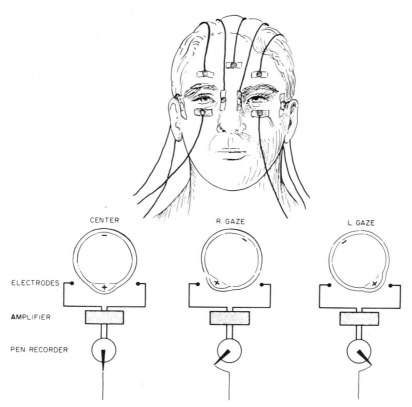

FIGURE 7–3. Recording of eye movements with ENG. See text for details. (From Baloh and Honrubia,[41] p 131, with permission.)

eye rotates in the opposite direction. Recordings are usually made with a three-electrode system, using differential amplifiers. Two of the electrodes (active) are placed on each side of the eye, and the reference electrode (ground) is placed in a remote location (e.g., on the forehead). The difference in potential between the active electrodes is amplified and used to produce a permanent record with the aid of a polygraph or similar device.

With properly designed amplification, ENG can consistently record eye rotations of 0.5 degree, although one occasionally encounters patients (particularly elderly patients) with a high noise-to-signal ratio, limiting the sensitivity to 1 to 2 degrees. Even at its best, the sensitivity of ENG is less than that of direct visual inspection (approximately 0.1 degree), and therefore visual search for small-amplitude eye movements (e.g., gaze-evoked vertical nystagmus) remains an important part of the examination.

Electrode Placement

Because of the genesis of the corneoretinal potential, ENG can monitor horizontal and/or vertical eye movements. Unfortunately, vertically aligned electrodes sense the voltage changes associated with both eye and lid movement, so that the recording represents an interaction of these two movements.[9] Thus, ENG is not suitable for quantitative analysis of vertical eye movements, for which purpose other methods must be used. Alternatively, vertical ENG recordings are useful in recognizing the existence of eye blinks, which affect the characteristics of horizontally recorded eye movements.

Interpreting the Recording

By convention, for horizontal recordings, eye movements to the right are displayed so that they produce upward pen deflections and those to the left produce downward pen deflections. For vertical recordings, upward and downward eye movements are made to produce upward and downward deflections, respectively. To interpret ENG recordings, a standard angle of eye deviation is represented by a known amplitude of pen deflection associated with the recorded change in ENG voltage. To calibrate ENG, the patient is asked to look at a series of dots or lights 10 to 15 degrees on each side of and above and below the central fixation point. The calibration should be performed frequently because the magnitude of the corneoretinal potential is affected by ambient light and changes in skin resistance. Once the calibration is established, the precise value of various nystagmus parameters, such as amplitude, duration, and velocity of recorded eye movements, can be easily calculated. Figure 7–1 illustrates the relationship between components of a typical beat of nystagmus. Scale values chosen for duration and amplitude are those commonly seen with vestibular nystagmus recorded in the dark. The fast component of the illustrated nystagmus moves to the left, so by convention the direction assigned to this nystagmus is to the left. A 10-degree fast component would have an average velocity of approximately 100 deg/sec. The slow component velocity is usually much slower—in this case, 10 deg/sec and is approximately the product of amplitude and frequency, as long as the fast duration is small compared to the slow duration. Although the magnitude of each nystagmus measurement, as shown in Figure 7–1, can be calculated directly from the polygraph recording, such a procedure is very tedious and time-consuming, and therefore subject to error. Digital computers are ideally suited for making such measurements. After analogue-to-digital conversion of the data, a digital computer, using a programmed algorithm, can measure the point-by-point position and velocity of the eye or can calculate the amplitude, duration, and velocity of each of the slow and fast components.[10,11] Plots of the nystagmus slow-component velocity versus time are particularly useful for quantifying the magnitude of induced nystagmus (as will be shown later).

Types of Pathologic Nystagmus

SPONTANEOUS NYSTAGMUS

Spontaneous nystagmus results from an imbalance of tonic signals arriving at the oculomotor neurons. The vestibular system is the main source of oculomotor tonus and is therefore the driving force of most types of spontaneous nystagmus (tonic signals arising in the smooth-pursuit and optokinetic systems may also play a role, particularly with congenital nystagmus).[12,13] Vestibular imbalance produces a constant drift of the eyes in one direction interrupted by fast components in the opposite direction. If the imbalance results from a peripheral vestibular lesion, the pursuit system can be used to cancel it. If the imbalance results from a central vestibular lesion, the pursuit system cannot suppress it because visual signals share some of the pathways of the vestibular signals in the vestibular nuclei.

Peripheral Spontaneous Nystagmus

Lesions of the peripheral vestibular system (labyrinth of eighth nerve) typically interrupt or diminish tonic afferent signals originating from all of the receptors of one labyrinth, so that the resulting peripheral vestibular spontaneous nystagmus has combined torsional, horizontal, and vertical components. The horizontal component dominates because the tonic activity from the intact vertical canals and otoliths partially cancel one another. Gaze in the direction of the fast component increases frequency and velocity, whereas gaze in the opposite direction has the reverse effect (Alexander's law). As noted earlier, peripheral spontaneous nystagmus is strongly inhibited by fixation. Unless the patient is seen within a few days of the acute episode, spontaneous nystagmus will not be present when fixation is permitted, even when gaze is in the direction of the fast component. On the other hand, when the slow component of spontaneous nystagmus is greater than 20 to 40 deg/sec, demonstrating any effect in the peripheral spontaneous nystagmus with any of the maneuvers is difficult. In addition, patient cooperation may be lacking because of the severity of symptoms.

Congenital Nystagmus

One type of spontaneous nystagmus is *congenital nystagmus*, which is almost always highly dependent on fixation, disappearing or decreasing with loss of fixation.[14] In some instances, a slow nystagmus in the reverse direction is recorded with eyes closed. One common variety, so-called latent congenital nystagmus, occurs only when either eye is covered, permitting monocular fixation. The resulting nystagmus beats toward the fixating eye. The frequency of congenital nystagmus is usually greater than 2 beats/sec and at times reaches 5 to 6 beats/sec. Such a high frequency is unusual in other types of nystagmus. Of course, most patients are aware that the nystagmus has been present since infancy.

Another form of spontaneous nystagmus is *periodic alternating nystagmus* (PAN), which periodically changes direction without a change in eye or head position.[15] Cycle length varies between 1 and 6 minutes, with null periods between each half-cycle varying from 2 to 20 seconds. The nystagmus slowly builds in intensity, reaching a peak slow component velocity near the center of each half-cycle before slowly decreasing. PAN has been reported to be a congenital disorder, but it has also been found in association with such varied conditions as encephalitis, brain-stem ischemia, demyelinating disease, syringobulbia, syphilis, and trauma.[15,16]

Central Spontaneous Nystagmus

Central spontaneous nystagmus is as prominent with as without fixation, as opposed to peripheral spontaneous nystagmus. This form of nystagmus may be purely vertical, horizontal, or torsional, or have some combination of torsional and linear components. As with peripheral spontaneous nystagmus, gaze in the direction of the fast component usually increases nystagmus frequency, but, unlike peripheral spontaneous nystagmus, gaze away from the direction of the fast component often changes the direction of nystagmus. In this case, there is a null region several degrees off center in the direction opposite to that of the fast component where nystagmus is minimal or absent. Gaze beyond this null region results in reversal of nystagmus direction.

Lesions involving the vestibular nuclear region can produce horizontal torsional nystagmus similar to that seen with peripheral lesions, but, unlike the latter, the direction of nystagmus does not reliably indicate the side where the lesion is located, and nystagmus persists with fixation owing to damage of visuovestibular interaction pathways.[17] Vertical nystagmus is of central origin and can have different presentations. *Spontaneous vertical downbeat nystagmus* may result from cerebellar atrophy, vertebrobasilar ischemia, multiple sclerosis, or Arnold-Chiari malformation.[18,19] *Spontaneous upbeat nystagmus* usually results from lesions of the dorsal central medulla in the region of the medial vestibular and prepositus hypoglossi nuclei.[18,20] Common causes include infarction, infiltrating tumors, and multiple sclerosis. Pure torsional spontaneous nystagmus is frequently associated with syringomyelia and syringobulbia. High-frequency, small-amplitude *pendular spontaneous nystagmus* commonly occurs in the late stages of multiple sclerosis.[21] This pendular nystagmus converts to a sawtooth pattern on lateral gaze to either side.

GAZE-EVOKED NYSTAGMUS

Patients with gaze-evoked nystagmus are unable to maintain stable, conjugate eye deviation away from the primary position. The eyes drift back toward the center with an exponentially decreasing waveform; corrective saccades (fast components) constantly reset the desired gaze position. Gaze-evoked nystagmus is therefore always in the direction of gaze. The site of abnormality can be anywhere from the neuromuscular junction to the multiple brain centers controlling conjugate gaze. Dysfunction of the so-called oculomotor integrator may be a common mechanism causing several types of gaze-evoked nystagmus.[13]

Symmetric gaze-evoked nystagmus (equal amplitude to the left and right) is most commonly produced by ingestion of drugs such as phenobarbital, phenytoin, diazepam, and alcohol. Symmetric gaze-evoked nystagmus can occur in patients with myasthenia gravis, advanced multiple sclerosis, and cerebellar atrophy.

Asymmetric horizontal gaze-evoked nystagmus always indicates a structural brain lesion. When caused by a focal lesion of the brain stem or cerebellum, the larger-amplitude nystagmus is usually directed toward the side of the lesion.[22] Large cerebellopontine angle tumors commonly produce asymmetric gaze-evoked nystagmus from compression of the brain stem and cerebellum (Bruns' nystagmus). Some patients with large acoustic neuromas develop a combination of asymmetric gaze-evoked nystagmus, from brainstem compression, and peripheral spontaneous nystagmus, from eighth nerve damage. Asymmetric gaze-evoked nystagmus may be present during the recovery from gaze paralysis (either cortical or subcortical in origin), in which case it is large in amplitude and low in frequency and present in only one direction of gaze (the direction of the previous gaze paralysis).[22]

A special type of gaze nystagmus is *rebound nystagmus*. When the eyes return to the primary position, a burst of nystagmus occurs in the direction of the return saccade. Rebound nystagmus occurs in patients with cerebellar atrophy and focal structural lesions of the cerebellum and is the only variety of nystagmus thought to be specific for cerebellar involvement.[23]

Lesions of the medial longitudinal fasciculus (MLF), so-called internuclear ophthalmoplegia, produce dissociated or disconjugate gaze-evoked nystagmus. With early MLF lesions, the eyes appear to move conjugately, but the abducting eye on the side opposite the MLF lesion develops regular, small-amplitude, high-frequency nystagmus in the direction of gaze. With more extensive MLF lesions, the adducting eye lags behind and develops low-amplitude nystagmus, while the abducting eye overshoots the target and develops large-amplitude nystagmus that has a characteristic "peaked waveform."[24] MLF nystagmus can be bilateral or unilateral, depending on the extent of MLF involvement. Bilateral MLF nystagmus is most commonly seen with demyelinating disease, while unilateral MLF nystagmus most often accompanies vascular disease of the brain stem.[25] Patients with myasthenia gravis develop dissociated gaze-evoked nystagmus, similar to MLF nystagmus (pseudo-MLF nystagmus), because of unequal impairment of neuromuscular transmission in adducting and abducting muscles. Unlike MLF nystagmus, the dissociated nystagmus with myasthenia gravis progressively increases in amplitude as gaze position is maintained.[26]

POSITIONAL NYSTAGMUS

Position-induced static nystagmus has been attributed to lesions of the otoliths and their connections in the vestibular nuclei and cerebellum, because these are the receptors sensitive to changes in the direction of gravity.[27-29] Recently, other mechanisms for the production of positional nystagmus have been proposed, forcing reexamination of traditional concepts. If the semicircular canal cupula were altered so that its specific gravity no longer equaled that of the surrounding endolymph, the organ would become sensitive to changes in the direction of gravity and would produce positional nystagmus. Several types of evidence suggest that both structural and metabolic factors can alter the specific gravity of the cupula and cause positional nystagmus.

Traditional classifications of positional nystagmus are often confusing and can be difficult to apply in clinical practice. Some classifications have been based on clinical observations obtained while the patient is fixating, whereas others have been based on ENG recordings with eyes closed or with eyes open in darkness. Some investigators use slow-positioning maneuvers, whereas others employ only rapid positioning. These different methods make comparing classifications difficult. Nylen[29] initially described three types of positional nystagmus based on visual inspection of nystagmus direction and regularity. Type I, direction-changing, and type II, direction-fixed, remained constant as long as the position was maintained. Type III was less clearly defined, comprising all paroxysmal varieties of positional nystagmus and some persistent varieties that did not fit into types I and II. Numerous modifications of Nylen's original classifications have subsequently been proposed, and the definition of each type has changed. Most investigators do agree that two general categories of positional nystagmus can be identified: paroxysmal and static.

Paroxysmal Positional Nystagmus

Paroxysmal positional nystagmus is induced by rapid change from erect sitting to supine head-hanging left, center, or right position—the so-called Hallpike maneuver (Fig. 7–4).[30] Movement is in the plane of the posterior semicircular canal of the ear on the downside of the head. Schuknecht[31] proposed that benign paroxysmal positional nystagmus results from a lesion in the posterior semicircular canal resulting in the formation of a precipitation in the cupula-endolymph of density greater than that of the surrounding fluid. This form of nystagmus is a common sequela of head injury, viral labyrinthitis, and occlusion of the vasculature of the inner ear. In the majority of cases, however, occurrence is an isolated sign of unknown cause. The nystagmus is initially high in frequency but dissipates rapidly within 30 seconds to a minute. The most common variety, benign paroxysmal positional nystagmus usually has a 3- to 10-second latency before onset and rarely lasts longer than 30 seconds.[32,33] The nystagmus has combined torsional and linear components (Fig. 7–5). Although infrequent bilateral cases have been reported, the nystagmus is usually prominent in only one head-hanging position, and a burst of nystagmus occurs in the reverse direction when the patient moves back to the sitting position.

The direction of nystagmus is consistent with the predictions of Ewald's third law for vertical canal function, whereby the posterior canal is excitatorily stimulated during

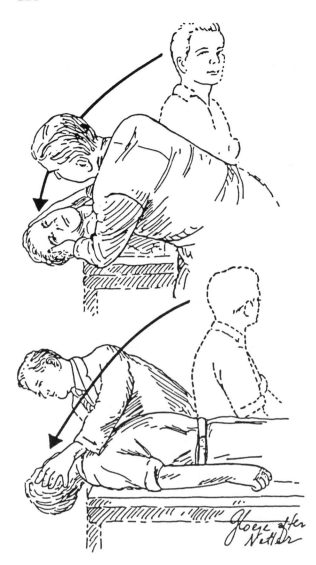

FIGURE 7–4. Technique for inducing paroxysmal positional nystagmus (Hallpike maneuver). Patient is taken rapidly from the sitting to head-hanging position. Note that head is turned 45 degrees to the side of the examiner for each test. (From Baloh and Honrubia,[41] p 124, with permission.)

backward motion, which produces ampullofugal endolymph and cupula motion. The eye movements are disconjugate, being predominantly vertical in the upper eye — the eye on the side opposite the one that induces the nystagmus — while the Hallpike maneuver is executed. This vertical motion of the upper eye is owing to the excitatory connection between the posterior canal and the contralateral inferior rectus. The nystagmus beats upward after the supine position is reached and downward after the sitting position is reached. The reversal in direction is owing to the reversal in direction of cupula motion. When the crista is higher than the canal while the body is supine and the head overextended, gravity pulls the cupula down, resulting in an ampullofugal cupular deviation, that is, excitation. In the opposite, downward eye, nystagmus is torsional, directed toward the upper eye when the body is supine, because of the excitatory connection between the posterior canal and the ipsilateral superior oblique muscle.[31] Also to be noted is that the patient experiences severe vertigo with the initial positioning,

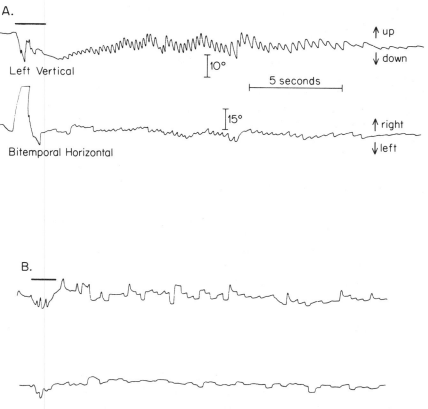

FIGURE 7–5. Benign positional nystagmus induced in the head-hanging-right position (vertical monocular and horizontal temporal recording). (*A*) Sitting to head-hanging. (*B*) Head-hanging to sitting. Solid bar indicates duration of rapid positioning maneuver. (From Baloh et al,[33] p 137, with permission.)

but with repeated positioning, vertigo and nystagmus rapidly diminish and may even disappear (so-called fatigability).

Benign paroxysmal positional nystagmus is a reliable sign of vestibular end-organ disease, can be the only finding in an otherwise healthy individual, or may be associated with other signs of peripheral vestibular damage, such as peripheral spontaneous nystagmus and unilateral caloric hypoexcitability. In those instances where abnormality is identified on caloric testing, nystagmus usually occurs when the patient is positioned with the damaged ear down.

Another type of nystagmus can also result from brain-stem and cerebellar lesions.[34,35] Central paroxysmal positional nystagmus does not decrease in amplitude or duration with repeated positioning, does not have a clear latency, and usually lasts longer than 30 seconds.[36] The direction is unpredictable and may be different in each position. It is often purely vertical, with the fast components directed downward, that is, toward the cheeks. The presence or absence of associated vertigo is not a reliable differential feature.

Static Positional Nystagmus

When the position of the head in relationship to gravity is changed, nystagmus may be produced that remains as long as the position is held but may fluctuate in frequency and amplitude. This nystagmus may be in the same direction in all positions or change directions in different positions. Often, patients with paroxysmal positional nystagmus will have static positional nystagmus after the paroxysmal positional nystagmus has disappeared or if the position is reached very slowly. We now generally accept that the two types, *direction-changing* and *direction-fixed static positional nystagmus*, are most commonly associated with peripheral vestibular disorders, although both occur with central lesions.[37,38] Their presence indicates only a dysfunction in the vestibular system without localizing value. As with spontaneous nystagmus, however, lack of suppression with fixation and signs of associated brain-stem dysfunction suggest a central lesion.

QUANTITATIVE VESTIBULAR TESTS

Tests of vestibular function should include evaluation of the operation of reflexes but should also include evaluation of the associated psychophysical experiences, as is the case, for example, with the auditory system. The psychophysical sensations more readily associated with vestibular system function are perception of self-motion or of relative motion between self and environment.

Subjective Vestibular Tests

Although simple in concept, the quantification of the sensation of self-motion, which is the most common problem of vestibular patients, has been a difficult task for clinicians. With vestibular stimulation, recognizing the beginning of motion and differentiating purely vestibular-derived information from that obtained through visual, tactile, or proprioceptive stimuli is often difficult. Indeed, because of these interactions, even normal humans experience a variety of illusions of motion that can lead to hazardous situations.

Of the vestibular system, the psychophysics of the semicircular canals have been the most intensively studied. The canals are thought to operate like velocity sensors in the frequency range of head movements; for example, when subjects are stimulated with angular rotations, they qualitatively describe the sensation as "moving" to the left or to the right. The characteristics of these psychophysical phenomena follow the prediction of the pendulum model of vestibular function in that perception of motion corresponds to velocity of head motion in a manner similar to the velocity component of eye movement being associated with this stimulus. In accordance with this model, the threshold for the perception of motion is approximately 1 deg/sec for all frequencies within the range of natural head movements (Fig. 7–6).[39] Unfortunately, the evaluation of these reactions is still in the experimental stage, and there is not yet a generally accepted method to overcome some of the technical difficulties mentioned earlier.

A recent study using physiologic stimulation of the horizontal semicircular canals showed that subjects fixating on a moving object judged the velocity of the object in a simple algebraic relationship to the eye velocity that would have acquired the eye movement (nystagmus slow component) produced during physiologic rotation in the dark.[40] That is, the object's velocity is evaluated as the difference between the "normal" slow component velocity — without interaction — and that of the object. This phenomenon occurs despite the subject's eye's fixation on the object. Because the velocity of the nystagmus slow component represents the brain's estimation of eye velocity necessary to

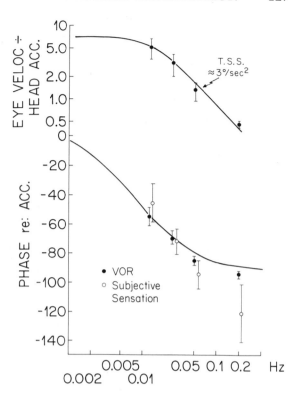

FIGURE 7–6. Summary of gain and phase measurements of VOR and of phase measurements of subjective sensation evaluations in normal subjects. Bars indicate 1 standard deviation around mean values. Abscissa indicates frequency of stimulus; ordinate indicates ratio of eye velocity to head acceleration (*top*) or phase of responses in relation to head acceleration (*bottom*). In the latter, all values are negative, indicating lag of reflex reactions to stimuli. Also indicated is the threshold for sensation in terms of acceleration for a sinusoidal stimulus of 0.05 Hz (~3.0 deg/sec). (From Honrubia et al,[39] p 498, with permission.)

compensate for head motion, it appears that during unsuspected rotation, while the subject tracks the object, the vestibular stimulation changes an internal reference somewhere in the brain by which a person determines motion of the environment in relation to self. A similar mechanism operating in patients with spontaneous nystagmus will result in an illusion of motion of the environment while the patient is stationary. The magnitude of the error should be related to the vestibular stimuli that will produce an equivalent eye movement. Furthermore, patients will have difficulty judging the relative motion of objects around them! Although more research needs to be conducted in this area, the examiner should be aware of and understand the disorientation experienced by patients and be appreciative of their difficulties.

Quantitative Vestibular Reflex Function Tests

The maintenance of gaze is one of the most important functions of human orientation and a relatively simple one to measure. Vestibular- and visual-dependent reflexes contribute to preserve gaze: those stemming from the inner ear, with its receptors for the perception of linear and angular acceleration, and those from the visual system, with the three major visuo-oculomotor systems—saccadic, smooth pursuit, and optokinetic. Hence, measurement of gaze following reflex stimulation is the ideal method to evaluate the function of these reflexes, and the study of vestibular disorders includes tests for their evaluation independently and during their interaction, the latter being the case during everyday conditions. For this purpose, a standardized test battery has been

TABLE 7–2 Standard ENG Test Battery

Recording for Pathologic Nystagmus

> Fixation at midposition
> Fixation inhibited with eyes open in darkness (constant mental alerting)
> Gaze held 30 degrees right, left up, and down
> Rapid and slow positional changes

Bithermal Caloric Test

> 30°C and 44°C water infused into each ear, eyes open in darkness, continuous mental alerting, allow at least 5 minutes between each

Visual Tracking Tests

> Saccades: 5–40 degrees, target can be series of dots or lights
> Smooth pursuit: target velocity 20–40 deg/sec
> Optokinetic nystagmus (OKN): stripe velocity 20–40 deg/sec
> Optokinetic afternystagmus (OKAN): lights turned off after 1-minute constant velocity OKN in each direction

developed in the laboratories at UCLA to quantify functions of the various systems (Table 7–2). This test allows the differentiation of pathology affecting peripheral vestibular end organs from that affecting vestibular pathways in the CNS. In many cases, the tests allow identification of the precise location of the lesion.

The design and interpretation of vestibular-function tests are predicated on understanding the anatomy and physiology of the vestibular and the visual systems. Even the caloric test, based on use of an unnatural stimulus and whose design and interpretation were of empirical nature, can now be interpreted in the context of physiologic principles. For example, contemporary understanding of vestibulo-ocular reflex (VOR) function substantiates the hypothesis initially advanced by Henriksson[42] that velocity of the slow component is the relevant vestibular parameter to evaluate the caloric test. The caloric test stimulates the horizontal semicircular canals, and the function of the horizontal canal ocular reflex is the production of eye movements to compensate for the angular rotation of the head. Measurements of duration or frequency of nystagmus have no direct physiologic correspondence and are only of empirical value. Furthermore, during the caloric test, theoretically, the magnitude of the reaction reflects sensitivity of the semicircular canals to a low-frequency physiologic stimulus of a period twice the duration of the irrigation. In patients, in particular, we can appreciate that the caloric response more closely approximates the reaction of the labyrinth to low-frequency than to high-frequency stimulation.[43]

Selection of stimuli in the test battery and interpretation of results of tests of vestibular and visual oculomotor function are likewise based on physiologic principles. Reports of measurements are interpreted in the context of parametric information using concepts borrowed from the field of control theory and the implications of heuristic models for description of various system reflex functions.[44,45]

THE BITHERMAL CALORIC TEST

Mechanism of Stimulation

The caloric test, introduced by Robert Bárány, uses a nonphysiologic stimulus (water or air) to induce endolymphatic flow in the semicircular canals by creating a temperature

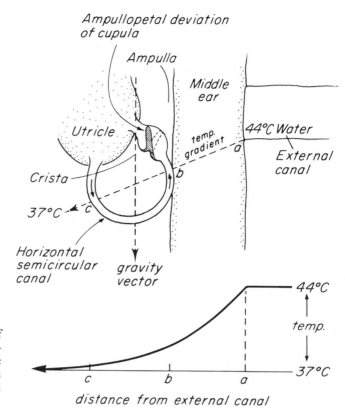

FIGURE 7–7. Mechanism of caloric stimulation of the horizontal semicircular canal (see text for details). (From Baloh and Honrubia,[41] p 138, with permission.)

gradient from one side of the canal to the other (Fig. 7–7).[46] Irrigation of the external auditory canal with water or air that is below or above body temperature transfers by conduction a temperature gradient from the external auditory canal to the inner ear. The largest temperature gradient develops in the horizontal semicircular canal: between the side of the canal closest to and that opposite to the source of temperature change. Because the vertical canals are relatively remote from the external ear, caloric stimulation of the vertical canals is unreliable.

The endolymph circulates because of the difference in its specific gravity on the two sides of the canal when the horizontal semicircular canal being investigated is in the vertical plane. Caloric testing of horizontal semicircular canal function is usually performed with the patient in the supine position, head tilted 30 degrees up, so that the horizontal semicircular canals are in the vertical plane. With warm caloric stimulation, the column of endolymph nearest the middle ear rises because of its decreased density. This movement causes the cupula to deviate toward the utricle (ampullopetal flow) and produces horizontal nystagmus, with the fast component directed toward the stimulated ear. A cold stimulus produces the opposite effect on the endolymph column, causing ampullofugal endolymph flow with nystagmus directed away from the stimulated ear (cold opposite, warm same [COWS]). If the same test is repeated with the patient lying on his or her abdomen so that the horizontal canal is reversed in the vertical plane (the direction of the gravity vector with relation to the head is reversed), the direction of nystagmus induced by warm and cold stimulation is reversed.[47]

Bárány received the Nobel prize for proposing the above-described mechanism of caloric stimulation. Other mechanisms, including differential pressure, electrokinetic effects from the temperature gradient, direct thermal effect on the nerve, and central otolith-canal interactions, have also been proposed as influencing caloric responses in abnormal situations.[48,49] From a clinical point of view, however, gravity is the main driving force behind the caloric response. The response can be effectively shut off (in instances when the patient becomes extremely uncomfortable) simply by positioning the head so that the horizontal canals are horizontal (i.e., tilted approximately 30 degrees downward while the patient sits).[47]

The caloric test is the most widely used clinical test of the VOR for two major reasons: (1) each labyrinth can be stimulated individually; and (2) the stimulus is easy to apply without requiring complex equipment. Several limitations of the test must be appreciated, however, if one is to assess the results properly. Slow component velocity and duration of caloric-induced nystagmus are dependent not only on the relationship between the temperature gradient vector and the gravity vector but also on blood flow to the skin, length of transmission pathway from the tympanic membrane to the horizontal canal, and heat conductivity of the temporal bone.[47,49,50] If local blood flow to the skin is decreased (from vasoconstriction owing to pain or anxiety), the velocity of the maximum slow component of the response decreases (from decreased heat conductivity through skin), but the duration is prolonged (from delayed heat transfer). Patients with infection or fluid in the middle ear and mastoid air cells may have increased caloric response (increased maximum slow component velocity) because of increased heat conductivity from the external to inner ear. Similarly, patients who have undergone mastoid surgery and reconstruction of the middle ear may have increased responses owing to shortening of the conduction pathway. A thickened temporal bone, on the other hand, would produce the opposite effect because of decreased bone heat conductivity. Some of these factors no doubt underlie the large variability of caloric responses in normal subjects and may explain the occasional unexpected increase or decrease in caloric responses from patients with temporal bone disease.

Test Methodology

With the bithermal caloric test introduced by Fitzgerald and Hallpike, each ear is irrigated for a fixed duration (30 to 40 seconds) with a constant flow rate of water that is 7°C below body temperature (30°C) and 7°C above body temperature (44°C).[51] A minimum period of 5 minutes must elapse from the end of one response to the beginning of the next stimulus to avoid addictive effects. The major advantages of this test methodology are that: (1) both ampullopetal and ampullofugal endolymph flow are serially induced in each horizontal semicircular canal; (2) the caloric stimulus is highly reproducible from patient to patient; and (3) the test is tolerated by most patients. The major limitation is the need for constant-temperature baths and plumbing to maintain continuous circulation of water through the infusion hose.

The magnitude of caloric-induced nystagmus is highly dependent on the degree of fixation permitted during the test procedure. Four different fixation conditions have been used for caloric testing: (1) eyes open, fixating; (2) eyes open, Frenzel glasses; (3) eyes open, total darkness; and (4) eyes closed. Without eye-movement-recording devices, obviously only the first two conditions can be used. Comparison of these four conditions in normal subjects reveals a consistently lower coefficient of variation (expressed as 100 × standard deviation/mean) for response measurements when the test is performed with eyes open, either behind Frenzel glasses or in total darkness.[51]

When caloric testing is performed with fixation (as it was initially conducted), two separate systems are being evaluated: the VOR and the smooth-pursuit system. Some normal subjects are very efficient in suppressing caloric-induced nystagmus with fixation; others are not. Patients with impaired smooth pursuit (such as those with cerebellar atrophy) may show no difference in caloric-induced nystagmus with or without fixation.[52] When measured with fixation, responses in these patients will appear hyperactive compared with those of subjects having a normal smooth-pursuit system. Eye closure and the associated upward deviation of the eyes can lead to suppression of both spontaneous and induced nystagmus[51] or can alter the nystagmus waveform, which then becomes more difficult to quantify with ENG. Patients with CNS lesions often have horizontal deviation of the eyes on closure that can also change the waveform of induced nystagmus.[53] To avoid these uncontrollable variables, we recommend that in such patients caloric testing be performed with eyes open, preferably in total darkness. For a brief period during the test, fixation can be permitted so that the functional status of the smooth-pursuit system can be evaluated.

Normative Data

With the application of computerized technology, multiple response measurements can be accurately recorded. The most useful information, however, is derived from measurements of the velocity of the slow component of nystagmus.[42,54] Figure 7–8 illustrates an ENG recording of a normal caloric response. The subject was supine, with head elevated 30 degrees and eyes open behind Frenzel glasses in a darkened room. Two hundred fifty milliliters of 44°C water were infused into the left ear during the 40 seconds as indicated in the figure, resulting in ampullopetal endolymph flow in the left horizontal semicircular canal, producing left-beating horizontal nystagmus. The nystagmus began just before the end of stimulation, reached a peak approximately 60 seconds post stimulus, and then slowly decayed over the next minute. Next to the ENG tracing on the left is shown a record of the velocity of the nystagmus slow component, and below, the amplitude and frequency, all plotted versus time. Each measurement

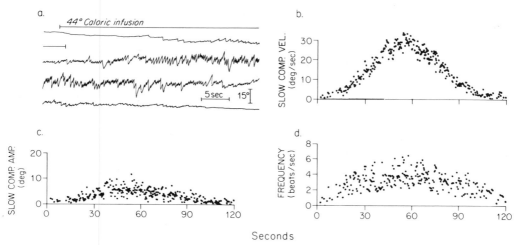

FIGURE 7–8. Caloric response produced by infusion of 250 ml of 44°C water into the left ear of a normal subject (a). Bitemporal ENG recording. Horizontal bar indicates duration of infusion. Plots of slow component velocity (b), slow component amplitude (c), and frequency (d) versus time generated by a digital computer. (From Baloh and Honrubia,[41] p 140, with permission.)

demonstrates beat-to-beat variability, but the velocity of the slow components shows the least amount of irregularity between successive nystagmus beats.

As suggested earlier, the absolute magnitude of caloric response depends on several physical factors unique to each subject that are unrelated to actual semicircular canal function. Maximum slow component velocity (MSCV) after caloric stimulation can be as low as 5 deg/sec and as high as 75 deg/sec and still be within the 95 percent confidence interval for normal subjects.[55] Mean values in our laboratory are 21 and 25 deg/sec for warm and cold irrigation, respectively. Because of the large intersubject variability, intrasubject measurements have been found to be more useful clinically, as shown in Figure 7–9.

To quantify caloric tests, two formulas are used. One is the vestibular paresis formula:

$$\frac{(R\ 30° + R\ 44°) - (L\ 30° + L\ 44°)}{R\ 30° + R\ 44° + L\ 30° + L\ 44°} \times 100$$

which compares MSCV of right-sided responses with that of left-sided responses. The second is the directional preponderance formula:

$$\frac{(R\ 30° + L\ 44°) - (R\ 44° + L\ 30°)}{R\ 30° + L\ 44° + R\ 44° + L\ 30°} \times 100$$

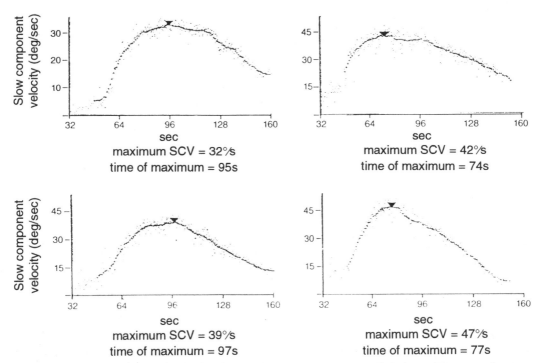

FIGURE 7–9. Plots of eye velocity during the slow component of the nystagmus reaction to caloric irrigation in a normal subject. The four traces correspond to irrigations of the left (L) and right (R) ears, each at water temperatures of 30° and 40°C (86° and 104°F). Arrows point to maximum intensity of each response. (From Honrubia,[120] p 83, with permission.)

which compares MSCV of nystagmus to the right with that of nystagmus to the left in the same subject.

A caloric fixation-suppression index is obtained by having the patient fixate on a target during the middle of the response. Because the slow-component velocity of caloric-induced nystagmus is constantly changing, the fixation period should occur near the time of maximum response to obtain the best estimate of fixation suppression. The fixation-suppression index is defined as MSCV with fixation ÷ MSCV without fixation × 100. With each of these formulas, the result is reported as a percentage of the total response. Dividing by the total response normalizes measurements to remove the large variability in absolute magnitude of normal caloric responses.

In our laboratory, vestibular paresis is defined as > 25 percent asymmetry between left-sided and right-sided responses and directional preponderance as > 30 percent asymmetry between left-beating and right-beating nystagmus; a fixation suppression index > 70 percent is abnormal. These values are comparable to those reported by other investigators, but each laboratory should establish its own normal range because of the many methodologic variables discussed earlier.

Results in Patients

The abnormalities found in caloric testing, their meaning in terms of location of lesion, and the mechanism by which each abnormality is produced are summarized in Table 7–3.

Peripheral Lesions. The finding of significant vestibular paresis with bithermal caloric stimulation suggests damage to the peripheral vestibular system that can be located anywhere from the end organ to the vestibular nerve root entry zone in the brain stem. This paresis almost certainly is a sign of unilateral peripheral vestibular disease if there are no associated brain-stem signs. Directional preponderance on caloric testing can occur with peripheral end organ and eighth nerve lesions as well as with CNS lesions (from brain stem to cortex). It indicates an imbalance in the vestibular system and is usually associated with spontaneous nystagmus; often, the velocity of slow components of spontaneous nystagmus adds to that of caloric-induced nystagmus in the same direction and subtracts from that of caloric-induced nystagmus in the opposite direction.[56] These interactions are nonlinear and unpredictable. Occasionally, directional preponderance will occur in patients without spontaneous nystagmus; in this case a central lesion is more likely.

The vestibular paresis and directional preponderance formulas are of little use in evaluating patients with bilateral peripheral vestibular lesions, since caloric responses

TABLE 7–3 Interpreting the Results of Bithermal Caloric Testing

	Location of Lesion	Mechanism
Vestibular paresis	Labyrinth, eighth nerve	Decreased peripheral sensitivity
Directional preponderance	Not localizing	Tonic bias in vestibular system
Hyperactive responses	Cerebellum	Loss of inhibitory influence on vestibular nuclei
Dysrhythmia	Cerebellum	Loss of inhibitory influence on pontine nuclei
Impaired fixation suppression	CNS pursuit pathways	Interruption of visual signals on way to oculomotor neurons
Perverted nystagmus	Fourth ventricular region	Disruption of vestibular commissural fibers

can be symmetrically highly depressed. Because of the wide range of normal values for MSCV, the patient's value may decrease severalfold before falling below the normal range. Serial measurements in the same patient are needed if one hopes to identify early bilateral vestibular impairment, such as that produced by ototoxic drugs.

Central Lesions. As suggested earlier, patients with CNS lesions may exhibit vestibular paresis on caloric testing if the lesion involves the root entry zone of the vestibular nerve. The most common neurologic disorders associated with this finding are multiple sclerosis, lateral brain-stem infarction, and infiltrating gliomas. Each disease produces other brain-stem signs so that the finding of vestibular paresis is not likely to be misinterpreted as a sign of peripheral vestibular disorder. In rare cases, massive brain-stem infarction or diffusely infiltrating glioma leads to bilaterally decreased caloric responses.

Lesions of the cerebellum can lead to heightened caloric responses. Because of the wide range of normal caloric responses, however, responses statistically exceeding the upper normal range are unusual. Patients with cerebellar atrophy syndromes demonstrate a wide range of caloric responses.[57] Those with Friedreich's ataxia often have bilaterally decreased responses because of associated atrophy of the vestibular nerve and ganglia, whereas those with olivopontocerebellar atrophy have decreased, normal, or even increased responses, depending on which areas of the medulla and pons are involved. Increased caloric responses, when they do occur, are usually found in patients with clinically pure cerebellar atrophy.

An abnormal fixation-suppression index on caloric testing typically occurs with lesions involving the smooth-pursuit system (from the parietal-occipital cortex to the pons and cerebellum).[52] Lesions of the midline cerebellum produce the most profound impairment of fixation suppression. When asymmetric, pursuit deficits in one direction correlate with suppression deficits in the opposite direction.

Dysrhythmia refers to a marked beat-to-beat variability in caloric-induced nystagmus amplitude without any change in slow-component velocity profile. This phenomenon has often been attributed to CNS lesions, mainly in the cerebellum. Unfortunately, from a diagnostic point of view, caloric dysrhythmia also occurs in normal subjects when they are tired and inattentive. As will be shown, rotatory stimuli are better suited than caloric stimuli for examining the pattern of induced nystagmus.

Vertical or oblique nystagmus produced by caloric stimulation of the horizontal semicircular canals is called *perverted nystagmus*. Normal subjects commonly exhibit a small vertical component on ENG recordings of caloric-induced nystagmus, but vertical components larger than horizontal components are clearly abnormal.[58] Perverted nystagmus with caloric stimulation has been reported with both peripheral and central lesions, the latter usually in the region of the floor of the fourth ventricle (near the vestibular nuclei).[59,60] Uemura and Cohen[61] found perverted caloric nystagmus in rhesus monkeys after producing unilateral focal lesions in the rostromedial vestibular nucleus. Warm caloric stimulation on the intact side produced downward nystagmus, and cold stimulation produced upward diagonal nystagmus. The investigators attributed their findings to disturbance of commissural fibers between vestibular nuclei.

ROTATIONAL TESTING OF THE HORIZONTAL SEMICIRCULAR CANAL

The most often used quantitative tests of vestibular function concentrate on the horizontal semicircular canal ocular reflex because it is the easiest reflex to induce and record. Tests of other VORs (from vertical semicircular canals and otolith organs) have yet to be shown useful and practical in the clinical setting.[62] Tests of several vestibulo-spinal reflexes are described in Chapters 2 and 3.

Rotational testing of the horizontal semicircular canal offers several advantages over caloric testing. Multiple graded stimuli can be applied in a relatively short period, and the testing is usually well tolerated by patients. Unlike caloric testing, rotatory stimulation of the semicircular canals is unrelated to physical features of the external ear or temporal bone, so that a more exact relationship between stimulus and response can be established. On the other hand, rotatory stimuli affect both labyrinths simultaneously, compared with the selective stimulation of one labyrinth with caloric testing.

According to the pendulum model, slow-component velocity of rotational-induced nystagmus should be proportional to deviation of the cupula, which, in turn, is proportional to magnitude of stimulation (i.e., angular movement of the head). As will be demonstrated in the following sections, this model's applicability to different forms of stimulation is remarkably consistent and provides a rational approach to the evaluation of clinical rotational testing.

Background

Three types of angular acceleration have been used to clinically evaluate the horizontal canal ocular reflex: (1) impulsive, (2) constant, and (3) sinusoidal. Historically, each type of stimulation has been popular at different times for different reasons. Bárány,[63] in 1907, introduced an impulsive rotational test in which the chair in which the patient was seated was manually rotated 10 turns in 20 seconds and then suddenly stopped with the patient facing the observer. The function of the horizontal semicircular canals was assessed by measuring duration of visually monitored nystagmus after clockwise and counterclockwise rotations. Montandon[64] introduced a constant acceleration test to investigate nystagmus threshold as the smallest stimulus at which nystagmus was first observed. A simple, reproducible method of generating sinusoidal angular acceleration in a clinical setting — the torsion swing test — was popularized in France as another method of rotatory stimulation. With this test, the patient is seated in a chair, the rotation of which is mechanically controlled by the action of a calibrated spring.[65] Because of technical limitations and limited understanding of the relevant physiology at the time, the most effective parameter for evaluation of vestibular reflex function was not used, that is, eye velocity. Instead, duration or frequency of nystagmus or threshold of fast-component production was measured. These test results, as could be anticipated by presently known mechanisms of vestibular function, were of limited value.

Contemporarily, among the various modalities of rotatory stimulation, impulsive and sinusoidal angular acceleration stimuli are preferred over constant acceleration. Sinusoidal stimulation is the most widely used because it is reproducible and easy to generate and can be defined by two simple variables: (1) period of oscillation, and (2) amplitude of oscillation.

Test Methodology

For rotational testing of the horizontal canal – ocular reflex, the patient is seated on a chair mounted on a motorized rotating platform that is under computer control inside a dark, acoustically and electrically shielded room.[66,67] An array of three lights (light-emitting diodes) spaced 10 or 15 degrees apart is attached to the chair directly in front of the subject. Frequent ENG calibrations are conducted throughout the testing procedure to correct for any fluctuations in corneoretinal potential. The ENG signals can be displayed on a polygraph recorder or the equivalent and digitized by a small laboratory computer for analysis. The patient is constantly questioned to maintain mental alertness. For sinusoidal testing, we use stimulus signals at frequencies ranging from 0.0125 to 1.6 Hz and several peak velocities with a maximum of 120 deg/sec. Impulse changes in velocity of 256 deg/sec can be produced with an acceleration of 140 deg/sec². This wide range of stimuli provides comprehensive information, but the procedure is time-consuming and tiring for most patients. Therefore, for screening purposes, and before exploring responses to other stimuli, we routinely use sinusoidal frequencies of 0.0125, 0.05, and 0.2 Hz, peak velocity of 60 deg/sec, and step change in velocity of 100 deg/sec. An example of responses obtained in a patient before and 1 month after left vestibular nerve section is shown in Figure 7–10.

Two types of measurement are typically used to quantify the response to rotational stimulation: timing and magnitude (gain) measurements. The timing measurement corresponds to evaluation of delays of the vestibular reflexes in responding to stimuli. In terms of the pendulum model, this corresponds to evaluation of the time constant of the (vestibular) system.

For a sinusoidal stimulus, timing refers to the phase measurement obtained by comparing the time of maximum head velocity (stimulus) with the time of maximum slow-component eye velocity (response). Responses from normal subjects show that maximum slow-component eye velocity leads maximum head velocity at low frequencies of sinusoidal rotation. More precisely, the response lags the stimulus — angular acceleration, the natural physiologic stimulus — but because the stimulus is conventionally

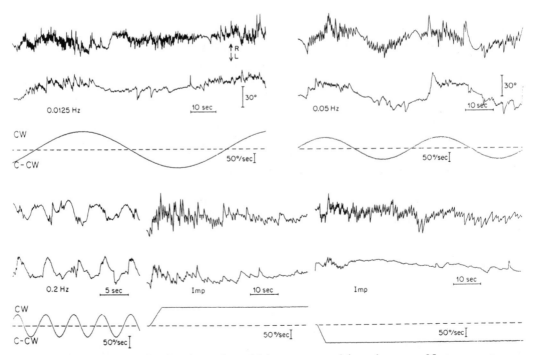

FIGURE 7–10. Records of various sinusoidal rotatory and impulse tests. Nystagmus traces were obtained before (*top*) and 1 month after (*bottom*) surgery for removal of a left acoustic neuroma. Stimulus velocity is indicated by the sinusoidal or step trajectory of the rotating platform. (From Honrubia et al,[71] p 16, with permission.)

expressed in terms of angular velocity, then the response, while lagging head accelera-tion, leads head velocity, which is 90 degrees, or a quarter cycle, behind acceleration. For impulse stimuli, the time constant is defined as the time required for the response to decay to $\frac{1}{e}$ or to 37 percent of the maximum value. The time constant (T_{COR}) measured after a step change in angular velocity and the phase lead at low frequencies of sinusoi-dal rotation are related by the following equation:

$$T_{COR} = \frac{1}{\omega \tan \theta}$$

where $\omega = 2\pi F$ is the angular frequency of rotation and θ the phase angle difference between stimulus and response.

Magnitude is traditionally defined as gain, which is obtained by dividing maximum slow-component eye velocity by maximum stimulus magnitude. The coefficient of varia-tion for gain values after sinusoidal and impulsive rotatory stimulation is about one half the coefficient of variation after caloric stimulation.[68,69] Even with this increased preci-sion, however, there is still large coefficient variation ($\simeq 30$ percent) in rotational responses of normal subjects. Factors such as stress, fatigue, level of mental alertness, and habituation contribute to variability.

Sinusoidal Rotational Tests. With sinusoidal rotational testing, gain of the canal-ocular reflex can be measured at multiple cycles after the subject has attained a "steady-state" response (i.e., after a half cycle of rotation). Because of the several values obtained in each test, sinusoidal rotational testing usually provides a more accurate assessment of gain than does impulsive testing. Its main disadvantage is the lengthy procedure required to test a broad frequency range.

Two standard computer plots generated during sinusoidal rotational testing in a normal subject are shown in Figure 7–11A. The subject was rotated at 0.05 Hz (peak velocity 60 deg/sec) with eyes open in the dark while performing continuous mental-alerting tasks. Each dot represents average slow-component velocity over a 25-msec interval. The plot on the left shows slow-component velocity versus time for two complete cycles of response. Gain (peak slow component velocity ÷ peak chair velocity) in each direction can be read directly from these plots, or average gain can be calculated by performing a curve-fitting analysis (Fourier analysis) of the data. From this analysis, one obtains gain, dc bias, and phase relationship between the fundamental of slow-com-ponent velocity and chair velocity.[66,70–72] If slow-component velocity data are symmetri-cal (as in normal subjects), phase can be read directly from these plots by comparing the time of zero eye velocity with that of zero chair velocity. The time difference (t), multiplied by 360° and by the frequency of the stimulus, gives the phase, θ ($\theta = t \cdot 360° \cdot f$). If, however, responses are asymmetric (as in Figure 7–11B), the computa-tions should be cautiously examined because often cycles also have asymmetric dura-tions. The time constant is computed objectively by using assessment of phase obtained with Fourier analysis of the data. Another view of response parameters is obtained with the second computer plot, a cartesian display of slow-component velocity versus stimu-lus velocity. This plot provides rapid visual assessment of dc bias and facilitates measure-ment of average gain in each direction (i.e., the slope of the line in each direction).

Gain and phase of the canal-ocular reflex vary with frequency in normal sub-jects,[44,70] consistent with the pendulum model (e.g., Fig. 7–6). Normal subjects exhibit approximately a 45-degree phase lead of eye velocity relative to chair velocity at 0.0125 Hz, but this phase lead is near zero by 0.2 Hz (see Table 7–4).

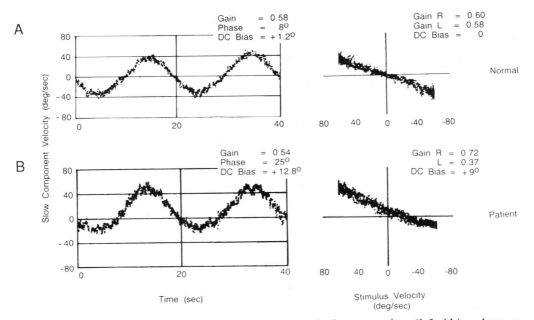

FIGURE 7–11. Plots of nystagmus slow component velocity versus time (*left side*) and versus chair velocity (*right side*) during sinusoidal angular rotation (0.05 Hz, 60 deg/sec peak velocity). The horizontal axis on the left indicates the time after the beginning of the cycle of stimulus velocity (period, 20 seconds), and on the right, the magnitude of the stimulus. The data in (*A*) are from a normal subject and in (*B*) from a patient with an acute right peripheral vestibular lesion. Gain, phase (lead), and dc bias (+rightward bias) were determined from frequency analysis (Fourier analysis) of the data. (From Baloh and Honrubia,[41] p 158, with permission.)

Variance associated with measurements comparing clockwise and counterclockwise responses in the same subject is less than variance between subjects. A normalized difference formula [(clockwise − counterclockwise) ÷ (clockwise + counterclockwise)] × 100 is analogous to the directional preponderance formula used with caloric testing. Asymmetry greater than 20 percent on this normalized difference formula is abnormal in our laboratory.

Impulse Rotational Tests. The impulse stimulus has the advantage of providing rapid assessment of gain and time constant of the canal-ocular reflex independently in each direction. Sinusoidal testing, on the contrary, provides a measure of only a single time constant, which represents the average value for responses in both directions of rotation. Since the impulse stimulus is so brief, however, if the subject is not maximally alert or attempts to suppress the response, the initial peak will be blunted and the estimate of gain inaccurate. The results of typical impulse responses in a normal subject are shown in Figure 7–12. Slow-component velocity is plotted versus time for four different stimuli of the indicated magnitudes; each dot in this illustration represents average slow-component velocity of one nystagmus beat. From these plots the peak slow-component velocity can be read directly as well as the time required for slow-component velocity to fall to 37 percent of its initial value, and gain and time constant can be computed. In our laboratory, these parameters are obtained by plotting the logarithm of the slow-component velocity versus time after start of the stimulus and curve-fitting the data to a straight line with a least-squares method. An example is shown in Figure 7–13B. Normal mean gain and T_{COR} values calculated from similar plots in 20 normal

TABLE 7–4 Gain, Phase, and Time-Constant Measurements for Sinusoidal (0.0125 to 2.0 Hz) and Impulse Rotation in Normal Subjects

Measurement	Frequency (Hz)*							Impulse[a]
	0.0125[a]	0.05[b]	0.2[b]	0.4[c]	1.0[d]	1.5[d]	2.0[d]	
Gain	0.40 ± 0.07	0.50 ± 0.15	0.59 ± 0.19	0.59 ± 0.18	0.94 ± 0.16	1.01 ± 0.12	1.14 ± 0.11	0.63 ± 0.18
Phase (degrees)	39 ± 7	10 ± 4	1 ± 4	0 ± 3				12.2 ± 3.6

Values are mean ± standard deviation.
*Stimulus magnitude in deg/sec: [a]100, [b]60, [c]30, [d]20.
Impulse time constant, equivalent to the time needed for the response to decline $1/e$ (i.e., as in a first-order system).

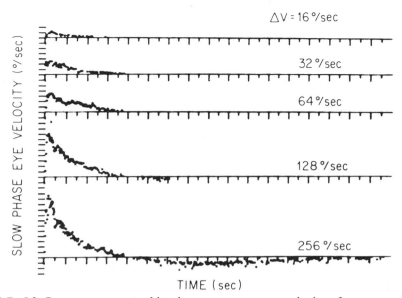

FIGURE 7–12. Responses measured by slow component eye velocity of nystagmus shown for progressively greater impulse stimuli (ΔV). Horizontal axis is marked every 5 seconds, and vertical axis is marked every 10 deg/sec. Axes are the same for all responses. Up to impulses of 64 deg/sec, responses behave as predicted by the damped pendulum model; above this, after nystagmus appears, beating in the direction opposite to that of the postrotatory response, as noted by change in signs of the last part of the eye velocity records. (From Sills and Honrubia,[121] p ORL81, with permission.)

subjects using step of velocity of 100 deg/sec were 0.63 ± 0.18 and 12.2 ± 3.6 sec, respectively. Asymmetry of more than 20 percent on the standard directional preponderance formula is considered abnormal for all frequencies and amplitudes of stimulation.

Results in Patients

Unilateral Peripheral Lesions. Patients who suddenly lose vestibular function on one side have asymmetric responses to rotational stimuli because of (1) the dc bias resulting from spontaneous nystagmus, and (2) the difference in response to ampullopetal and ampullofugal stimulation of the remaining intact labyrinth.[70–74] These features are readily seen in impulsive and sinusoidal data in the records of eye movements in Figure 7–10 and in the reproduction of data analysis from the same patient in Figure 7–13. The data were obtained shortly before and after surgery for removal of a left acoustic nerve tumor. At the time of postoperative testing, the patient exhibited spontaneous nystagmus (with eyes open in the dark), with average slow-component velocity of 7 deg/sec. This spontaneous nystagmus was added to rotational-induced nystagmus in the same direction and subtracted from that in the opposite direction, contributing to asymmetry in the response or the dc bias. That is, peak values are different, and the data do not cross the coordinates of the plot at the intersection. Another effect, however, is shown in the difference in gain of the responses obtained from ampullopetal and ampullofugal stimulation of the intact labyrinth, as predicted by Ewald's second law of labyrinthine function. This gain asymmetry is particularly obvious in differences in the

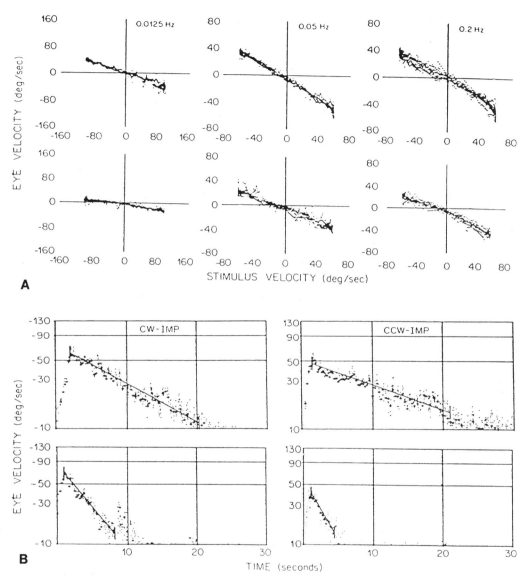

FIGURE 7–13. Computer outputs used to quantify results of sinusoidal and impulse tests. (*A*) Scatter plots of the relationship between slow component eye velocity and table velocity for three frequencies after the phases of the two signals were aligned. The set of records shown in the top row was obtained before surgery; that shown in the bottom row, after surgery. (*B*) Scatter plots, using semilog coordinates, of the magnitude of slow component eye velocity during the postrotatory nystagmus response following an impulse of acceleration. (From Honrubia et al,[71] p 17, with permission.)

slopes of the lines describing the relationship between eye velocity and stimulus velocity (Fig. 7–13), especially following rotations at 0.0125 and 0.2 Hz. (Counterclockwise-induced rotations produced smaller responses than those of clockwise-induced rotations.) On impulse stimulation, changes in gain and time constant of responses resulting from unilateral lesions are very impressive in this patient (Figure 7–13*B*).

After compensation by the CNS for vestibular loss, clinically important changes take place in VOR responses, even in patients with complete unilateral paralysis. An example is illustrated in Figure 7–14. These responses were obtained 1 year after surgical resection of the vestibular nerve. With compensation, spontaneous nystagmus diminishes, dc bias gradually disappears, gain asymmetry between ampullopetal and ampullofugal stimulation decreases, and responses to low frequencies of rotation become symmetrical.[44,72] Differences in impulse stimuli responses are more resistant to change than are differences in sinusoidal stimuli responses (Fig. 7–14).

Theoretical computations based on the pendulum model of vestibular function postulate four conditions following unilateral labyrinthectomy that contribute to asymmetric responses.[73,75] First, a decrease of gain of approximately 50 percent should occur owing to removal of input from one ear. Second, asymmetry should occur in responses to each of the half-cycles of stimuli with magnitudes much less than 100 deg/sec owing to the difference in sensitivity of primary neurons to excitatory and inhibitory stimulation. (Theoretically, the ratio of ampullopetal to ampullofugal response should be 1.3 at low frequencies and less at higher frequencies, according to Ewald's first law.) Third, for higher stimulus magnitudes, there should be differences among ampullopetal and ampullofugal responses of another nature. These differences are owing to cancellation of

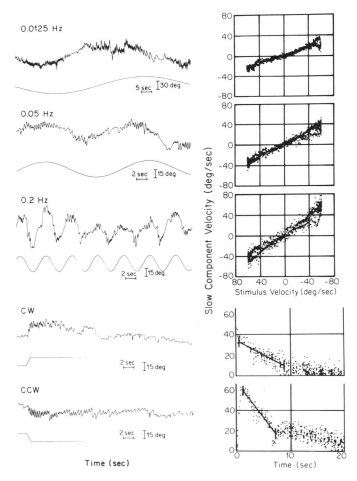

FIGURE 7–14. Responses of a patient (history of Ménière's disease, 1 year postoperative, right vestibular nerve section) to different vestibular rotatory stimulations. (From Honrubia et al,[44] p 66, with permission.)

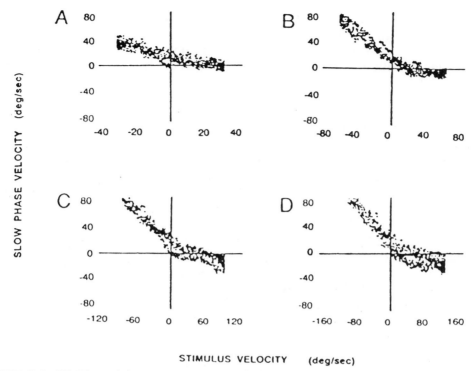

FIGURE 7–15. Plots of slow component eye velocity versus stimulus velocity from one patient (right-sided lesion) at four peak stimulus velocities (30, 60, 90, 120 deg/sec, 0.05 Hz). (From Baloh et al,[77] with permission.)

spontaneous activity with inhibitory stimuli of large magnitude; the ampullofugal response will reach a limit value of zero while the ampullopetal response will increase with increased stimulus, making the difference more obvious, as illustrated in Figure 7–15. The canal's transduction process, however, is more sensitive (relative to velocity) to high than to low frequencies of rotation; hence ampullofugal stimulation should completely inhibit the vestibular nerve's spontaneous activity with a smaller stimulus at high frequencies of rotation. Theoretically, this effect will be noticeable for high frequencies of stimulation at stimulus velocities of approximately 100 deg/sec and greater, but only at much greater velocity at low frequencies, below 0.05 Hz (much greater than 300 deg/sec). These three predictions have been demonstrated experimentally.[75,76] Fourth and finally, although time constants and phase relationships should be expected to remain approximately constant, instead there are changes that continue for years (e.g., Fig. 7–14). The reason for this finding is unclear. The changes in the time constant and phase relationship represent a functional change in the CNS associated with unilateral disappearance of inputs to the second-order neurons in the vestibular nuclei.[75,76]

The process of compensation leads to the production of more symmetric responses at moderate stimulus magnitudes at all frequencies. At high stimulus values and, particularly, high frequencies, however, we can still demonstrate asymmetries long after labyrinthectomy (Fig. 7–14 and 7–15).[77] This phenomenon is probably owing to a combination of circumstances. First, the process of compensation is highly dependent on visuovestibular interactions, and at high frequencies visual modulation of VOR is minimal (see below). Second, the end-organ conditions mentioned earlier, contributing to the asymmetries at high frequencies, are still operational—there is no evidence that compensation affects vestibular nerve and hair-cell function.

In patients with a partial unilateral lesion, as would be expected from the above discussion, the changes depend on the degree of involvement and the time since the inception of the lesion.[44] In a study of rotatory responses from two groups of patients, one with total unilateral labyrinthine paralysis, as judged by caloric testing, and another with partial but statistically significant (>20 percent) paralysis, only among the first group were differences in gain and phase from those of normal subjects found to be significant.[68] Because of limited availability of data and the variable pathologic conditions studied, interpretation of rotatory test data remains a subject of debate. Nevertheless, for the purpose of identification of a unilateral lesion, clearly the caloric test is more sensitive than the rotatory test, and this test remains a highly valuable diagnostic tool.

Bilateral Peripheral Lesions. Rotational stimuli are ideally suited for testing patients with bilateral peripheral vestibular lesions. Because both labyrinths are stimulated simultaneously, the degree of remaining physiologic function can be accurately quantified[67,71] (Fig. 7-16). Several other observations support the value of rotational tests in these patients. Frequently, patients with absent response to bithermal caloric stimulation have decreased but recordable rotational-induced nystagmus, particularly at higher

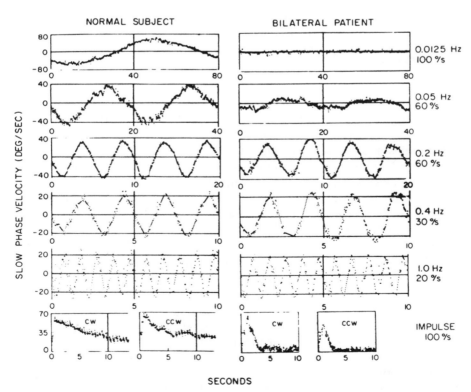

FIGURE 7-16. Plots of slow component eye velocity versus time for sinusoidal (0.0125 to 1.0 Hz) and impulse stimulation in a normal subject and a patient with bilateral peripheral vestibular lesion. (From Baloh et al,[70] Reprinted with permission from Annals of Neurology, 16:222-228, 1984.)

frequencies of sinusoidal rotation (see below). Diminished bilateral function is identified earlier because variance associated with normal rotational responses is less than that associated with caloric responses. Changes in gain are also associated with changes in phase—an important parameter that has the smallest variance among normal subjects and contributes to identification of abnormality. Furthermore, artifactually decreased caloric responses occasionally occur in patients with angular, narrow external canals or with thickened temporal bones, whereas the intensity of rotational stimuli is unaffected by these physical features. Results of rotatory responses in two groups of patients with bilateral labyrinthine disorders are shown in Fig. 7–17 (gain) and 7–18 (phase). Patients in the first group had received ototoxic drugs for treatment of bacterial infections. The second group consisted of patients with various inner-ear pathologies. All patients had either complete absence of caloric response to ice water or responses to the four caloric irrigations that averaged less than 20 percent of normal—below the 95 percent confidence limits from our laboratory. None had spontaneous nystagmus with eyes open in the dark.

The ability to identify remaining vestibular function, even if minimal, is an important advantage of rotational testing, particularly when the physician is contemplating ablative surgery or monitoring the effects of ototoxic drugs. By using precisely graded rotational stimuli on a serial basis, ototoxic effects are recognized earlier than by using the quantitatively less precise caloric stimulus.

The patients whose VOR responses are shown in Figures 7–17 and 7–18 had normal optokinetic nystagmus (OKN) and smooth-pursuit responses; consequently, when they were rotated in the light, their vestibulovisual ocular responses were perfectly normal—a finding of significant behavioral difference. Because of the normal visual oculomotor responses, most of these patients were able to maintain fixation during head rotations and were unaware of their VOR pathology.

Central Vestibular Lesions. As with lesions of peripheral vestibular structures, lesions of central VOR pathways can lead to a variety of abnormalities, including

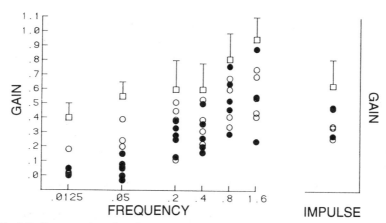

FIGURE 7–17. Scatter plot showing normal subjects' mean and standard deviation values (*squares*) and data from individual patients (*circles*). In the plot on the left, the ordinate indicates the gain of the VOR. In the plot on the right, the ordinate indicates the gain for the single impulse of 100 deg/sec. Gain is defined as the ratio of the response amplitude to the stimulus amplitude. Filled circles represent data from ototoxic patients. Frequency is in Hz. (From Honrubia et al,[122]p 345, with permission.)

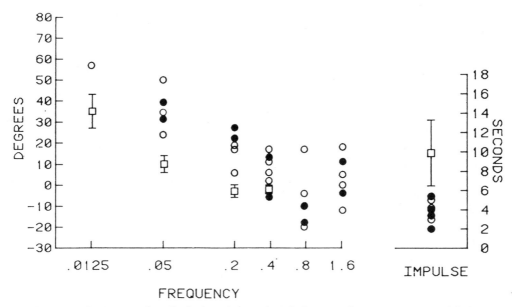

FIGURE 7–18. Scatter plot displaying the results of phase angle measurements (*left*) and the time constant following impulse testing (*right*). Phase was measured in relation to the velocity of the rotation of the table. For convenience, 180 degrees have been subtracted from the data. Frequency is in Hz. (From Honrubia et al,[122] p 345 with permission.)

asymmetries in gain of rotational-induced nystagmus. Lesions involving the nerve root entry zone and vestibular nuclei may produce responses indistinguishable from those produced by peripheral vestibular lesions. The spectrum of abnormalities associated with central lesions, however, is much more diverse than a simple decrease in slow-component velocity. Gain may be increased in some patients with cerebellar lesions.[78] The highly organized pattern of the nystagmus seen in normal subjects may be disorganized, resulting in so-called dysrhythmic nystagmus.[79] If the production of fast components is impaired, the nystagmus waveform is distorted or there may be only a slow tonic deviation of eyes from side to side. Finally, central lesions often interfere with the integration of visual and vestibular signals, producing abnormalities on tests of visuo-vestibular interaction (see below).

Sinusoidal rotational tests are ideally suited for studying the specific pattern of induced nystagmus because they produce nystagmus beating in opposite directions during each half cycle, enabling immediate comparison. Figure 7–19 illustrates responses to sinusoidal rotation (eyes open in darkness) in (*A*) a normal subject, and patients with (*B*) cerebellar atrophy, (*C*) left pontine lesion (astrocytoma), and (*D*) bilateral lesion of the MLF. In the normal subject, the eyes alternately deviate in the direction of the slow component for each half cycle of induced nystagmus. In humans, the average eye position in the orbit for initiation of fast components is near the midline, from which the eyes take a countercompensatory direction (Fig. 7–19*A*), contrary to what happens in afoveate animals (e.g., rabbits).[80] Fast components (saccades) are generated in the paramedian pontine reticular formation, and the cerebellum controls (fine tunes) the amplitude of both voluntary and involuntary saccades. In the patient with cerebellar atrophy

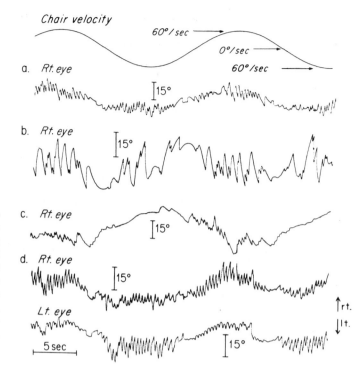

FIGURE 7-19. ENG recordings of nystagmus response to sinusoidal rotation at 0.05 Hz, peak velocity 60 deg/sec in a normal subject (a) and in patients with cerebellar atrophy (b), left pontine glioma (c), and bilateral MLF lesions caused by multiple sclerosis (d). (From Baloh and Honrubia,[41] p 162, with permission.)

(Fig. 7-19B), the nystagmus pattern is disorganized, with fast components occurring in random fashion, causing marked beat-to-beat variability in amplitude. This type of abnormality has been termed *dysrhythmia* and commonly occurs in patients with varieties of cerebellar lesions. Patients with dysrhythmic vestibular nystagmus also demonstrate dysmetria of voluntary saccades.

The patient with a left pontine lesion (Fig. 7-19C) could not produce voluntary or involuntary saccades (fast components) to the left, so that during the half cycle that normally produces left-beating nystagmus, the eyes tonically deviated to the right. In patients with bilateral pontine lesions, the eyes tonically deviate to the right and left with each half cycle of rotation because of the complete absence of fast components.[81] One might mistakenly interpret this abnormality as an absent vestibular response.

The patient with a bilateral MLF lesion (Fig. 7-19D) demonstrates dissociation in fast components between the two eyes. When either "paretic" abducting eye is required to produce a fast component, nystagmus beats are rounded because of a decrease in frequency of action potentials arriving at the medial rectus motor neurons via the damaged MLF. Abducting fast components, however, are normal, because the abducting muscles (abducens nuclei) receive their innervation for fast components directly from the paramedian pontine reticular formation, with no involvement of the MLF. Frequently, the abducting fast components are actually too large, and the oculomotor control centers attempt to overcome the block at the MLF by increasing the innervation transmitted from the paramedian pontine region to the paretic oculomotor neurons.[82,83] Because, according to Herring's law, this increased innervation is transmitted equally to the two synergistic muscles — the medial and lateral rectus — the difference in amplitude between adducting and abducting fast components is further magnified.

TESTS OF VISUO-OCULAR CONTROL

Three major visuo-oculomotor systems contribute to the production of eye movements: the saccadic, the smooth-pursuit, and the optokinetic systems. The saccadic system responds to an error in the direction of gaze with respect to the position of an object of interest by initiating a rapid eye movement — a saccade — to bring objects into the fovea in the shortest possible time. The reflex arc involves cortical centers as well as centers in the midbrain and brain stem. Saccades are stereotyped in that their trajectory and velocity cannot be voluntarily altered.

The two other systems allow the eye to maintain gaze on moving objects. The smooth-pursuit system has rapid dynamics, depends primarily on foveal activation, and requires voluntary participation involving the cerebral cortex.[84,85] This negative feedback system minimizes velocity difference between the eye and the object selected for fixation and operates quite effectively to maintain objects within a visual angle even smaller than that of the fovea for object velocities below 90 deg/sec. The optokinetic system has rather sluggish dynamics, depending mainly on activation of direction-sensitive neurons scattered through the retina. It produces involuntary, reflexive fixation eye movements — more effective with objects that cover large portions of the visual field and that move with velocities of less than 20 to 30 deg/sec. Visually generated signals of the optokinetic system travel through short subcortical neural pathways — the accessory optic system — to reach the vestibular nuclei. Here they are integrated with afferent vestibular signals[84,86] and participate in the maintenance of gaze and equilibrium.

Central vestibulo-ocular connections are highly integrated with visuo-ocular stabilizing pathways, and both systems share the final common pathway of oculomotor neurons. If the efferent limb of the VOR arc is damaged, visually controlled eye movements are abnormal, whereas if the afferent limb of the reflex is damaged, visually controlled eye movements are usually normal.

Saccadic Eye Movements

Methods of Testing and Results in Normal Subjects. Saccadic eye movements can be induced by a series of dots or lights separated by specific angular degrees, or by a dot of light moving on a screen through a series of stepwise jumps of different amplitudes. The ENG recording in Figure 7–20A illustrates the high speed and accuracy of saccadic eye movements induced in a normal subject by a target moving in steps of random amplitude. Normal subjects consistently undershoot the target for jumps larger than 20 degrees, requiring a small corrective saccade to achieve the final position.

Computer algorithms have been developed to rapidly quantify these saccade parameters.[10,87] Saccades are easily evaluated based on their characteristic relationship between peak velocity and amplitude (the so-called main sequence). This relationship is nonlinear, with larger but relatively decreasing peak velocities for higher-amplitude saccades (Fig. 7–20B).[87] For example, the average peak velocity for a 15-degree saccade is 400 deg/sec, whereas that for a 30-degree saccade is 550 deg/sec. Saccade accuracy is defined as the ratio of saccade amplitude to target displacement amplitude times 100. Mean saccade accuracy for normal subjects on the random saccade test is 88 percent. Overshooting of the target rarely occurs in normal subjects. The mean delay time on the same test is 0.180 second.

Results in Patients. Slowing of saccadic eye movements can be caused by lesions anywhere in the widely scattered central pathways involved in generating saccades. The most pronounced slowing occurs with lesions of pretectal and paramedian pontine gaze centers, oculomotor neurons, and extraocular muscles. Lesions involving these pathways

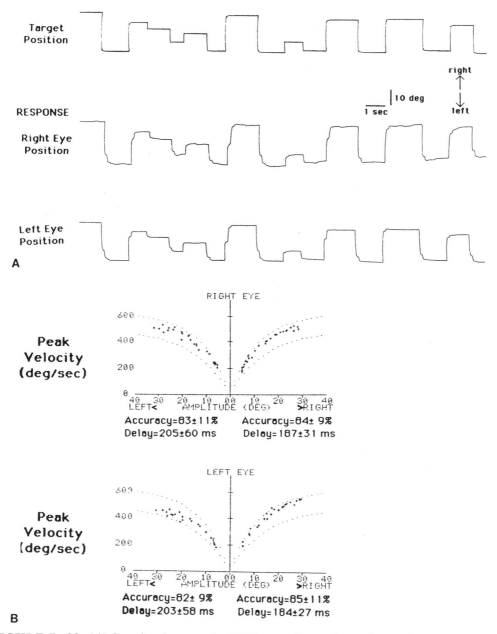

FIGURE 7–20. (A) Sample of monocular ENG recordings of saccades produced by random steps of target position in a normal subject. (B) Graphs showing the relationship between the saccade maximum velocity and its amplitude from the same subject.

impair both voluntary and involuntary saccades. Damage to oculomotor neurons, oculomotor nerves, and extraocular muscles causes slowing of saccades when the paretic muscle is the agonist required to generate the sudden force necessary to move the globe rapidly. In early lesions of the MLF, saccade slowing is identified on ENG testing,[88,89] before clinical examination reveals the presence of strabismus (Fig. 7–21).[90,91] In myas-

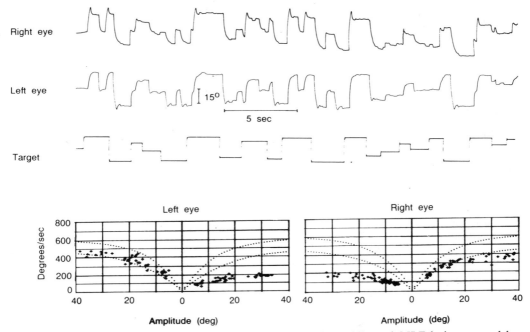

FIGURE 7–21. Saccadic eye movements in a patient with a bilateral MLF lesion caused by multiple sclerosis. Recordings as in Figure 7–20. Adducting saccades are markedly slow; abducting saccades have normal velocity but overshoot the target. (From Baloh and Honrubia,[41] p 145, with permission.)

thenia gravis, saccades begin with normal velocity, but within a short time the transmitters at the myoneural junction are depleted, and the remainder of the saccade is markedly slow.[92] Patients with Huntington's disease and progressive supernuclear palsy develop slowing of saccades, apparently owing to diffuse degeneration of supranuclear pathways.[93,94] Lesions of one paramedian pontine center produce ipsilateral saccade slowing. Reversible saccade slowing is produced by fatigue or by ingestion of alcohol or tranquilizers.[95–97]

Impaired saccade accuracy commonly occurs with cerebellar disorders.[97,98] Overshooting of the target (saccade overshoot dysmetria) is apparent, as overshoots rarely occur in normal subjects. Saccade dysmetria is most prominent with Friedreich's ataxia.[99] Monocular overshoots in the abducting eye are characteristic of MLF lesions. Disorders of cortical and subcortical supranuclear centers also affect accuracy of saccades.[100,101] Patients with Parkinson's disease exhibit delayed saccade reaction time and hypometria of voluntary saccades. Complete removal of one hemisphere or the presence of a large frontal parietal lesion results in hypometria of horizontal saccades in the contralateral direction.[102] Vertical saccades are unaffected.

Impaired reaction time for initiation of voluntary saccades occurs in patients with acquired and congenital oculomotor apraxia[103] and ataxia telangiectasia.[104] Nystagmus fast components (involuntary saccades) are also abnormal, so that the eyes deviate in the direction of the slow component rather than in the direction of the fast component.

Smooth Pursuit

Methods of Testing and Results in Normal Subjects. Precise control of a visual target can be achieved over a series of velocities by projecting a dot on a screen with a

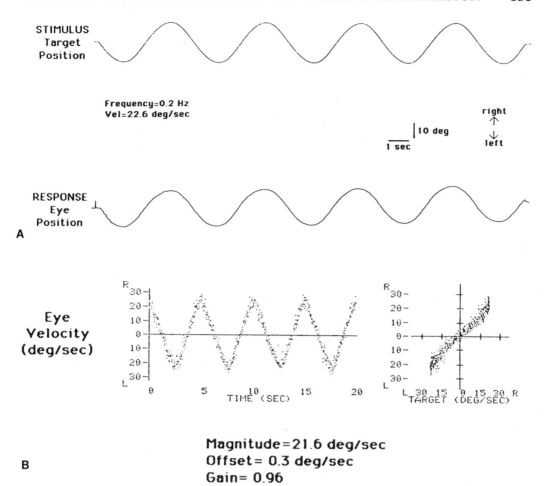

FIGURE 7–22. (*A*) Sample of binocular ENG recordings of smooth pursuit reflex response to a sinusoidally moving light at 0.2 Hz and ±18 degrees amplitude. (*B*) Graphs illustrating eye velocity during four consecutive cycles of target trajectory, as in Figure 7–22A (*left*), and of the relationship between eye and target velocity (*right*).

motor-controlled device. Figure 7–22*A* is a polygraph recording of smooth pursuit in a normal subject who follows a sinusoidally moving dot on a white screen (0.2 Hz, maximum amplitude 18 degrees). Accuracy of smooth pursuit is quantified by repeatedly sampling eye and target velocity and plotting the two velocities against each other (Fig. 7–22*B*). A computer algorithm compares eye and target velocities after saccade waveforms have been removed, if necessary[10] (e.g., as in Fig. 7–23). The slope of this eye-target velocity relationship represents the gain of the smooth-pursuit system (in this case, the slope of a normal subject is 0.96). The mean gain determined from similar plots in 25 young normal subjects was 0.95 ± 0.07. Elderly normal subjects (> 70 years of age) show marked variability in pursuit ability, and therefore pursuit testing must be interpreted with caution in elderly patients.[105,106] Also, smooth-pursuit gain decreases with both increasing frequency and increasing velocity of the target. Each laboratory must establish normative data for their standard test protocol.

Results in Patients. Patients with impaired smooth pursuit require frequent correc-

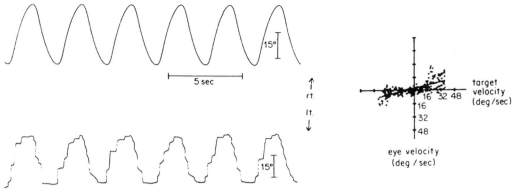

FIGURE 7–23. Smooth pursuit of a target moving with a sinusoidal waveform in a normal subject and in a patient with cerebellar atrophy. Eye velocity is plotted against target velocity (both samples 10 times per second) after saccades have been removed for the normal subject and the patient, respectively. (From Honrubia, V and Luxon, L: Optokinetic nystagmus with reference to the smooth-pursuit system. In Oosterveld, WJ (ed): Otoneurology. John Wiley & Sons, Chichester, 1984, p 195. ©1984 John Wiley & Sons. Reprinted by permission of John Wiley & Sons, Ltd.)

tive saccades to keep up with the target, producing so-called cogwheel or saccadic pursuit (Fig. 7–23). As expected, gain (given by the slope of the plot of eye velocity versus target velocity) of the smooth-pursuit system is markedly decreased in such patients.

Abnormalities of smooth pursuit occur with disorders throughout the CNS. Acute lesions of the peripheral labyrinth or vestibular nerve transiently impair smooth pursuit contralateral to the lesion when the eyes are moving against the slow component of spontaneous nystagmus.[107] This asymmetry in smooth pursuit disappears within a few weeks despite the continued presence of spontaneous nystagmus in darkness. Just as they affect saccadic eye movements, tranquilizing drugs, alcohol, and fatigue impair smooth-pursuit eye movements.[107,108] Smooth pursuit is also affected by retinal lesions.[109] Patients with diffuse cortical disease[110] (degenerative or vascular); basal ganglia disease[93,100] (Parkinson's and Huntington's disease); and diffuse cerebellar disease[57,98] consistently have bilaterally impaired smooth-pursuit eye movements. Focal disease of one cerebellar hemisphere or one side of the brain stem usually produces ipsilateral impairment of smooth pursuit, although large cerebellopontine angle tumors are frequently associated with bilaterally impaired smooth pursuit. Focal cortical lesions in the parieto-occipital region impair ipsilateral smooth pursuit[111,112] (Fig. 7–24).

Optokinetic Nystagmus

Methods of Testing and Results in Subjects. Optokinetic testing should be conducted by using an optokinetic full visual field moving at constant or sinusoidal velocities. Figure 7–25A shows such a recording of optokinetic nystagmus (OKN) induced by a striped drum completely surrounding a subject and moving at a constant velocity of 30 deg/sec (top) and with a sinusoidal trajectory of 60 deg/sec peak velocity (bottom). A plot of nystagmus slow-component velocity is provided in Figure 7–25B. Typically, OKN slow-component velocity approaches that of drum velocity as long as the latter does not exceed 30 to 40 deg/sec.[69,113] Following constant-velocity stimulation, if the lights are extinguished and optokinetic afternystagmus (OKAN) is recorded, OKAN

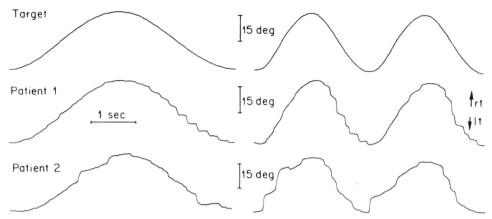

FIGURE 7–24. Smooth pursuit records of patients with left temporal lesions. Tests were conducted at two frequencies: 0.4 and 0.2 Hz. Stimulus excursions are of equal amplitude (±18 degrees) (upper trace) and hence the stimuli have different peak velocities: 45 and 22.5 deg/sec for the 0.4 and 0.2 Hz frequencies, respectively. (From Honrubia, V and Luxon, L: Optokinetic nystagmus with reference to the smooth-pursuit system. In Oosterveld, WJ (ed): Otoneurology. John Wiley & Sons, Chichester, 1984, p 195. ©1984 John Wiley & Sons. Reprinted by permission of John Wiley & Sons, Ltd.)

velocity is more variable than OKN velocity, even in young normal subjects. Usually, a rapid exponential dropoff is followed by gradual decay. Mean OKAN slow-component velocity (after the initial rapid dropoff) and mean OKAN duration in 20 normal subjects after 1 minute of 30 deg/sec optokinetic stimulation was 6.3 deg/sec ± 4.5 deg/sec and 23.75 seconds ± 23.1 seconds, respectively.[114]

Results in Patients. As a general rule, abnormalities of optokinetic slow components parallel abnormalities of smooth pursuit, while abnormalities of fast components parallel abnormalities of voluntary saccades.[114] Symmetrically decreased slow-component velocity is produced by diffuse disease of the cortex, diencephalon, brain stem, or cerebellum (Fig. 7–26).[57,69,100,103,109,111] As with smooth pursuit, focal lateralized disease of the parietal region, brain stem, and cerebellum result in impaired OKN when the stimulus moves toward the damaged side.[115] Lesions of the occipital lobe, even though associated with hemianoptic visual field defect, are not associated with impaired smooth pursuit or OKN, presumably because each parietal lobe receives oculomotor signals from each occipital lobe. Some patients with severely impaired smooth pursuit exhibit gradual buildup in OKN slow-component velocity (Fig. 7–27).[115] This feature of OKN normally occurs in afoveate animals, which have only a subcortical OKN system. Presumably, in normal humans, the cortical pursuit system dominates the subcortical OKN system, so that normal OKN exhibits features of normal pursuit. When the cortical pursuit system is lesioned, however, the remaining OKN may exhibit features of the subcortical system. The precise anatomic and physiologic mechanisms responsible for these observations in humans are yet to be elucidated.

Patients who are unable to produce saccadic eye movements produce only slow tonic deviation of the eyes in the direction of an optokinetic stimulus. Although patients with slow saccades produce OKN, the waveform is rounded, and amplitude and slow-component velocity are decreased. The delayed ending of the impaired fast component subtracts from the initial part of the slow component in the opposite direction.

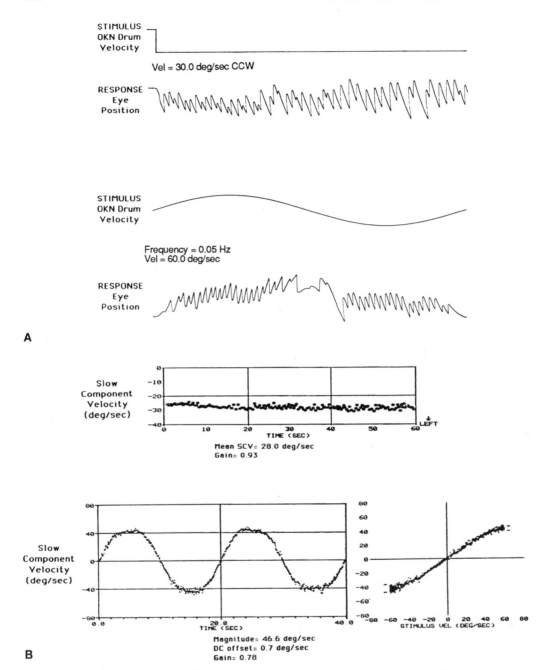

FIGURE 7–25. (*A*) Sample of binocular ENG recordings of optokinetic reflex responses to constant (*top*) and sinusoidal (*bottom*) stimuli of the specified characteristics as indicated. (*B*) Graphs showing the results of analysis of the data shown in (*A*). Top plot shows slow component eye velocity in response to the constant OK stimulus. Bottom plots show the eye velocity during two cycles of stimulus (*left*) and the relationship between eye and stimulus velocity (*right*). Note the amplitude saturation of the response to the large stimulus (60 deg/sec).

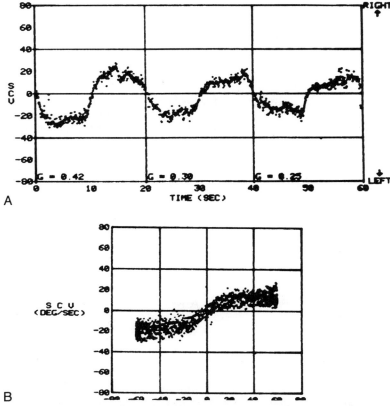

FIGURE 7–26. (A) Sinusoidal OKN in patient with cerebellar degeneration, slow component velocity (SCV) versus time. Drum is rotating at 0.05 Hz and 60 deg/sec peak velocity. Note that peak SCV is low compared with peak drum velocity. G is peak SCV gain. (B) Sinusoidal OKN in patient with cerebellar degeneration, slow component velocity (SCV) versus drum velocity. Drum is rotating at 0.05 Hz and 60 deg/sec peak velocity. Three cycles are overlaid. Velocity + (right); − (left). Note that SCV increases to a peak of only 20 deg/sec. (From Yee et al,[109] pp 256–257, with permission.)

Abnormalities of OKAN typically occur with peripheral vestibular lesions.[116] Unilateral lesions result in asymmetric OKAN (present only in the direction of spontaneous nystagmus) while bilateral lesions (e.g., owing to ototoxic drugs) result in diminished or absent OKAN.[113]

Test of Visuovestibular Interaction

The maintenance of gaze and posture is accomplished by interaction of inputs from the vestibular, visual, and proprioceptive systems. Daily activity requires normal functioning of the three reflexes. Vestibular nuclei are crucial integrators of these multiple sensory inputs. The same vestibular neurons that respond to vestibular stimulation also respond to smooth-pursuit and optokinetic stimuli. The interaction of the reflexes is the result of complex mechanisms that can be explained on the basis of elementary control theory principles. The VOR is an open-loop reflex; that is, it does not have the capacity to monitor and appropriately adjust its own performance and depends on visual input to provide feedback. The smooth pursuit and optokinetic systems function as closed-loop reflexes. An example of the interaction occurs during low-frequency head movements.

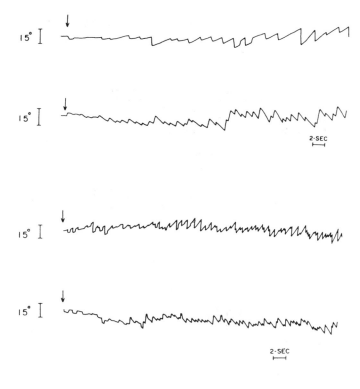

FIGURE 7–27. Slow build-up of OKN in two patients with down-beat vertical nystagmus. Deflections upward are to the right, downward to the left. Lights were turned on at arrows. Drum velocity was always 30 deg/sec whether in the clockwise or counterclockwise direction. (From Honrubia, V and Luxon, L: Optokinetic nystagmus with reference to the smooth-pursuit system. In Oosterveld, WJ (ed): Otoneurology. John Wiley & Sons, Chichester, 1984, p 195. ©1984 John Wiley & Sons. Reprinted by permission of John Wiley & Sons, Ltd.)

Below about 0.5 Hz, visual reflexes are dominant, while at higher frequencies, input from the vestibular system alone is sufficient to maintain retinal stability.

There is clear experimental evidence of how these interactions take place. The optokinetic and smooth-pursuit signals reach vestibular nuclei interacting with peripheral vestibular inputs in second-order neurons. Visual inputs arrive by different pathways that involve several brain centers from the cerebral cortex to the medulla. Among these, the cerebellar flocculus is known to relay smooth-pursuit signals to vestibular nucleus cells. Tests of visuovestibular interaction take advantage of these different anatomic connections in acquiring data for the purpose of topologic diagnosis. Diagnostic interpretation of the results should be based on and is strengthened by using predictions of heuristic models of visuovestibular interaction,[4] as described in the basic physiologic chapters.

Methods of Testing and Results in Normal Subjects. Despite some theoretical limitations, clinical experience during the 1980s has demonstrated important applications of tests of visuovestibular interaction. Of the many possible combinations of stimuli that can be applied to study visual-VOR (VVOR) function, the one most commonly used in our laboratory is the following. The patient is first tested independently for smooth pursuit, optokinetic, and VOR functions, as described earlier, and then with synergistic and antagonistic stimuli. For these, the subject is rotated either sinusoidally or with a step change in velocity while (1) the surrounding optokinetic drum is stationary (to induce the VVOR—a synergistic interaction of visual and vestibular systems) or (2) drum and chair are coupled so that they move together (to accomplish fixation suppression of the VOR: VOR-FIX—an antagonistic interaction between visual and vestibular systems). Fixation suppression can also be tested by rotating the subject in the dark with a single-fixation light attached to the chair.

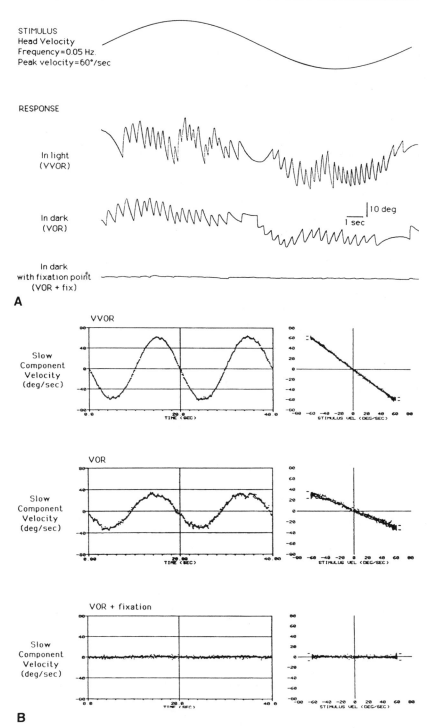

FIGURE 7–28. (*A*) Illustration to show three typical eye movement responses to a sinusoidal rotatory stimulus as indicated in the frequency under three test conditions: in the light (VVOR), in the dark (VOR), and in the dark with a fixation point that moves with the subject (VOR + FIX). (*B*) Illustrations of computer analysis of the slow component velocity for the three responses during the rotatory test illustrated in Figure 7–28A.

Typical responses of a normal subject to low-frequency sinusoidal (0.05-Hz) VOR, VVOR, and VOR-FIX stimulation are shown in Figure 7–28. In each case, peak stimulus velocity is 60 deg/sec. At this low frequency and peak velocity, the normal subject has a VVOR gain of 1 (i.e., slow-component eye velocity is equal and opposite to head velocity) and a VOR-FIX gain of 0 (i.e., the subject is able to suppress completely the VOR with fixation). Gain (mean ± 1 standard deviation) for the complete test battery in 20 normal subjects was smooth pursuit, 0.96 ± 0.06 (0.2 Hz ± 18 degrees); OKN, 0.83 ± 0.13; VOR, 0.50 ± 0.15; VVOR, 0.99 ± 0.05; and VOR-FIX, 0.03 ± 0.02.

Results in Patients. Examples of responses from tests of visuovestibular interaction reflexes in patients with different inner-ear pathologies are shown in Figure 7–29. Patients with *peripheral* vestibular lesions have decreased and/or asymmetric VOR gain, but visuovestibular responses are usually normal at low-stimulus frequencies and velocities (Fig. 7–29, center and right). Even with complete bilateral loss of vestibular function, the visuomotor system can provide good ocular stability. At high frequencies and velocities, however, VVOR gain decreases if VOR gain decreases.[117]

Three abnormal patterns of visuovestibular interaction seen on low-frequency sinusoidal testing in patients with *central* lesions are shown in Fig. 7–30.[67] Patients with lesions involving the vestibular nucleus region (e.g., Wallenberg's syndrome) exhibit prominent oculomotor abnormalities. OKN and VOR responses are asymmetric but in opposite directions. Despite decreased OKN gain, VVOR gain is normal in both direc-

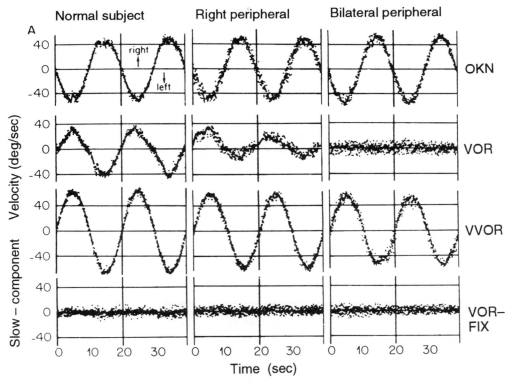

FIGURE 7–29. Plots of slow component velocity versus time from the four standard sinusoidal rotatory tests (0.05 Hz, peak velocity 60 deg/sec) in a normal subject and patients with peripheral vestibular lesions. (From Baloh et al,[118] p 233, with permission.)

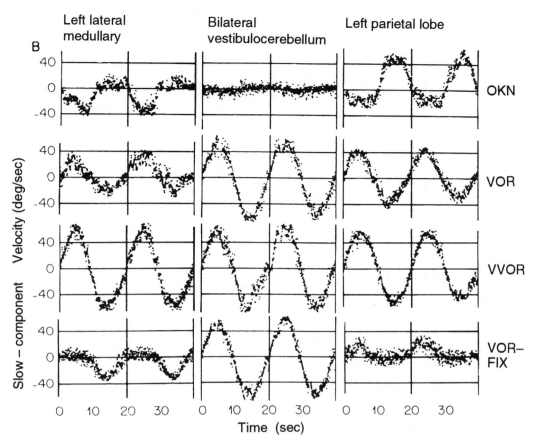

FIGURE 7 – 30. Plots of slow component velocity versus time from the four standard sinusoidal rotatory tests (0.05 Hz, peak velocity 60 deg/sec in a variety of patients with CNS lesions. (From Baloh et al,[118] p 233, with permission.)

tions. Fixation suppression of VOR slow components toward the side of the lesion is impaired. A similar pattern of abnormalities was found in six other patients with infarction in the lateral medulla.[82]

Patients with lesions involving the vestibulocerebellum are unable to modify vestibular responses with vision. This inability is illustrated by the patient data shown in Figure 7 – 30 (center), in which VOR, VVOR, and VOR-FIX gains are approximately the same (nearly 1) and OKN gain is markedly decreased in both directions.

Lesions of the visuomotor pathways from the parieto-occipital cortex to the pons lead to impaired smooth-pursuit and optokinetic slow components toward the side of the lesion.[111-113] The abnormal visuoocular control does not impair VOR responses but does alter visuovestibular interaction. Typical responses to the four sinusoidal rotatory test conditions in a patient with a deep parietal lobe lesion are shown in Figure 7 – 30 (right). OKN gain is normal to the right and markedly decreased to the left. VOR gain is normal in both directions, but the patient was unable to inhibit VOR slow components to the right with fixation (i.e., VOR-FIX gain is increased to the right). VVOR gain is slightly asymmetric, with lower gain to the left than to the right.

As noted earlier, in patients with minimal or absent sinusoidal OKN and smooth

TABLE 7–5 Summary of Diagnostic Implications of the Visuovestibular Interaction Test

Location of Lesion	OKN		VOR		VVOR		VOR-FIX	
	Gain[a]	Phase	Gain[a]	Phase	Gain[a]	Phase	Gain[a]	Phase[b]
Labyrinth or eighth nerve unilateral	Normal	Normal	Decreased contralaterally[c] acutely	Increased phase lead	Normal	Normal	Normal	—
Bilateral	Low normal	Normal	Decreased bilaterally	Increased phase lead	Low normal	Normal	Normal	—
Lateral medullary	Decreased bilaterally ipsilaterally > contralaterally	Normal	Asymmetric variable direction	Increased phase lead	Low normal	Normal	Increased bilaterally ipsilaterally > contralaterally	—
Bilateral vestibulo-cerebellum	Decreased bilaterally	Normal	Increased bilaterally	Normal	Normal	Increased phase lead	Increased bilaterally	—
Unilateral parietal lobe	Decreased ipsilaterally[c]	Normal	Normal	Normal	Decreased ipsilaterally[c]	Normal	Increased contra-laterally	—

[a]Peak slow-phase eye velocity/peak stimulus velocity.
[b]Normal subjects completely inhibit the VOR at this frequency and peak velocity.
[c]Direction of slow-component eye movement.
Source: From Honrubia and Brazier,[118] p 231, with permission.

pursuit, sinusoidal VOR, VVOR, and VOR-FIX responses are almost identical (Fig. 7–30, center).

SUMMARY

Modern rotational testing examines the VOR as well as visuovestibular interaction. Lesions of the peripheral vestibular system typically impair only the VOR, whereas lesions of the CNS impair OKN and visuovestibular interaction. The pattern of abnormal responses can help localize lesions within central pathways. A summary of diagnostic possibilities offered by combined use of the visuovestibular interaction battery is shown in Table 7–5.

REFERENCES

1. Baloh, RW: Pathologic nystagmus: A classification based on electro-oculographic recordings. Bull LA Neurol Soc 41:120, 1976.
2. Fenn, WO and Hursh, JB: Movements of the eyes when lids are closed. Am J Physiol 118:8, 1937.
3. Pousner, ER and Lion, KS: Testing eye muscles. Electronics 23:96, 1950.
4. Barber, HO and Stockwell, CW: Manual of Electronystagmography. CV Mosby, St Louis, 1976.
5. Coats, AC: Electronystagmography. In Bradford, L, (ed): Physiological Measures of the Aduio-Vestibular System. Academic Press, New York, 1975, p 37.
6. Barber, HO, and Wright, G: Positional nystagmus in normals. Adv Otol Rhinol Laryngol 19:276, 1973.
7. Kamei, T and Kornhuber, HH: Spontaneous and head shaking nystagmus in normals and in patients with central lesions. Can J Otolaryngol 3:372, 1974.
8. Lin, J, et al: Direction-changing positional nystagmus: Incidence and meaning. Am J Otolaryngol 7:306, 1986.
9. Barry, W and Melvill Jones, G: Influence of eye lid movement upon electro-oculographic recording of vertical eye movements. Aerospace Med 36:855, 1965.
10. Baloh, RW, et al: On-line analysis of eye movements using a digital computer. Aviat Space Environ Med 51:563, 1980.
11. Honrubia, V, et al: Computer analysis of induced vestibular and optokinetic nystagmus. I. Computer analysis of induced vestibular nystagmus. Rotatory stimulation of normal cats. Ann Otol Rhinol Laryngol 80 (suppl 3):7, 1971.
12. Lorente de Nó, R: Observations on nystagmus. Acta Otolaryngol (Stockh) 21:46, 1935.
13. Leigh, RJ and Zee, DS: The Neurology of Eye Movements. FA Davis, Philadelphia, 1983.
14. Cogan, DG: Congenital nystagmus. Can J Ophthalmol 2:4, 1967.
15. Baloh, RW, Honrubia, V, and Konrad, HR: Periodic alternating nystagmus. Brain 99:11, 1976.
16. Davis, DG, and Smith, JL: Periodic alternating nystagmus. Am J Ophthalmol 72:757, 1971.
17. Baloh, RW, Yee, RD, and Honrubia, V: Eye movements in patients with Wallenberg's syndrome. Ann NY Acad Sci 374:600, 1981.
18. Baloh, RW and Yee, RD: Spontaneous vertical nystagmus. Rev Neurol (Paris) 145:527, 1989.
19. Halmagyi, GM, et al: Downbeating nystagmus. Arch Neurol 40:777, 1983.
20. Fisher, A, et al: Primary position upbeat nystagmus: A variety of central positional nystagmus. Brain 106:949, 1983.
21. Aschoff, JC, Conrad, B, and Kornhuber, HH: Acquired pendular nystagmus with oscillopsia in multiple sclerosis: A sign of cerebellar nuclei disease. J Neurol Neurosurg Psychiatry 37:570, 1974.
22. Baloh, RW, et al: Cerebellar-pontine angle tumors. Results of quantitative vestibulo-ocular testing. Arch Neurol 33:507, 1976.
23. Hood, JD: Further observations on the phenomenon of rebound nystagmus. Ann NY Acad Sci 374:352, 1981.
24. Baloh, RW, Yee, RD, and Honrubia, V: Internuclear ophthalmoplegia. I. Saccades and dissociated nystagmus. Arch Neurol 35:484, 1978.
25. Cogan, DG, Kubik, SC, and Smith, WL: Unilateral internuclear ophthalmoplegia: Report of eight clinical cases and one post-mortem study. Arch Ophthalmol 44:783, 1950.
26. Spooner, JW and Baloh, RW: Eye movement fatigue in myasthenia gravis. Neurology 29:29, 1979.
27. Bárány, R: Neue Untersuchungsmethoden, die Beziehungen zwischen Vestibular-apparat, Kleinhirn, Grosshirn und Rückenmark betreffend. Wien Med Wchnschr 60:2033, 1910.
28. Jongkees, LBW: On positional nystagmus. Acta Otolaryngol 159 (suppl): 78, 1961.

29. Nylen, CO: Positional nystagmus. A review and future prospects. J Laryngol Otol 64:295, 1950.
30. Dix, M and Hallpike, C: The pathology, symptomatology and diagnosis of certain common disorders of the vestibular system. Ann Otol Rhinol Laryngol 61:987, 1952.
31. Schuknecht, HF: Pathology of the Ear. Harvard University Press, Cambridge, Mass, 1974.
32. Baloh, RW, Sakala, SM, and Honrubia, V: Benign paroxysmal positional nystagmus. Am J Otolaryngol 1:1, 1979.
33. Baloh, RW, Honrubia, V, and Jacobson, K: Benign positional vertigo: Clinical and oculographic features in 240 cases. Neurology 37:371, 1987.
34. Grand, W.: Positional nystagmus: An early sign of medulloblastoma. Neurology 21:1157, 1971.
35. Gregorius, FK, Crandall, PH, and Baloh, RW: Positional vertigo in cerebellar astrocytoma. Report of two cases. Surg Neurol 6:283, 1976.
36. Cawthorn, T and Hinchcliffe, R: Positional nystagmus of the central type as evidence of subtentorial metastases. Brain 84:415, 1961.
37. Barber, HO: Positional nystagmus: Testing and interpretation. Ann Otol Rhinol Laryngol 73:838, 1964.
38. Lin, J, et al: Direction changing positional nystagmus: Incidence and meaning. Am J Otolaryngol 7:306, 1986.
39. Honrubia, V, et al: Comparison of vestibular subjective sensation and nystagmus responses during computerized harmonic acceleration tests. Ann Otol Rhinol Laryngol 91:493, 1982.
40. Honrubia, V, et al: Optokinetic and vestibular interactions with smooth pursuit: Psychophysical responses. Acta Otolaryngol (Stockh) 112:163, 1992.
41. Baloh, RW and Honrubia, V: Clinical Neurophysiology of the Vestibular System, ed. 2. FA Davis Philadelphia, 1990.
42. Henriksson, NG: The correlation between the speed of the eye in the slow phase of nystagmus and vestibular stimulus. Acta Otolaryngol (Stockh) 45:120, 1955.
43. Honrubia, V, et al: Vestibulo-ocular reflexes in peripheral labyrinthine lesions: II. Caloric testing. Am J Otolaryngol 5:93, 1984.
44. Honrubia, V, et al: Evaluation of rotatory vestibular tests in peripheral labyrinthine lesions. In Honrubia, V and Brazier, MAB (eds): Nystagmus and Vertigo: Clinical Approaches to the Patient with Dizziness. UCLA Forum in Medical Sciences, No. 24. Academic Press, New York, 1982, p 57.
45. Lau, CGY, et al: A linear model for visual-vestibular interaction. Aviat Space Environ Med 49:880, 1978.
46. Schmaltz, G: The physical phenomena occurring in the semicircular canals during rotatory and thermic stimulation. Proc Roy Soc Med 25:359, 1932.
47. Baertschi, AJ, Johnson, RN, and Hanna, GR: A theoretical and experimental determination of vestibular dynamics in caloric stimulation. Biol Cybern 20:175, 1975.
48. Paige, G: Caloric vestibular responses despite canal inactivation. Invest Ophthalmol Vis Sci 25 (suppl): 229, 1984.
49. Scherer, H and Clarke, AH: The caloric vestibular reaction in space. Physiological considerations. Acta Otolaryngol 100:328, 1985.
50. Zangemeister, WH and Bock, O: The influence of pneumatization of mastoid bone on caloric nystagmus response. Acta Otolaryngol 88:105, 1979.
51. Baloh, RW, et al: Caloric testing. I. Effect of different conditions of ocular fixation. Ann Otol Rhinol Laryngol (suppl 43) 86:1, 1977.
52. Takemori, S: Visual suppression test. Ann Otol Rhinol Laryngol 86:80, 1977.
53. Cogan, DG: Neurologic significance of lateral conjugate deviation of the eyes on forced closure of the lids. Arch Ophthalmol 39:37, 1948.
54. Sills, AW, Baloh, RW, and Honrubia, V: Caloric testing. II. Results in normal subjects. Ann Otol Rhinol Laryngol (suppl 43) 86:7, 1977.
55. Honrubia, V, et al: Optokinetic and Vestibular Interactions with Smooth Pursuit: Psychophysical Responses. Acta Otolaryngol (Stockh) 112:163, 1992.
56. Baloh, RW, Sills, AW, and Honrubia, V: Caloric testing. III. Patients with peripheral and central vestibular lesions. Ann Otol Rhinol Laryngol (suppl 43) 86:24, 1977.
57. Baloh, RW, Konrad, HR, and Honrubia, V: Vestibulo-ocular function in patients with cerebellar atrophy. Neurology 25:160, 1975.
58. Elidan, J, Gay, I, and Lev, S: On the vertical caloric nystagmus. J Otolaryngol 14:287, 1985.
59. Fredrickson, JM and Fernández, C: Vestibular disorders in fourth ventricle lesions. Arch Otolaryngol 80:521, 1964.
60. Norre, ME: Caloric vertical nystagmus: The vertical semicircular canal in caloric testing. J Otolaryngol 16:1, 1987.
61. Uemura, T and Cohen, B: Effects of vestibular nuclei lesions on vestibulo-ocular reflexes and posture in monkeys. Acta Otolaryngol (suppl) 315:1, 1973.
62. Furman, JMR and Baloh, RW: Otolith-ocular testing in human subjects. Ann NY Acad Sci 656:431, 1992.
63. Bárány, R: Physiologie und Pathologie des Bogengangsapparates beim Menschen. Deuticke, Vienna, 1907.
64. Montandon, A: A new technique for vestibular investigation. Acta Otolaryngol 39:594, 1954.
65. Van de Calseyde, P, Ampe, W, and Depondt, M: The damped torsion swing test. Quantitative and qualitative aspects of the ENG pattern in normal subjects. Arch Otolaryngol 100:449, 1974.

66. Sills, AW, Honrubia, V, and Kumley, WE: Algorithm for the multiparameter analysis of nystagmus using a digital computer. Aviat Space Environ Med 46:934, 1975.
67. Baloh, RW, et al: Quantitative vestibular testing. Otolaryngol Head Neck Surg 92:145, 1984.
68. Baloh, RW, Sills, AW, and Honrubia, V: Impulsive and sinusoidal rotatory testing. A comparison with results of caloric testing. Laryngoscope 89:646, 1979.
69. Honrubia V, and Luxon, L: Optokinetic nystagmus with reference to the smooth-pursuit system. In Oosterveld, WJ, (ed): Otoneurology. John Wiley & Sons, Chichester, 1984, p 195.
70. Baloh, RW, et al: Changes in the human vestibulo-ocular reflex after loss of peripheral sensitivity. Ann Neurol 16:222, 1984.
71. Honrubia, V, et al: Vestibulo-ocular reflexes in peripheral labyrinthine lesions: I. Unilateral dysfunction. Am J Otolaryngol 5:15, 1984.
72. Jenkins, HR, Honrubia, V, and Baloh, RW: Evaluation of multiple frequency rotatory testing in patients with peripheral labyrinthine weakness. Am J Otolaryngol 3:182, 1982.
73. Baloh, RW, Honrubia, V, and Konrad, HR: Ewald's second law reevaluated. Acta Otolaryngol 83:475, 1977.
74. Wolfe, JW, Engelken, EJ, and Olson, JE: Low-frequency harmonic acceleration in the evaluation of patients with peripheral labyrinthine disorders. In Honrubia, V and Brazier, MAB (eds): Nystagmus and Vertigo: Clinical Approaches to the Patient with Dizziness. UCLA Forum in Medical Sciences, No. 24. Academic Press, New York, 1982, p 95.
75. Honrubia, V, et al: Ewald's second law of labyrinthine function and the vestibulo-ocular reflex. In Gualtierotti, T (ed): The Vestibular System: Function and Morphology. Springer-Verlag, Berlin, 1981, p 509.
76. Honrubia, V, et al: Vestibulo-ocular reflex changes following peripheral labyrinthine lesions. In Ruben, RW, et al (eds): The Biology of Change in Otolaryngology. Excerpta Medica International Congress Series, Elsevier, Amsterdam, 1986, p 155.
77. Baloh, RW, et al: Horizontal vestibulo-ocular reflex after acute peripheral lesions. Acta Otolaryngol (Stockh) (suppl)468:323, 1989.
78. Thurston, SF, et al: Hyperactive vestibulo-ocular reflex in cerebellar degeneration. Neurology 37:53, 1987.
79. Honrubia, V, et al: The patterns of eye movements during physiologic vestibular nystagmus in man. Trans Am Acad Ophthalmol Otolaryngol 84:339, 1977.
80. Lau, CGY and Honrubia, V: Fast component threshold for vestibular nystagmus in the rabbit. J Comp Physiol 160:585, 1987.
81. Baloh, RW, Furman, J, and Yee, RD: Eye movements in patients with absent voluntary horizontal gaze. Ann Neurol 17:283, 1985.
82. Baloh, RW, Yee, RD, and Honrubia, V: Internuclear ophthalmoplegia. I. Saccades and dissociated nystagmus. Arch Neurol 35:484, 1978.
83. Baloh, RW, Yee, RD, and Honrubia, V: Internuclear ophthalmoplegia. II. Pursuit, optokinetic nystagmus, and vestibulo-ocular reflex. Arch Neurol 35:490, 1978.
84. Lisberger, SG, Morris, EJ, and Tychsen, L: Visual motion processing and sensory-motor integration for smooth pursuit eye movements. Ann Rev Neurosci 10:97, 1987.
85. Collewijn, H and Tamminga, EP: Human smooth and saccadic eye movements during voluntary pursuit of different target motions on different backgrounds. J Physiol 351:217, 1984.
86. Cohen, B, Matsuo, V, and Raphan, T: Quantitative analysis of the velocity characteristics of optokinetic nystagmus and optokinetic after-nystagmus. J Physiol 270:321, 1987.
87. Baloh, RW and Honrubia, V: Reaction time and accuracy of the saccadic eye movements of normal subjects in a moving-target task. Aviat Space Environ Med 47:1165, 1976.
88. Crane, TB, et al: Analysis of characteristic eye movement abnormalities in internuclear ophthalmoplegia. Arch Ophthalmol 101:206, 1983.
89. Meienberg, O, Muri, R, and Rabineau, PA: Clinical and oculographic examinations of saccadic eye movements in the diagnosis of multiple sclerosis. Arch Neurol 43:438, 1986.
90. Metz, HS, et al: Ocular saccades in lateral rectus palsy. Arch Ophthalmol 84:453, 1970.
91. Solingen, LD, et al: Subclinical eye movement disorders in patients with multiple sclerosis. Neurology 27:614, 1977.
92. Yee, RD, et al: Rapid eye movements in myasthenia gravis. II. Electro-ocular analysis. Arch Ophthalmol 94:1465, 1976.
93. Leigh, RJ, et al: Abnormal ocular motor control in Huntington's chorea. Neurology 33:1268, 1983.
94. Troost, BT and Daroff, RB: The ocular motor defects in progressive supranuclear palsy. Ann Neurol 2:397, 1977.
95. Baloh, RW, et al: The effect of alcohol and marijuana on eye movements. Aviat Space Environ Med 50:18, 1979.
96. Gentles, W, and Llewellyn-Thomas, E: Effect of benzodiazepines upon saccadic eye movements in man. Clin Pharmacol Ther 12:563, 1971.
97. Wilkinson, IMS, Kime, R, and Purnell, M: Alcohol and human eye movement. Brain 97:785, 1974.
98. Zee, DS, et al: Ocular motor abnormalities in hereditary cerebellar ataxia. Brain 99:207, 1976.
99. Furman, JM, Perlman, S, and Baloh, RW: Eye movements in Friedreich's ataxia. Arch Neurol 40:343, 1983.

100. Dejong, JD, and Melvill Jones, G: Akinesia, hypokinesia, and bradykinesia in the oculomotor system of patients with Parkinson's disease. Exp Neurol 32:58, 1971.
101. White, OB, et al: Ocular motor deficits in Parkinson's disease. II. Control of the saccadic and smooth pursuit systems. Brain 106:925, 1983.
102. Sharpe, JA, Lo, AW, and Rabinovitch, HE: Control of the saccadic and smooth pursuit systems after cerebral hemidecortication. Brain 102:387, 1979.
103. Zee, DS, Yee, RD, and Singer, HS: Congenital ocular motor apraxia. Brain 100:581, 1977.
104. Baloh, RW, Yee, RD, and Boder, E: Ataxia-telangiectasia. Quantitative analysis of eye movements in six cases. Neurology 28:1099, 1978.
105. Spooner, JW, Sakala, SM, and Baloh, RW: Effect of aging on eye tracking. Arch Neurol 37:575, 1980.
106. Zackon, DH, and Sharpe, JA: Smooth pursuit in senescence: Effects of target velocity and acceleration. Acta Otolaryngol 104:290, 1987.
107. Holzman, PS, et al: Smooth-pursuit eye movements, and diazepam, CPZ, and secobarbital. Psychopharmacologia 44:111, 1975.
108. Rashbass, C: The relationship between saccadic and smooth tracking eye movements. J Physiol 159:326, 1961.
109. Yee, RD, et al: Pathophysiology of optokinetic nystagmus. In Honrubia, V and Brazier, MAB (eds): Nystagmus and Vertigo: Clinical Approaches to the Patient with Dizziness. UCLA Forum in Medical Sciences, No. 24. Academic Press, New York, 1982, p 251.
110. Fletcher, WA and Sharpe, JA: Smooth pursuit dysfunction in Alzheimer's disease. Neurology 38:272, 1988.
111. Baloh, RW, Yee, RD, and Honrubia, V: Optokinetic nystagmus and parietal lobe lesions. Ann Neurol 7:269, 1980.
112. Leigh, RJ and Tusa, RJ: Disturbance of smooth pursuit caused by infarction of parieto-occipital cortex. Ann Neurol 17:185, 1985.
113. Baloh, RW, Yee, RD, and Honrubia, V: Clinical abnormalities of optokinetic nystagmus. In Lennerstrand, G and Zee, D (eds): Functional Basis of Ocular Motility Disorders. Pergamon Press, New York, 1982, p 311.
114. Zasorin, NL, et al: Influence of vestibulo-ocular reflex gain on human optokinetic responses. Exp Brain Res 51:271, 1983.
115. Yee, RD, et al: Slow build-up of optokinetic nystagmus associated with downbeat nystagmus. Invest Ophthalmol Vis Sci 18:622, 1979.
116. Lafortune, S, et al: Human optokinetic after nystagmus. Acta Otolaryngol 101:183, 1986.
117. Hydén, D, Istl, YE, and Schwartz, DWF: Human visuovestibular interaction as a basis for quantitative clinical diagnosis. Acta Otolaryngol 94:53, 1982.
118. Baloh, RW, et al: Quantitative assessment of visual-vestibular interaction using sinusoidal rotatory stimuli. In Honrubia, V and Brazier, MAB (eds) Nystagmus and Vertigo: Clinical Approaches to the Patient with Dizziness. UCLA Forum in Medical Sciences, No. 24. Academic Press, New York, 1982, p 231.
119. Baloh, RW and Honrubia, V: Clinical Neurophysiology of the Vestibular System. FA Davis, Philadelphia, 1979.
120. Honrubia, V: Auditory disorders, evaluation and diagnosis of: Vestibular examination. In Gaullaudet Encyclopedia of Deaf People and Deafness, vol 1. McGraw-Hill, New York, 1986, p 82.
121. Sills, AW and Honrubia, V: A new method for determining impulsive time constants and their application to clinical data. Otolaryngology 86:81, 1978.
122. Honrubia, V, et al: Vestibulo-ocular reflexes in peripheral labyrinthine lesions: III. Bilateral dysfunction. Am J Otolaryngol 6:342, 1985.

CHAPTER 8

Audiologic Assessment and Management

M. Cara Erskine, MEd
Hiroshi Shimizu, MD

AUDIOLOGIC ASSESSMENT

The vestibular apparatus is connected with the cochlear duct, which holds the sensory organ of hearing. Pathologic processes, therefore, can affect both the vestibular and cochlear organs, causing dizziness and hearing impairment. For example, the typical triad of Ménière's disease consists of episodic vertigo, fluctuating hearing loss, and tinnitus.[1] Labyrinthine fistula, ototoxicity, and acoustic neuroma are other examples that are often presented with both dizziness and hearing loss. Consequently, the audiologic evaluation is required for early diagnosis in many cases of dizziness. The purpose of this chapter is to describe:

1. The basic components of an audiologic assessment as well as the more sophisticated measures of the auditory system used in diagnosis
2. The clinical application of the test results
3. Various methods used for auditory rehabilitation

More than 21.9 million Americans are afflicted with hearing loss in one or both ears.[2] The real hearing-impaired population probably exceeds 22 million if undetected mild hearing losses or losses in high frequencies are included. Hearing loss is one of the major disabling conditions; however, some types of hearing loss can be prevented, treated, or improved by surgery or a hearing device. Therefore, accurate audiologic evaluation is essential for differential diagnosis and appropriate intervention. Audiologists are professionals who have been trained in the assessment, habilitation, and rehabilitation of individuals with a hearing impairment, including the use of hearing aids and assistive listening devices. They are required to have at least a Master's degree and to be certified by the American Speech-Language-Hearing Association. In some states, they are licensed to practice audiology. Many audiologists are also engaged in a wide variety of scientific research.

Measurement of Behavioral Hearing Threshold

Hearing threshold is the faintest audible sound level and is expressed by the decibel (dB) notation. The decibel may be referred to as sound pressure level (SPL) or hearing level (HL). The unit to describe the magnitude of the sound wave is called pascal (Pa), and the weakest sound pressure audible to the human being at the frequency of 1000 hertz (Hz) is 20 micropascals (μPa). The decibel is not a fixed unit like the meter or gram but an expression of a certain number of times greater than the reference level, which is 20 μPa. The decibel is defined as the logarithm of the ratio between a given sound pressure and the reference pressure. Namely,

$$dB\ SPL = 20\ \log \frac{P1}{P2}.$$

where P1 is sound pressure of a given sound, and P2 is the reference sound pressure (20 μPa). For example, 20 dB SPL means a 10-fold increase (200 μPa), and 60 dB SPL corresponds to a 1000-fold increase (20,000 μPa). As the minimal audible SPL is different from frequency to frequency, 0 dB dial reading on the audiometer was designed to present a pure tone of the minimal audible pressure under a given earphone regardless of frequency and is expressed in dB HL.

Hearing thresholds for pure tones are usually recorded on a graph called an *audiogram* (Fig. 8–1). Although the audible frequency range of young human ear is from 20 to 20,000 Hz, hearing thresholds are measured mostly from 250 to 8000 Hz for diagnostic objectives. The abscissa of the audiogram indicates dB HL, and the ordinate indicates the frequencies for pure tones. Different symbols are used for the results obtained by *air conduction* (AC) and *bone conduction* (BC) with and without masking, in sound field where pure tones are presented from the loudspeaker and for no response. Those symbols are usually shown on the audiogram form.

Because the behavioral hearing threshold depends on the patient's subjective response, the results are influenced by many factors such as attention, motivation, instruction, patient's physical condition, age, testing procedure, response criteria, and the audiologist's skill.

Air conduction threshold is measured by presenting pure tones either through the headphone or loudspeaker in the sound field. For bone conduction testing, a bone conduction oscillator is placed on the mastoid process behind the pinna. Because the sound reaches the cochlea, directly bypassing the external and middle ear conduction system, BC audiometry measures the function of the cochlea. The maximum BC threshold which can be measured is 65 to 70 dB HL.

Types of Hearing Loss

CONDUCTIVE HEARING LOSS

This hearing loss is caused by a pathologic condition that exists in the external ear canal or the middle ear. Case 2 in Figure 8–1 shows a typical audiogram of a conductive

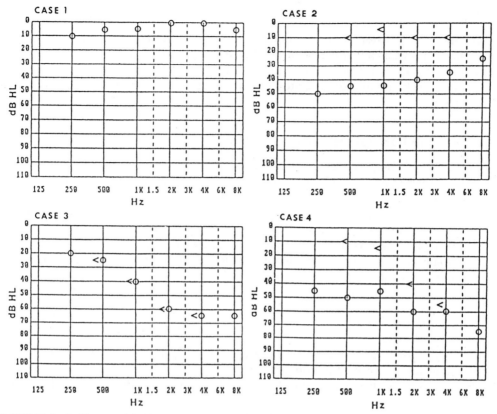

FIGURE 8–1. Types of audiogram. Case 1: Normal hearing; Case 2: Conductive hearing loss; Case 3: Sensorineural hearing loss; Case 4: Mixed type hearing loss. O = air condition; < = bone conduction.

hearing loss characterized by elevated AC thresholds with normal BC threshold. Audiograms showing significant gaps between AC and BC thresholds indicate the involvement of the external and/or middle ear. The main causes of conductive hearing loss include impact cerumen; foreign bodies in the external ear canals; acquired stenosis and closure of the external ear canal; and disconnection of ossicular chain owing to injuries, otosclerosis, otitis media, cholesteatoma, barotrauma, genetic disorders, and neoplasms.

SENSORINEURAL HEARING LOSS

Hearing loss owing to pathologic conditions in the cochlea and/or the eighth nerve is called sensorineural hearing loss. The audiogram shows no gaps between AC and BC thresholds (case 3 in Fig. 8–1) The pathogenesis of sensorineural hearing loss includes injuries to the cochlea owing to temporal bone fracture, barotrauma or noise, labyrinthitis, ototoxicity, Ménière's disease, aging process (presbyacusis), genetic process, some vascular and metabolic disorders, eighth nerve schwannoma, and meningioma in the cerebellopontine angle. Premature birth, hyperbilirubinemia, congenital infections such as toxoplasmosis, syphilis, rubella, cytomegalovirus and herpes, craniofacial anomalies, bacterial meningitis, hypoxia at birth, and prolonged mechanical ventilation are high-risk factors for prelinguistic sensorineural hearing loss.

MIXED-TYPE HEARING LOSS

When both the external and/or middle ear and sensorineural system are involved, the audiogram reveals an elevation of BC thresholds but with AC-BC gaps as shown in Figure 8–1 (case 4). This type of loss is called *mixed-type hearing loss*. Mixed-type hearing loss can be seen in advanced otosclerosis, severe chronic otitis media, and some genetic hearing losses.

CLASSIFICATION OF HEARING LOSS

The degree of hearing loss is often expressed by *pure tone average* (PTA), which is the average hearing level of AC thresholds at 500, 1000, and 2000 Hz (Table 8–1). The frequency range between 500 and 2000 Hz is referred to as the *speech frequencies*.

The classification shown in Table 8–1 may be adequate for adults who developed a hearing loss later but is not necessarily appropriate for young children. For example, a loss of 30 dB PTA is classified as a mild hearing loss but is serious enough to cause a delay in speech and language development or difficulty understanding the teacher's speech in the classroom.

Speech Audiometry

Ordinary speech audiometry typically consists of *speech reception threshold* (SRT) measurement and word recognition testing. The SRT is defined as the lowest level of speech at which the listener is able to repeat 50 percent of the two syllable words (spondee) presented. If the patient is a young child, the SRT is sometimes estimated by presenting only familiar words to the child or letting the child identify pictures or toys on a tray. SRT measurement is essential to validate the reliability of PTA, since the SRT should be within the 6-dB range of PTA. If no agreement is found between SRT and PTA, the reliability of the pure tone audiogram needs to be examined.

The *word recognition score* is expressed by the percentage of the *phonetically balanced* (PB) words that the listener can repeat correctly at a given level above the listener's SRT. By measuring the score at different speech intensity levels, starting from a low level to a high level, a word recognition score curve can be drawn (performance intensity function). The curve provides valuable information regarding the maximum score, called PB Max, and site of lesion. The PB Max is 88 to 100 percent and is usually obtained at 30 to 40 dB above SRT in normal listeners and patients with a conductive hearing loss. On the other hand, many patients with a cochlear hearing loss show PB Max at only 15 to 20 dB

TABLE 8–1 Classification of Hearing Loss

PTA (dB)	Classification
<15	Normal
16–25	Slight
26–40	Mild
41–55	Moderate
56–70	Moderately severe
71–90	Severe
>91	Profound

above the SRT with a score lower than normal. The PB Max is usually obtained at the most comfortable level (MCL) for speech. Abnormally narrowed range between the SRT and the MCL (dynamic range) is often referred to as *loudness recruitment*, which is one of the characteristics of cochlear sensorineural hearing loss. Patients with a precipitously downward-sloping high-frequency hearing loss perform poorly in speech recognition testing because of their inability to hear consonants. The PB Max, which is unproportionately poor for the degree of hearing loss and the configuration of audiogram, is often found in patients with a retrocochlear lesion, such as an acoustic neuroma. The speech recognition test is very important for differential diagnosis, assessment of the patient's communication ability, and evaluation for a hearing aid.

Acoustic Immittance Measurements

When a traveling sound wave reaches the tympanic membrane, a small portion of the sound energy is reflected at the tympanic membrane. The amount of reflection depends on the acoustic impedance (resistivity to the flow of acoustic energy) of the middle ear system. The middle ear analyzer is a device to measure a change in the acoustic impedance of the middle ear system by feeding the reflected sound received by a probe microphone to an impedance bridge. The measurement is called *acoustic immittance measurement* or *immittance audiometry* and typically consists of *tympanometry* and *acoustic reflex measurement*.

Tympanometry measures a change in the compliance of the tympanic membrane and ossicular chain as a function of the air pressure in the external ear canal. When the air pressure in the external ear canal is matched to that in the middle ear, the compliance (mobility) of the tympanic membrane is highest. The testing results are depicted in a graph, referred to as a *tympanogram*, which reports the magnitude of acoustic transmission in terms of acoustic millimhos (mmhos) or as an equivalent volume of air in cubic centimeters or millimeters. The tympanogram is most commonly obtained with a single-probe tone frequency of 226 Hz, but multiple-frequency tympanometry (678 or 1000 Hz in addition to 226 Hz) has been found to identify different types of ossicular chain disruptions.[3,4]

Five typical tympanograms are shown in Figure 8–2; each type is associated with various middle ear disorders:

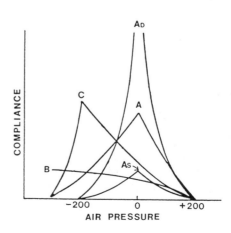

FIGURE 8–2. Types of tympanogram.

Type A: Normal middle ear air pressure and normal mobility of the tympanic membrane
Type As: Ossicular chain fixation, adhesive fixation, thickened or heavily scarred tympanic membrane, cholesteatoma, polyps, or granuloma
Type Ad: Ossicular chain discontinuity or flaccid tympanic membrane
Type B: Middle ear effusion, adhesive otitis media, tympanic membrane perforation, PE tube, impact cerumen, or artifact
Type C: Serous otitis media, or blocked eustachian tube

The acoustic reflex measurement has been used to identify site of lesion[5] or to identify and estimate hearing sensitivity.[6] The acoustic reflex occurs when the stapedius muscle contracts in response to a loud signal. A stimulus applied to either ear will cause muscles to contract binaurally. The reflex is tested at the point of maximum compliance of the middle ear and can be seen on the middle ear analyzer as a change in compliance. When an acoustic signal is presented continuously at 10 dB above the reflex threshold, the magnitude of the reflex is usually sustained for 10 seconds at 500 and 1000 Hz. The measurement of the magnitude of reflex for the 10 seconds is called the *acoustic reflex decay test*. This test is primarily used to identify a lesion in the eighth nerve.

The acoustic reflex occurs at 70 to 100 dB HL in individuals with normal hearing. However, the reflex is often seen at only 30 to 50 dB above hearing threshold in patients with a sensorineural hearing loss. The narrow range between the reflex threshold and the hearing threshold indicates a cochlear lesion. On the other hand, the patient with an acoustic tumor may show elevated acoustic reflex thresholds and also rapid reflex decay. The absence or elevation of reflex thresholds can be seen in stapes fixation as in otosclerosis, disarticulation of the middle ear ossicles, conductive hearing losses, and brain-stem pathway disorders.

The acoustic immittance measurements have also been used as a screening tool to identify middle ear disorders and hearing loss in young children.[7,8]

Auditory Brain-Stem Response Testing

By means of an average response computer, a series of time-locked electrical potentials evoked by acoustic stimuli, can be recorded with a regular EEG electrode placed on the top of the head (vertex) or on the forehead below the hairline and another electrode placed on each earlobe. The electrode on the earlobe ipsilateral to the ear stimulated is used as a reference electrode and the other as a ground electrode. The broad-band click-elicited auditory brain-stem response (ABR) typically consists of a series of five or more evoked electrical potentials generated within the eighth nerve and the central auditory pathways of the brain stem (Fig. 8–3). At 70-dB nHL (70 dB above the mean value of click thresholds obtained from a group of normally hearing young adults), the wave I occurs at around 1.6 msec after the click onset and is then followed by wave II at 2.8 msec, wave III at 3.8 msec, wave IV at 5.1 msec, and wave V at around 5.7 msec. The wave I and II arise primarily from the auditory nerve, but because of the complexity of the neuroanatomy of the auditory system in the brain stem, the later wave appears to be the summation of the electrical activity in more than one auditory source between the cochlear nucleus and inferior colliculus. The latency values get longer as the intensity is decreased, but the interwave interval is relatively[9] unaffected by the intensity of the acoustic signal.

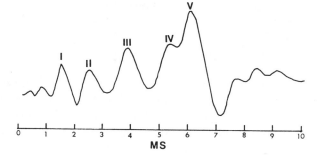

FIGURE 8–3. Basic morphology of auditory brainstem response (ABR). Wave I corresponds to the cochlea, acoustic N; wave II—acoustic N, cochlear Nu; wave III—superior olivary complex; wave IV—lateral lemniscus; wave V—inferior colliculus.

Because the recording technique is noninvasive and the responses are highly sensitive and reproducible, ABR testing became an important clinical tool in audiology, otology, and neurology.

CLINICAL APPLICATIONS OF ABR

Estimation of Hearing Sensitivity

Assessment of hearing of difficult-to-test young children is crucial but requires special techniques. Brain-stem response audiometry is a powerful tool to assess hearing in those children because it can be done in natural and sedated sleep. The click-elicited ABR estimates hearing sensitivity at 3000 to 4000 Hz.[10–12] The morphology of the ABR with a conductive hearing loss is characterized by prolonged latency of each wave with normal or near-normal interwave intervals. The latency values are greatly influenced by the pathology of the cochlea and the configuration of audiogram. Sloping high-frequency cochlear hearing losses usually cause prolonged latencies without greatly affecting the wave I–V interval.[13] The prediction of hearing threshold in low and middle frequencies requires the use of tone bursts, although the sensitivity is not as high as that with click stimuli.

ABRs can be obtained even in neonates (Fig. 8–4), and the effectiveness of ABR screening in the neonatal intensive care unit and in any neonates at risk for hearing

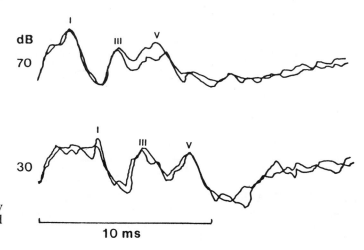

FIGURE 8–4. Auditory brainstem responses obtained from a 3-day-old baby.

impairment has been well recognized.[14-18] Significant contributions of ABR screening in neonates at risk lie in early identification of hearing-impaired infants and early intervention. Portable battery-operated ABR screeners, which are now commercially available, will further improve the cost-effectiveness of neonatal ABR screening.

Identification of Lesions in the Auditory Nerve and Brain Stem

The morphology, the absolute latency, and interwave intervals of the ABR provide significant information regarding the condition of the eighth nerve and auditory pathway within the brain stem. Inconsistent morphology, abnormally prolonged latencies and/or interwave intervals, reversed wave IV/V amplitude, and the absence of wave V or the entire response are indicative of lesions in the eighth nerve or the brain stem. The abnormal ABR can be found in acoustic tumors (Fig. 8–5), brain-stem tumors, demyelinating disorders such as multiple sclerosis and leukodystrophy, brain death, coma, head trauma, stroke or ischemia, hydrocephalus, sudden infant death syndrome, alcoholism, sleep apnea, and spastic dysphonia.[19,20] A general relationship between the level

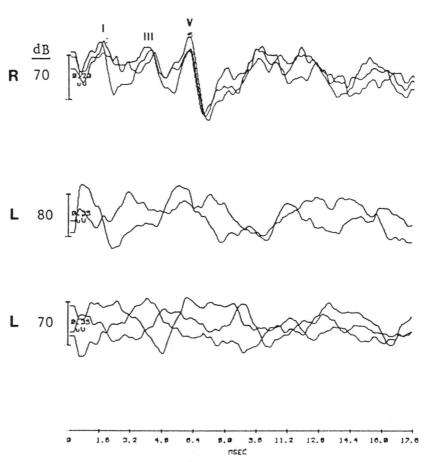

FIGURE 8–5. ABRs obtained from a 46-year-old patient who had a surgically confirmed acoustic neuroma on the left side. She had a moderate sensorineural hearing loss in the left ear. Repeated ABR on the left side at 70 dB and 80 dB nHL showed no discernible responses, but clear responses were obtained when the right ear was stimulated.

of the lesion and its effect on the ABR has been well recognized, but the abnormality of the ABR is not uniquely characteristic for a given pathology. For example, the complete absence of ABR can be seen in both acoustic tumor and multiple sclerosis.

Diagnostic and Prognostic Applications in the Intensive Care Unit for Cases of Severe Head Injury

ABR, often combined with somatosensory and visual evoked potentials, has been used for severely brain-damaged patients in the intensive care unit to monitor neurologic status, to localize the lesion, to evaluate the effectiveness of medical and surgical treatment, to determine brain death, or to predict the prognosis of the patient.[21] Because the patient is in critical condition, the interpretation of the evoked potential data requires careful considerations of the effects of various pharmacologic agents, hypothermia, intracranial pressure, and arterial blood gases.

Intraoperative Monitoring

Recent development of electrophysiologic and evoked potential monitoring during surgery has made a significant contribution in the improved intraoperative patient management and reduction of postoperative complications. The monitoring by ABR has proved useful for surgical procedures on the eighth nerve and brain stem, such as acoustic tumor resection, retrolabyrinthine vestibular nerve section, trigeminal nerve section, brain-stem tumor resection, microvascular decompression of cranial nerves V or VII, and posterior fossa decompression.[22]

Electrocochleography

Electrocochleography (ECoG) is the recording of acoustically evoked electrical potentials arising from the cochlea and the eighth nerve: *cochlear microphonic* (CM), *summation potential* (SP) and *whole action potential* (AP) of the eighth nerve.

The CM is an alternating current (AC) potential that is generated by the hair cells. CM mimics the waveform of sound stimulation like the AC voltage from a microphone. For example, if a 1000-Hz pure tone is presented to the ear, the recorded CM is also a 1000-Hz sinusoidal wave and is maintained for the duration of the stimulation. However, the CM is not symmetric about the baseline, indicating a shift of a direct current (DC). This shift of the baseline (DC shift) is called *SP*. It is not well known how the SP is generated, but it is believed to reflect the distortion in the hair-cell transduction process. The whole eighth nerve AP is the summation of synchronized discharge from many auditory neurons. The wave I of the ABR represents the AP.

Those stimulus-related electrical potentials can be recorded with a needle electrode placed on the promontory through the tympanic membrane (TM) or by an electrode placed on the TM or the wall of the external ear canal near the TM. The shorter the distance between the electrode and cochlea, the larger the amplitude of the potentials. However, the TM or ear canal electrode is more popular than the transtympanic electrode in the United States because of its noninvasiveness. The reference electrode is preferably placed on the contralateral earlobe, mastoid, or ear canal. The potentials can be elicited by either clicks or tone bursts at moderately high intensities. Because the CM mimics the waveform of the acoustic stimulus, it can be canceled out by alternating the polarity of clicks during the stimulation or adding the averaged CMs obtained with condensation and rarefaction clicks. When the CM is canceled out, the SP appears as

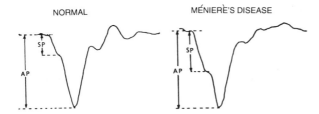

FIGURE 8-6. Electrocochleograms from the normal ear and the ear with Ménière's disease. The responses in Ménière's disease shows large summation potential (SP). AP represents the magnitude of the whole nerve action potential.

steplike voltage on the leading edge of the AP waveform (Fig. 8-6). The AP is not affected by the polarity of the click.

CLINICAL APPLICATIONS OF ELECTROCOCHLEOGRAPHY

Attempts had been made using ECoG to predict hearing threshold and to identify the cite of lesion until the ABR was accepted as being more sensitive and useful than the ECoG.[24-27] Recently, ECoG has attained the popularity as identifying and monitoring endolymphatic hydrops or Ménière's disease.[23,28-30] Normally, the amplitude of SP is very small compared with the AP amplitude. The range of SP/AP amplitude ratio is normally 10 to 50 percent but exceeds 50 percent in many patients with Ménière's disease (Fig. 8-6). Because Ménière's disease is characterized by episodic attacks of vertigo and fluctuating sensorineural hearing loss, whether or not ECoG is performed during the active stage of endolymphatic hydrops may alter the results. The "hit rate" of ECoG seems to be poor with a mild or severe hearing loss in high frequencies.[31] Consequently, the absence of abnormally enlarged SP does not necessarily rule out Ménière's disease.

An enlargement of SP has also been found in both humans and experimental animals with perilymphatic fistula.[32] Perilymphatic fistula may result in secondary endolymphatic hydrops owing to a decrease in perilymph causing an enlarged SP. The symptoms of perilymphatic fistula often mimic Ménière's syndrome. Another clinical application of ECoG has been to monitor the functional integrity of the eighth nerve and the auditory pathway in the brain stem during posterior fossa surgery.[33-36] One of the advantages of promontory ECoG with a transtympanic electrode is the significantly improved signal-to-noise ratio resulting from recording in the proximity of the eighth nerve.

Otoacoustic Emission

During the past decade, a dramatic change has evolved in our knowledge of the physiology of the cochlea by the discoveries of *otoacoustic emission*,[37] the *sharp basilar membrane tuning*,[38,39] and the *motility of the outer hair cells*.[40] We now know that the cochlea has both passive and active mechanisms and that the cochlea emits sounds that can be recorded in the external ear canal. There are two types of otoacoustic emissions (OAEs). The one is the OAE that can be recorded in the absence of acoustic stimulation and is called *spontaneous otoacoustic emission* (SOAE). SOAEs are low-intensity narrowband sounds that are present in 40 to 60 percent of healthy ears.

The other type of OAE is evoked by acoustic stimuli, called *evoked otoacoustic emission* (EOAE). They can be elicited by clicks or tone pips (transiently evoked

OAE:TEOAE), single, continuous pure tones (stimulus frequency OAE), and by two continuous pure tones that are separated by a prescribed frequency distance (distortion product OAE). EOAEs can be detected in nearly all normal human ears.

To measure the OAEs, a small-probe tip, which contains a sensitive microphone and a sound source, is inserted into the external ear canal in a similar fashion used in acoustic immittance measurement. The emitted sound energy is amplified and fed into the computer-based dynamic signal analyzer. For details of the recording technique and to understand the waveforms of the OEAs, the reader is referred to Kemp, Ryan, and Bray.[41] Because of the objectivity of OAE measurement, noninvasiveness of the recording procedure, its frequency-specific nature, and the specificity for outer hair cells, the OAE has great potential to provide clinically significant information on cochlear function and pathology.[42-44] Because of the recent development of instrumentation, we can record OAEs for patients in clinical situations. However, the clinical application is still in the early stage of development. The most promising clinical application has been the use of TEOAE for hearing screening of infants including neonates.[42,45-47] The ideal hearing screening for the difficult-to-test young infants requires that the test be fast, easy, noninvasive, highly sensitive, and low in the false-positive and false-negative rates. The TEOAE are present in virtually all normal neonates[41,45,48,49] and are not present in adults with a mild hearing loss. The test time is reportedly only 12 minutes on the average versus 26 minutes by ABR screening.[50] With these findings, the transient evoked otoacoustic emission (TEOAE) appears to meet the requirements for infant hearing screening. However, the long-term follow-up results remain to be evaluated.

MANAGEMENT OF HEARING IMPAIRMENT

Selection of the best amplification system for an individual must be based on thorough, individualized assessment of hearing function. The greatest potential benefits from a hearing aid are best achieved by those with moderate-to-severe hearing losses (30 through 85 dB). Although most people with a hearing loss may enjoy an assistive listening device and/or hearing aid in selected situations, people with profound losses (no benefit from a hearing aid) may benefit from a cochlear implant. Clinicians generally agree that hearing-impaired people would benefit from aural rehabilitation, speech reading, and/or auditory training.

Hearing Aids

As of 1990, in this country alone, 11 million people over the age of 65 require the use of amplification.[51] Bogenshaw-Jensen[52] estimated that 5 percent of the world's population are hearing impaired. Hearing impairment is the third most common health problem of the elderly behind arthritis and hypertension. The Hearing Aid Industries Association Consumer Survey of 1984[53] showed that the elderly do not obtain a hearing aid because they believe that:

1. Their hearing loss is not significant enough to warrant the use of a hearing aid.
2. A hearing aid will not help them.
3. The professional fees for obtaining a hearing aid are too expensive.
4. A hearing aid is bulky and unsightly.

The function of a hearing aid is to amplify sound to help the hearing-impaired person use his or her residual hearing to the maximum. The first amplification system was the cupped ear, which gave an increase of about 10 dB in the high frequencies. Horns and speaking tubes were first used in the late 1800s as aids to hearing. The transistor hearing aids currently in use have greater flexibility, reduced size, and low battery cost.

The electronic hearing aid (Fig. 8–7) is a miniature telephone with three basic parts: the microphone that picks up the sound and converts it to an electrical signal, the amplifier that increases the strength of the electrical signal, and the receiver that converts the amplified sound back into acoustic energy.

TYPES OF HEARING AIDS

1. Behind the ear (BTE) (Fig. 8–7, center). This hearing aid fits behind the pinna, is considered fairly rugged, and is available in a wide variety of amplification configurations and can be fit to the most severe hearing losses.
2. In the ear (ITE) (Fig. 8–7, left): This aid is the most popular type now available and can be used with hearing losses up to 70 dB. In 1973 ITE aids constituted only 2.3 percent of the hearing aids being used, but by 1987 were almost 80 percent of the market.[53,54]
3. In the canal (ITC) (Fig. 8–7, right). These hearing aids are very small and fit directly into the ear canal. Usually they are fit on people with mild losses who have large ear canals.
4. Eyeglass hearing aid. This hearing aid is manufactured in the temporal piece of an eyeglass frame. This type of hearing aid accounted for 50 percent of the market in 1959 but now is rarely used.[54]
5. Body hearing aid: Up to 1955, this hearing aid was the only wearable one available but now accounts for less than 2 percent of the market. The body hearing aid usually is worn by people with a very profound hearing loss.
6. Contralateral routing of sound (CROS). A hearing aid shell is worn by each ear; one contains a hearing aid and the other a microphone emitter. The sound is picked up on the side with no usable hearing and routed to the better side by a radio frequency.

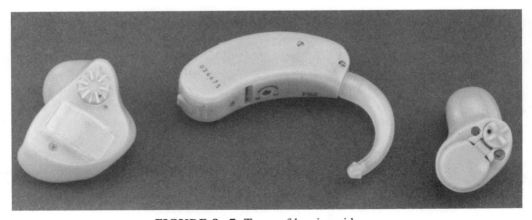

FIGURE 8–7. Types of hearing aids.

This aid is helpful for people with profound unilateral hearing loss and near-normal hearing in the better ear and helps users to understand speakers when they stand on the impaired side.

7. Bilateral contralateral routing of sound (BICROS). This system is the same as the CROS but two microphones are connected to the same amplifier. BICROS is used when there is no hearing in one ear and a hearing loss in the other.

8. Bone conduction hearing aid. This hearing aid conducts the sound directly to the inner ear by bone vibration and bypasses the middle ear system. It is used when bone conduction is near normal or mildly depressed and when the patient is unable to wear conventional hearing aids owing to aural atresia or medical problems. This aid can be attached to a headband and placed tightly against the mastoid or it can be surgically implanted. The microphone and receiver are encased in a BTE device.

Hearing aids can be equipped with a telephone coil, which is an induction coil to pick up electromagnetic signals directly from a telephone or a loop amplification system.

Hearing aids are now available with a variety of circuits, such as automatic signal processing, digitally programmable hearing aids, and K-AMP. These circuits help to improve their aided function in noise, the localization of sound, and when individuals experience sensitivity to loud sounds.

If the patient has a bilateral hearing loss, the consensus has been to recommend two hearing aids to benefit from binaural hearing. Ross[55] reviewed 19 studies on monaural and binaural hearing aid use, and 15 of them showed binaural superiority. Users set the volume lower when wearing two hearing aids and were able to function better in noise. However, in a comparison trial of binaural and monaural hearing aid use, two hearing aids were preferred in everyday quiet situations, but one aid was more effective in a noisy environment.[56]

Aural Rehabilitation

An aural rehabilitation program is always recommended as part of the hearing aid selection. Such a program is designed to help individuals integrate the use of the hearing aid with the proper adjustments in the environment to maximize their performance. Hearing aid users are taught how to manipulate background noise and select favorable seating. In addition, emphasis is placed on incorporating the auditory and visual modalities.[57] The goal of an aural rehabilitation program is to orient each person to a specific hearing aid and to provide strategies for coping in all environments with the hearing aid.[58]

ASSISTIVE LISTENING DEVICES

Assistive listening devices (ALDs) are a significant adjunct to the rehabilitation and habilitation process for the hearing impaired. The term ALD is broadly used to encompass the equipment designed to improve the communication ability of the hearing-impaired population. The equipment primarily consists of: (1) ALD as in a loop-amplifying system, hardware system, or infrared system; (2) assistive alerting device (AADs), such as bells and buzzers; (3) assistive signaling device (ASDs) referring to a signaling device, such as in flashing lights; and (4) telecommunication devices for the disabled or TDDs and closed-captioning units for television.[59]

These devices are needed because a hearing aid has limitations. Most individuals are dissatisfied with their hearing aid, and few hearing aid users have no complaints. The ALDs bypass the background noise so that the signal goes directly from the speaker to the listener.

Aids can be categorized according to their commonality. This categorization includes: (1) Hard-wired devices in which the microphone is near the sound source and the signal is sent electronically to the ear of the listener. These devices include the Pocket Talker and a system called direct audio input, which attaches directly to the hearing aid with a boot; and (2) *wireless listening systems,* including the *loop system,* which is based on the principle of magnetic induction in which a signal from an amplifier is fed into a coil of wire that is placed around the room. The wire generates an audiofrequency magnetic field that is picked up by the telephone switch on the hearing aid. Also included is the *infrared system,* in which sounds are picked up by a microphone and are transferred to an infrared beam that is emitted by a special list-emitting diode (LED). The listener wears a battery-operated infrared receiver with a volume control. These devices are popular in theaters, concert halls, and places of worship.

AADs emit an alerting signal by converting a normal alerting sound to a low-frequency loud sound for the hearing-impaired person to hear. Smoke detectors, door bells, and telephone bells are some of the most frequently used units.

ASDs transform the acoustic signal by transmitter to a visual or tactile sound. For example, a light can be activated when the doorbell rings or a vibrating unit under the pillow can be attached to an alarm clock.

An informing device is a *telecommunication device* (TDD, formerly TTY) for the severely hearing impaired and deaf that allows them to communicate by telephone. This device allows for an acoustic coupler to convert the typed messages into sequences of tones. The signal is then converted into a readout enabling use of the phone lines.

Close-captioning TV is a decoding device that provides readable messages for the hearing impaired and deaf.

ALDs and these other systems enrich the lives of the hearing impaired and the deaf and allow for greater security and independence.[59,60]

Cochlear Implants

Cochlear implants are a viable choice for the profoundly hearing impaired population. They are appropriate only for those people who cannot achieve any benefit from a hearing aid. Cochlear implants produce a sensation of hearing by direct electrical stimulation of the acoustic nerve. This technique is not novel and was first reported by the Romans as a way to treat headache. The earliest report of direct electrical stimulation to the ear was reported in 1790 when Volta inserted metal rods into each ear and connected them to a circuit of 50 volts. He experienced the sensation of a blow to the head.[61] It did not receive mention again until the 1900s. In 1957, Djourno and Eyries became the first group to stimulate the acoustic nerve of a deaf patient.[61]

Cochlear implants are implanted either outside the cochlea (round window, mastoid) and are referred to as *extracochlear* or within the cochlea and called *intracochlear.* They are further defined by the number of channels: single or multiple. The multichannel devices are the only ones that are being manufactured in the United States. They are

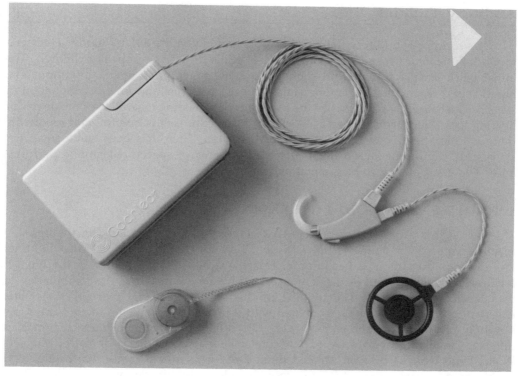

FIGURE 8–8. A multichannel cochlear implant, processor, and microphone.

reported to provide superior information over the single-channel units because they provide frequency-specific information about the signal.[62]

The main components of the cochlear implant (Fig. 8–8) are: (1) the microphone that sends an electrical equivalent of an acoustic stimulus to the signal processor; (2) the signal processor that transforms the electrical input into the desired electrical stimuli; and (3) the surgically implanted system, in which the signal goes to one or more electrodes depending on the design of the device.

Of the 2900 adults and 1400 children currently using cochlear implants worldwide, about 50 percent are able to understand some open-set information (no clues are provided to the patient).[63] Although outstanding results, such as being able to talk on the telephone, do occur, they are rare. Most patients, however, can carry on controlled conversations with visual cues.

The technology for the cochlear implant is considered to be in the early stages at this time. Under the current selection process, it cannot be predicted who will function well with the cochlear implant, but those who do best seem to be generally younger, motivated individuals who have good lip-reading skills and have only very recently lost their hearing.

The rehabilitation process is a lengthy but vital one to the success of the cochlear implant. The procedure involves tuning the speech processor by computer hookup, orientation to the device, aural rehabilitation, and experiencing new environments while using the device.

Auditory Training

The concept of auditory training was originally noted in 1802 by Itard.[64] He began to work systematically on improving auditory skills in hearing-impaired children. The initial work usually begins with sound awareness tasks, gross sound discrimination, broad sound discrimination among simple speech patterns, and fine discrimination of speech. The concept is to maximize the use of residual hearing regardless of the degree of hearing loss. Controversy exists as to whether this approach is helpful, and reportedly there is little scientific evidence to support its value. There has been some small but statistically significant improvement noted in the area of speech recognition performance. The gains appear to be maintained over time.[65]

SPEECH READING AND LIP READING

This skill is a multifactor process that involves how sounds look on the lips. Lip reading requires combining visual attention, situational and contextual cues, lighting, and distance from the speaker in order to achieve maximum benefit.[58] In the English language, about one third of the sounds are visible on the lips; thus the combination of these factors is essential. The training of this skill is aimed at teaching systematic observation of visual symbols combined with optimal environmental factors and topic selection. The most common methods are: (1) Synthetic (Nitchie) which uses materials in differing linguistic contexts (words to conversational speech); (2) analytic (Mueller-Walle, Jena) which works on isolated sounds and nonsense syllables that begins with visible sounds (/p/, /th/, /f/) and proceeds to low-visibility sounds (/k/, /g/, /h/); and (3) eclectic (Kinzie) which combines both methods of using sounds in isolation and words in context.[64]

Speech reading is considered an important component of the aural rehabilitation process, particularly for those individuals with significant hearing impairment.

SUMMARY

The auditory and vestibular systems are often affected by the same disorders. Evaluation of auditory function in cases in which dizziness is a complaint; therefore, contributes to the diagnosis of the patient's problem. This chapter reviewed the numerous procedures for evaluating auditory function that can be incorporated into the total workup. Information obtained from tests about auditory function not only aids in diagnosis but is the basis for treatment and rehabilitation of the hearing loss itself.

REFERENCES

1. Pfaltz, CZ and Matefi, L: Ménière's disease or syndrome? A critical review of diagnostic criteria. In Vosteen, KH, et al (eds): Ménière's Disease: Pathogenesis, Diagnosis and Treatment. Thieme-Stratton, New York, 1981, p 1.
2. Shewan, CM: The prevalence of hearing impairment. American Speech, Language, and Hearing Association 32:62, 1990.
3. Lilly, DJ: Multiple frequency, multiple component tympanometry: New approachs to an old diagnostic problem. Ear Hearing, 5:300, 1986.
4. Van Camp, KJ and Vogeleer, M: Normative multi-frequency tympanometric data on otosclerosis. Scand Audiol, 15:187, 1986.

5. Stach, BA and Jerger, JF: Acoustic reflex patterns in peripheral and central auditory system disease. Semin Hearing 8:369, 1987.
6. Silman, S, et al: Prediction of hearing loss from the acoustic reflex threshold. In Silman, S (ed): The Acoustic Reflex Basic Principles and Clinical Application. Academic Press, New York, 1984, p 187.
7. Guidelines for screening for hearing impairment and middle ear disorders. American Speech, Language, and Hearing Association (suppl) 2:17, 1990.
8. Walters, RJ and Shimizu, H: Acoustic immittance screening of infants. Semin Hearing 11:177, 1990.
9. Coats, AC and Martin, JL: Human auditory nerve action potentials and brainstem evoked responses. Arch Otolaryngol 103:605, 1977.
10. Jerger, J and Mauldin, L: Prediction of sensorineural hearing level from the brain stem evoked response. Arch Otolaryngol 104:456, 1979.
11. McDonald, JM and Shimizu, H: Frequency specificity of the auditory brain stem response. Am J Otolaryngol 2:36, 1989.
12. Shimizu, H: Some considerations on standardizing measurement and interpretation of brainstem response audiometry. In Starr, A, et al (eds): Sensory Evoked Potentials. Centro Ricerche e Studi Amplifon, Milan, Italy, 1984.
13. Bauch, CD and Olsen, WO: The effect of 2000-4000 Hz hearing sensitivity on ABR results. Ear Hear 7:314, 1986.
14. Gorga, MP, Kaminski, JR, and Beauchaine, KA: Auditory brain stem responses from graduates of an intensive care nursery using an insert earphone. Ear Hear 9:144, 1988.
15. ASHA Guidelines on audiologic screening of newborn infants who are at risk for hearing impairment. American Speech, Language, and Hearing Association 31:89, 1989.
16. Hyde, LM, et al: Audiometric accuracy of the click ABR in infants at risk for hearing loss. J Am Acad Audiol 1:59, 1990.
17. Shimizu, H, et al: Identification of hearing impairment in neonatal intensive care unit population: Outcome of a five-year project at the Johns Hopkins Hospital. Semin Hearing 11:150, 1990.
18. Markowitz, RK: Cost-effectiveness comparisons of hearing screening in the neonatal intensive care unit. Semin Hearing 11:161, 1990.
19. Rowe, MJ: The brainstem auditory evoked response in neurological disorders: A review. Ear Hear 2:141, 1981.
20. Stockard, JJ and Hecox, K: Brainstem auditory evoked potentials in sudden infant death syndrome (SIDS), "near-miss-SIDS", and infant apnea syndromes. Electroencephalogr Clin Neurophysiol 51:43, 1981.
21. Hall, JW, III and Tucker, DA: Sensory evoked responses in the intensive care unit. Ear Hear 7:220, 1986.
22. Dennis, JM and Earley, DA: Monitoring surgical procedures with the auditory brainstem response. Semin Hearing 9:113, 1988.
23. Coats, AC: The summating potential and Ménière's disease. Arch Otolaryngol 107:199, 1981.
24. Ruben, RJ, Bordley, JE, and Lieberman, AP: Cochlear potentials in man. Laryngoscope 71:1141, 1961.
25. Cullen, JK, et al: Human acoustic nerve action potential recordings from the tympanic membrane without anesthesia. Acta Otolaryngolgica 4:15, 1972.
26. Sohmer, H and Feinmesser, M: Electrocochleography in clinical-audiological diagnosis. Arch Otolaryngol 206:91, 1974.
27. Aran, JM: Contributions of electrocochleography to diagnosis in infancy. An eight year survey. In Gerber, SE and Mencher, GT (eds): Early Diagnosis of Hearing Loss. Grune & Stratton, New York, 1978, p 215.
28. Gibson, WPR and Prasher, DKL: Electrocochleography and its role in the diagnosis and understanding of Ménière's disease otolaryngol. Clin North Am 16:59, 1983.
29. Ferraro, JA, Arenberg, IK and Hassanein, RS: Electrocochleography and symptoms of inner ear dysfunction. Arch Otolaryngol 111:71, 1985.
30. Dauman, R, et al: Clinical significance of the summating potential in Ménière's disease. Am J Otology 9:31, 1988.
31. Coats, AC, Jenkins, HA, and Monroe, B: Auditory evoked potentials—The cochlear summating potential in detection of endolymphatic hydrops. Am J Otol 5:443, 1984.
32. Arenberg, IK, et al: ECoG results in perilymphatic fistula: Clinical and experimental studies. Otolaryngol Head Neck Surg 99:435, 1988.
33. Levine, RA, et al: Monitoring auditory evoked potentials during acoustic neuroma surgery: Insights into the mechanism of hearing loss. Ann Otol Rhinol Laryngol 93:116, 1984.
34. Ojemann, RG, et al: Use of intraoperative auditory evoked potentials to preserve hearing in unilateral acoustic neuroma removal. J Neurosurg 61:938, 1984.
35. Silverstein, H, Norrell, H, and Hyman, S: Simultaneous use of CO_2 laser with continuous monitoring of eight cranial nerve action potentials during acoustic neuroma surgery. Otolaryngol Head Neck Surg 92:80, 1984.
36. Silverstein, H, et al: Retrolabyrinthine vestibular neurectomy with simultaneous monitoring of eight nerve and brainstem auditory evoked potentials. Otolaryngol Head Neck Surg 93:736, 1985.
37. Kemp, DT: Stimulated acoustic emission from within the human auditory system. J Acoust Soc Am 64:1386, 1978.
38. Khana, SM and Leonard, DGB: Basilar membrane tuning in the cat cochlea. Science 215:305, 1982.

39. Sellick, PM, Patuzzi, R, and Johnston, BM: Measurement of basilar membrane motion in the guinea pig using the Mossbauer technique. J Acoust Soc Am 72:131, 1982.
40. Brownell, WE: Observations on a motile response in isolated outer hair cells. In Webster, WR and Aitken, LM (eds): Mechanisms of Hearing. Monash University Press, 1983, p 5.
41. Kemp, DT, Ryan, S, and Bray, P: A guide to the effective use of otoacoustic emissions. Ear Hear 11:93, 1990.
42. Elberling, C, et al: Evoked acoustic emission: Clinical application. Acta Oto-Laryngologica (suppl) 421:77, 1985.
43. Kemp, DT, et al: Acoustic emission cochleography—Practical aspects. Scand Audiol 15:71, 1986.
44. Tanaka, Y, Suzuki, M, and Inoue, T: Evoked otoacoustic emissions in sensorineural hearing impairment: Its clinical implications. Ear Hear 11:134, 1990.
45. Johnsen, NJ, et al: Evoked acoustic emissions from the human ear. IV. Final results in 100 neonates. Scand Audiol 17:27, 1988.
46. Bonfils, P, et al: Clinical significance of otoacoustic emission: A perspective. Ear Hear 11:155, 1990.
47. Stevens, JC, et al: Click evoked otoacoustic emissions in neonatal screening. Ear Hear 11:128, 1990.
48. Bonfils, P, Uziel, A, and Pujol, R: Evoked oto-acoustic emissions from adults and infants: Clinical applications. Acta Otolaryngol 105:445, 1988.
49. Norton, SJ and Widen, JE: Evoked otoacoustic emissions in normal-hearing infants and children: Emerging data and issues. Ear Hear 11:121, 1990.
50. White, KR: The Rhode Island Project: Otoacoustic emissions and neonatal hearing screening. Presented at International Symposium on Otoacoustic Emissions, Kansas City, Missouri, May 9–11, 1991.
51. Goldstein, BA: Factors contributing to the changing hearing aid scene. Ear Hear 2:260, 1981.
52. Bogeskov-Jensen. O: World report on hearing aids. Hearing Aid J 32:6, 1978.
53. Smriga, DJ, Huber TP, and Paparella, MM: Developments in hearing aid fitting and delivery. Otolaryngol Clin North Am 22:105, 1989.
54. Wernick, JS: Using of hearing aids. In Katz, J (ed): Handbook of Clinical Audiology, ed 3. Williams & Wilkins, Baltimore, 1985, p 911.
55. Ross, M: Binaural vs. monoaural hearing aid amplification for hearing impaired individuals. In Libby, ER (ed): Binaural Hearing and Amplification, vol 2. Zenetron, Chicago, 1980, p 1.
56. Schureurs, KK and Olsen, WO: Comparison of monaural and binaural hearing aid use on a trial period basis. Ear Hear 6:198, 1985.
57. Lowe, AD: Integrating the hearing aid into the audiological rehabilitation process. American Speech, Language, and Hearing Association 32(4):32, 1990.
58. Sims, DG: Audlts with hearing impairment. In Katz, J (ed): Handbook of Clinical Audiology. Williams & Wilkins, Baltimore, 1985, p 1017.
59. Pehringer, JL: Assistive devices: technology to improve communication. Otolaryngol Clin North Am 22:143, 1989.
60. Vaughn, GR, Lightfoot, RK, and Teter, DL: Assistive devices and systems (ALDS) enhance the lifestyles of hearing impaired persons. Am J Otology 9:101, 1988.
61. Luxford, WM and Brackmann, DE: The history of cochlear implants. In Gray, RF (ed): Cochlear Implants. College-Hill, San Diego, 1985, p 1.
62. NIH Consensus Development Conference Statement/Program Cochlear Implants, US Dept. of Health and Human Services, V 7, May 1988.
63. Osberger, MJ: Audiological rehabilitation with cochlear implants and tactile aids. American Speech, Language, and Hearing Association 32(4):38, 1990.
64. Rodel, MJ: Children with hearing impairment. In Katz, J (ed): Handbook of Clinical Audiology, ed 3. Williams & Wilkins, Baltimore, 1985, p 1004.
65. Rubinstein, A and Boothroyd, A: Effect of two approaches to auditory training on speech recognition by hearing impaired adults. Journal of Speech and Hearing Disorders 30:153, 1987.

SECTION III

Medical Management

Pharmacologic and Optical Methods of Treating Vestibular Disorders and Nystagmus

R. John Leigh, MD

Patients with vestibular disease may complain of vertigo, oscillopsia, or the visual consequences of nystagmus.[1] *Vertigo* consists of the illusion of turning and implies vestibular imbalance. *Oscillopsia* consists of illusory to-and-fro, movements of the seen environment; when it occurs with head movements, oscillopsia usually implies bilateral loss of vestibular function. Patients with spontaneous nystagmus owing to vestibular or other processes may also complain of oscillopsia when their heads are still. This chapter discusses pharmacologic and optical treatment measurements for vertigo, oscillopsia, and the visual consequences of nystagmus and attempts to base therapies on known pathophysiology.

In trying to understand and treat the symptoms resulting from labyrinthine disorders, we must bear in mind the nature of the demands placed on the vestibular system *during natural activities, especially locomotion.* The purpose of the vestibulo-ocular reflex (VOR) is to maintain clear and stable vision during natural head movements. A major threat to clear vision is the head perturbations occurring during locomotion. Figure 9–1 summarizes the peak velocities and predominant frequencies of head rotations measured in 20 normal subjects as they walked or ran in place. Note that although peak head velocity is generally below 150 deg/sec, the predominant frequencies range above 5 Hz. The latter value is much above the frequencies that vestibular physiologists conventionally use to test patients with vestibular disorders, and recent studies of natural locomo-

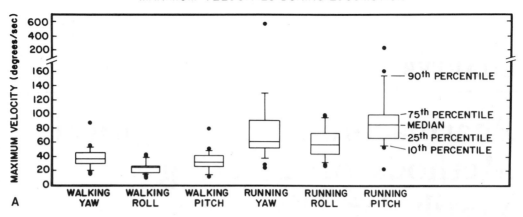

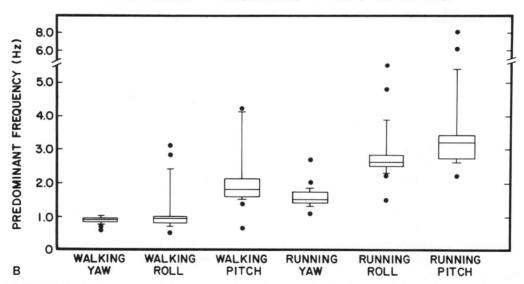

FIGURE 9–1. Summary of the ranges of maximum velocity (*top*) and frequency (*bottom*) of rotational head perturbations occurring during walking or running in place. Distribution of data from 20 normal subjects are displayed as Tukey box graphs, which show selected percentiles of the data. All values beyond the 10th and 90th percentiles are graphed individually as points (From King, Seidman, and Leigh[29] p. 569, with permission).

tion have shown similar results.[2] Furthermore, in designing exercises to rehabilitate vestibular patients, strategies should be developed to use head movements that contain these sort of frequencies, which mainly result from transmitted heel-strike. Thus, in thinking about methods to improve vestibular symptoms, we should identify the functional goal for which the patient strives and define physiologic demands that can be made on the vestibular system to achieve that goal.

VERTIGO

Pathophysiology of Vertigo

As distinct from one's perception of self-motion during natural locomotion, vertigo is a distressing, illusory sensation of turning that is linked to impaired perception of a stationary environment. The mismatch between the actual multisensory inputs and the expected pattern of sensory stimulation with the head stationary produces vertigo.[3] While rotational vertigo connotes disturbance of the semicircular canals or their central projections, sensations of body tilt or impulsion (e.g., lateropulsion, levitation) imply otolithic disturbance.

Vertigo should be differentiated from other causes of "dizziness," such as presyncopal faintness, loss of stable balance, light-headedness, or psychologic disorders (such as agoraphobia, acrophobia, or phobic vertigo syndrome).[4] Clearly, accurate identification of symptoms is essential before starting therapies although, in practice, diagnosis is often difficult.[5] Furthermore, even when patients do experience true vertigo, this feeling may not be due to organic disease. So, for example, certain individuals are prone to develop vertigo, unsteadiness, or malaise with motion, at height, or when assuming certain postures.[3]

Besides causing vertigo, sudden loss of tonic neural input from one labyrinth or vestibular nerve causes nystagmus and unsteadiness.[1] The nystagmus is typically mixed horizontal-torsional with slow phases directed toward the side of the lesion. The nystagmus is more marked on looking in the direction of the quick phases, a phenomenon known as Alexander's law. Past-pointing to the side of the lesion reflects imbalance of vestibulo-spinal reactions.[3] Patients with rotational vertigo owing to acute peripheral vestibular lesions are often uncertain as to the direction of their vertiginous illusions. This uncertainty is due to their vestibular sense indicating self-rotation in one direction, but their eye movements (slow phases of vestibular nystagmus) causing visual image movements that, when self-referred, connote self-rotation to the opposite side. It is therefore worthwhile to evaluate the vestibular sense alone by asking specifically about the perceived direction of self-rotation with the eyes closed, thus eliminating any possibly confounding visual stimuli. Although most patients with acute peripheral lesions recover within a month or two, some are left with persistent vestibular symptoms, and others develop benign paroxysmal positional vertigo.

Treatment of Vertigo

In *acute vertigo* owing to a peripheral vestibular lesion, functional recovery is the rule in the ensuing weeks. Recent evidence suggests that drugs that have a "sedative effect" on the vestibular system should only be used for the first 24 hours;[6] examples of some commonly used agents are summarized in Table 9–1. After this period, these drugs should be used sparingly, and patients should be encouraged to get up and increase their activities, as there is evidence that failure to do so will limit the recovery.[7] During this period, a course of specific vestibular exercises may be indicated (see Chapter 14). Those patients who develop enduring vestibular symptoms may have an underlying central nervous system (CNS) disorder, typically of the cerebellum,[8] and imaging studies are indicated. Other patients who complain of persistent symptoms may have either developed a phobic disorder,[4] or have the potential for secondary gain as a consequence of their injury.

TABLE 9–1 Some Commonly Used Vestibular Sedatives

Class of Drugs	Generic Name (Proprietary Name)	Common Side Effects
Antihistamines	Meclizine (Antivert)	Blurred vision, dry mouth, fatigue, sedation
	Promethazine (Phenergan)	Sedation; may cause dystonic reactions
Antidopaminergic	Prochlorperazine (Compazine)	May cause dystonic reactions
	Thiethylperazine (Torecan)	Dry mouth, blurred vision; may cause dystonic reactions
Anticholinergic	Scopolamine	Blurred vision, dry mouth, tachycardia, confusion
GABA-ergic	Diazepam (Valium)	Drowsiness; may become habit-forming
Amphetamines	Dextroamphetamine	May be habit-forming

Treatment of *recurrent vertigo* depends on the nature of the underlying disorder. For example, vertigo owing to migraine (including migraine without a headache) can usually be successfully managed medically. Recurrent vertigo owing to a perilymph fistula usually recovers spontaneously, although some patients require surgical repair (see Chapter 10).

On the other hand, vertigo owing to Ménière's disease is often difficult to manage, although a low-salt diet and diuretics help some patients.[9] Because the vestibular imbalance may be in a continuous state of flux, use of "vestibular sedatives" such as meclizine on a chronic basis is justified in some of these patients. Although systemic aminoglycoside administration to abolish residual vestibular function is now less commonly used in the treatment of Ménière's disease, injection of gentamicin into the middle ear is currently undergoing re-evaluation (Dr. J. M. Nedzelski, University of Toronto, personal communication, 1991).

Central neurologic conditions, such as multiple sclerosis, vertebrobasilar ischemia, and posterior fossa mass lesions, may cause severe, recurrent vertigo. When treatment of the underlying condition does not produce improvement, then "vestibular sedatives" are justified. Often a combination of agents, such as an anticholinergic (e.g., scopolamine) and an antidopaminergic agent (e.g., prochlorperazine) will bring more relief than a single agent.

Benign paroxysmal positional vertigo is effectively treated in most cases by specific vestibular exercises;[10,11] drugs are not indicated in this condition. A small percentage of patients do not improve with exercises, and in them either surgical section of the nerve to, or plugging of, the posterior semicircular canal is effective.[12,13]

OSCILLOPSIA

Pathogenesis of Oscillopsia

Oscillopsia brought on or accentuated by head movement is usually of vestibular origin and reflects an inappropriate VOR gain or phase. Vision becomes blurred so that,

TABLE 9–2 Etiology of Oscillopsia

Oscillopsia with head movements: Abnormal VOR*
  Peripheral vestibular hypofunction:
    Aminoglycoside toxicity
    Surgical section of eighth cranial nerve
    Congenital ear anomalies
    Hereditary vestibular areflexia
    Cisplatin therapy
    Idiopathic
  Central vestibular dysfunction:
    Decreased VOR gain
    Increased VOR gain
    Abnormal VOR phase

Oscillopsia due to nystagmus
  Acquired nystagmus (especially pendular, upbeat, downbeat, see-saw, dissociated nystagmus)
  Saccadic oscillations (psychogenic flutter/voluntary nystagmus, ocular flutter, microsaccadic flutter and opsoclonus)
  Superior oblique myokymia (monocular oscillopsia)
  Congenital nystagmus (uncommon under natural illumination)

Central oscillopsia
  With cerebral disorders: seizures, occipital lobe infarction

Source: From Leigh and Zee.[1]
*VOR = vestibulo-ocular reflex.

for example, fine print on grocery items can only be read if the patient stands still in the store aisle. Oscillopsia is usually caused by excessive motion of images of stationary objects on the retina (Table 9–2). Excessive retinal slip not only causes oscillopsia but also impairs vision. Oscillopsia with head movements may also occur as a result of weakness of an extraocular muscle (e.g., abducens nerve palsy). Oscillopsia owing to nystagmus and other ocular oscillations occurs when the head is stationary.

An abnormal VOR may lead to oscillopsia during head movements in three possible ways: abnormal gain, abnormal phase shift between eye and head rotations, and a directional mismatch between the vectors of the head rotation and eye rotation. Disease of either the vestibular periphery or its central connections may be the cause (see Table 9–2).

Typically, oscillopsia is worse during locomotion but may be noticed during chewing food and, in the severest cases, can occur owing to transmitted cardiac pulsation.[14] In addition, visual acuity declines during head movements, and this loss can be easily demonstrated at the bedside by testing visual acuity first with the patient's head stationary and then while rotating it side to side at 1 to 2 cycles/sec.[1]

Oscillopsia may also occur with disorders of the CNS that change the gain or phase of the VOR.[15,16] Thus, disease of the vestibulocerebellum may cause "vestibular hyperresponsiveness," particularly in the vertical plane. This is common in patients with the Arnold-Chiari malformation[17] and, occasionally, patients are reported with increased gain of both the horizontal and vertical VOR.[18] In some patients with vestibulocerebellar dysfunction, the gain of the VOR is normal, but the phase relationship between head and eye movements is abnormal and causes retinal image slip.[15] Lesions of the medial longitudinal fasciculus (internuclear ophthalmoplegia in multiple sclerosis) may cause a low gain of the vertical VOR[15,16] and produce oscillopsia with vertical head movements.

Treatment of Oscillopsia

With time, compensation takes place in patients with oscillopsia owing to vestibular loss. This compensation is owing to a variety of factors that include potentiation of the cervico-ocular reflex, preprogramming of compensatory eye movements, and perceptual changes.[14,19–21] Thus, drugs have little to offer, and exercises (see Chapter 13) and encouragement of the patient to resume activities such as walking are of key importance. Rarely can oscillopsia owing to a hyperactive VOR be treated pharmacologically.[18]

NYSTAGMUS AND ITS VISUAL CONSEQUENCES

Pathogenesis of Nystagmus

As indicated earlier, acquired nystagmus commonly causes impaired vision and oscillopsia—illusory movement of the environment. These symptoms, which are due to drift of images of stationary objects on the retina, interfere with reading and watching television, and the oscillopsia is often distressing to the patient. The relationship between retinal image velocity and visual acuity is a direct one: image motion in excess of about 4 deg/sec impairs vision. On the other hand, the relationship between retinal image velocity and the development of oscillopsia is less consistent; the magnitude of oscillopsia is usually less than the magnitude of nystagmus. For example, in patients with downbeat nystagmus, oscillopsia is, on average, about one third of the amplitude of the nystagmus. This latter finding suggests that the brain compensates for the excessive retinal image motion by monitoring an internal ("efference") copy of the eye movement signal, and so partly maintains visual constancy. Nevertheless, if retinal image drift in patients with nystagmus can be reduced below about 5 deg/sec, then oscillopsia is usually abolished and vision is improved.[22]

Treatment of Nystagmus

Of the various drugs reported to suppress nystagmus (Table 9–3), only a few reliably improve symptoms. Baclofen is usually effective in treating acquired periodic alternating nystagmus (PAN). Acquired PAN is a spontaneous horizontal nystagmus, present in primary gaze, that reverses its direction approximately every 2 minutes.[1] Acquired PAN has been reported in association with a variety of conditions, many of which involve the cerebellum. Experimental ablation of the nodulus and uvula of the cerebellum in monkeys causes PAN when they are put into darkness; baclofen abolishes this nystagmus. Although baclofen has been tried in a variety of other forms of nystagmus, its effect is unreliable.

A second drug that usually reduces nystagmus is acetazolamide in the rare syndrome of familial periodic ataxia with nystagmus. Other reports of drug treatments of nystagmus mainly concern success in one or two individuals. Clonazepam has been reported to be useful in the treatment of downbeat nystagmus.[23] Isoniazid has been reported to suppress acquired nystagmus in some patients.[24]

Reports of controlled trials of drugs in the treatment of nystagmus are rare. However, we have recently conducted a randomized, double-blind crossover trial of two *anticholinergic agents,* trihexyphenidyl (Artane), and tridihexethyl chloride (Pathilon, a

TABLE 9–3 Treatments for Nystagmus and Its Visual Consequences

Drugs	Optical Devices	Invasive Procedures
Baclofen	Base-out prisms	Operative treatment of Arnold-
Acetazolamide	Other prism arrangements	Chiari malformation
Clonazepam	Spectacle lens–contact lens	Botulinum toxin
Isoniazid	combination (for retinal image	
Trihexyphenidyl	stabilization)	
Valproic acid		
Carbamazepine		
Barbiturates		
Alcohol		

quarternary anticholinergic that does not cross the blood–brain barrier) in patients with acquired nystagmus.[25] We measured visual acuity and nystagmus before and at the end of 1 month on each of these medications. We found that trihexyphenidyl is not a reliable treatment for acquired nystagmus, although occasional patients may benefit. Furthermore, the side effects of anticholinergic agents limit their effectiveness in the treatment of nystagmus.

A number of optical devices have been suggested for treatment of nystagmus. Patients whose nystagmus suppresses with convergence may benefit by wearing base-out prisms.[26] In some patients, acquired nystagmus may be less prominent in one gaze angle (e.g., upgaze for some cases of downbeat nystagmus); in these individuals, prisms that turn the eyes toward the gaze direction of least nystagmus may be useful.

Another approach has been the development of an optical system to stabilize images on the retina during eye movements.[22,27] This system consists of a high-plus spectacle lens worn in combination with a high-minus contact lens (Fig. 9–2). Stabilization can be achieved if the power of the spectacle lens focuses the primary image close to the center of rotation of the eye. A contact lens is then required to extend back the focus onto the retina. Because the contact lens moves with the eye, it does not negate the effect of retinal image stabilization produced by the spectacle lens. With such a system, it is possible to achieve up to about 90 percent stabilization of images on the retina. This system has the disadvantage of disabling the VOR (so causing oscillopsia during head movements) and voluntary eye movements.

We have attempted to treat 10 patients with nystagmus with the optical stabilization device. In practice, only two patients were able to persevere for more than a few months, and none for more than a year. One reason was that the hard contact lens is not well tolerated. Recently, however, we have been able to develop a gas-permeable contact lens of powers up to −58 diopters that is more comfortable for patients to wear.

Invasive procedures, such as the Kestenbaum operation, which effectively treats certain patients with congenital nystagmus, are of uncertain value in the treatment of acquired forms of nystagmus.[1] Neurosurgery does have a clear role in the therapy of the Arnold-Chiari syndrome; suboccipital decompression is reported to improve downbeat nystagmus and to prevent progression of other neurologic deficits. Attempts to stop the eyes from moving, either by detaching the extraocular muscles or by injecting them with botulinum toxin,[28] are measures that may help in some cases, but they require further evaluation.

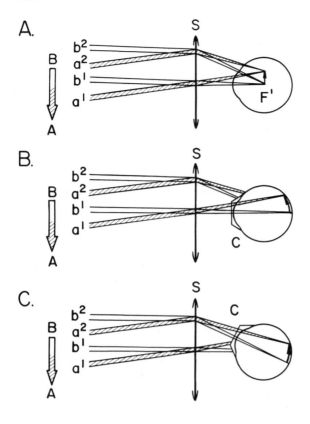

FIGURE 9–2. An optical method for stabilizing images of stationary objects on the retina. (*A*) When viewing a distant object, AB, a convergent spectacle lens, S, will focus rays of light (b¹, b²) from a point of interest B, on its focal point F¹, which is close to the center of rotation of the globe. Thus, if the eyeball were to rotate, light rays from point B would remain focused at the same point as in the eye. (*B*) A strongly divergent contact lens, C, extends back the focus from the center of the globe to the retina. (*C*) Because the contact lens moves with the eye, it does not negate the effect of retinal image stabilization produced by the spectacle lens, and rays of light from point B remain focused on the foveal region of the retina. (From Leigh et al,[22] p 124, with permission).

SUMMARY

Disruption of the vestibular system often results in vertigo, oscillopsia, and nystagmus. Acute vertigo from peripheral vestibular lesions usually recovers spontaneously, and vestibular suppressant medications, although appropriate during the first 24 hours, should be used sparingly after that initial period. The use of medications in recurrent vertigo is dependent on the specific disorder affecting the vestibular system. As with acute vertigo, oscillopsia usually recovers spontaneously, and medications do not help the recovery. In contrast, medications such as baclofen, acetazolamide, and clonazepam may occasionally reduce nystagmus. Several different optical devices have also been developed for the treatment of various types of nystagmus. We must remember, however, that none of these medications or optical devices can be applied uniformly to all patients, and careful diagnosis of the problem must be made before one of these treatments is attempted.

ACKNOWLEDGMENTS

Supported by USPHS grant EY06717, the Department of Veterans Affairs, and the Evenor Armington Fund.

REFERENCES

1. Leigh, RJ and Zee, DS: The Neurology of Eye Movements, ed 2. FA Davis, Philadelphia, 1991.
2. Pozza T, Berthoz A, and Lefort, L: Head stabilization during various locomotor tasks in humans. I. Normal subjects. Exp Brain Res 82:97, 1990.
3. Brandt, T and Daroff, RB: The multisensory physiological and pathological vertigo syndromes. Ann Neurol 7:195, 1980.
4. Brandt, T and Dieterich, M: Phobic postural vertigo attacks: New syndrome. München Med Wochenschr 128:247, 1986.
5. Nedzelski, JM, Barber, HO, and McIlmoyl, L: Diagnoses in a dizziness unit. J Otolaryngol 15:101, 1986.
6. Leigh, RJ and Zee, DS: Episodic vertigo. In Rakel, RE (ed): Conn's Current Therapy. WB Saunders, Philadelphia, 1984, p 722.
7. Zee, DS: Perspectives on the pharmacotherapy of vertigo. Arch Otolaryngol 111:609, 1985.
8. Rudge, R and Chambers, BR: Physiological basis for enduring vestibular symptoms. J Neurol Neurosurg Psychiatry 45:126, 1982.
9. Zee, DS: The management of patients with vestibular disorders. In Barber, HO and Sharpe, JA (eds): Vestibular Disorders. Year Book, Chicago, 1988, p 254.
10. Brandt, T and Daroff, RB: Physical therapy for benign paroxysmal positional vertigo. Arch Otolaryngol 106:484, 1980.
11. Semont, A, Freyss, G, and Vitte, E: Curing the BPPV with a liberatory maneuver. Adv Oto-Rhino-Layrng 42:290, 1988.
12. Gacek, RR: Pathophysiology and management of cupulolithiasis. Am J Otolaryngol 6:66, 1985.
13. Parnes, LS and McClure, JA: Posterior semicircular canal occlusion for intractable benign paraoxysmal positional vertigo. Ann Otol Rhinol Laryngol 99:330, 1990.
14. JC: Living without a balancing mechanism. N Engl J Med 246:458, 1952.
15. Gresty, MA, Hess, K, and Leech, J: Disorders of the vestibulo-ocular reflex producing oscillopsia and mechanisms compensating for loss of labyrinthine function. Brain 100:693, 1977.
16. Ranalli, PJ and Sharpe, JA: Vertical vestibulo-ocular reflex, smooth pursuit and eye-head tracking dysfunction in internuclear ophthalmoplegia. Brain 111:1299, 1988.
17. Zee, DS, Friendlich, AR, and Robinson, DA: The mechanism of downbeat nystagmus. Arch Neurol 30:227, 1974.
18. Thurston, SE, et al: Hyperactive vestibulo-ocular reflex in cerebellar degeneration: Pathogenesis and treatment. Neurology 37:53, 1987.
19. Bronstein, AM and Hood, JD: The cervico-ocular reflex in normal subjects and patients with absent vestibular function. Brain Res 373:399, 1986.
20. Bronstein, AM and Hood, JD: Oscillopsia of peripheral vestibular origin. Acta Otolaryngol (Stockh) 104:307, 1987.
21. Kasai, T and Zee, DS: Eye-head coordination in labyrinthine-defective human beings. Brain Res 144:123, 1978.
22. Leigh RJ, et al: Effects of retinal image stabilization on acquired nystagmus due to neurological disease. Neurology 38:122, 1988.
23. Currie, JN and Matsuo, V: The use of clonazepam in the treatment of nystagmus-induced oscillopsia. Ophthalmology 93:924, 1986.
24. Traccis, S, et al: Successful treatment of acquired pendular elliptical nystagmus in multiple sclerosis with isoniazid and base-out prisms. Neurology 40:492, 1990.
25. Leigh, RJ, et al: The effect of anticholinergic agents upon acquired nystagmus: A double-blind study of trihexyphenidyl and tridihexethyl chloride. Neurology 41:1737, 1991.
26. Lavin, PJM, et al: Downbeat nystagmus with a pseudocycloid waveform: Improvement with base-out prisms. Ann Neurol 13:621, 1983.
27. Rushton, D and Cox, N: A new optical treatment for oscillopsia. J Neurol Neurosurg Psychiatry 50:411, 1987.
28. Leigh, RJ, et al: Effectiveness of botulinum toxin administered to abolish acquired nystagmus. Ann Neurol 32:633, 1992.
29. King, OS, Seidman, SH and Leigh, RJ: Control of head stability and gaze during locomotion in normal subjects and patients with deficient vestibular function. In Berthoz, A, Graf, W, and Vidal, PP (eds): Second Symposium on Head-Neck Sensory-Motor System. Oxford University Press, New York, 1991.

CHAPTER 10

Surgical Management of Vestibular Disorders

Douglas E. Mattox, MD

The diagnosis of vestibular disorders is complicated by overlapping symptoms among the various disorders and the lack of pathognomonic diagnostic tests. At times, it may even be difficult to determine which inner ear is causing the symptoms. Most patients' symptoms can be managed with the medical and physical therapy measures described elsewhere in this book. However, surgical intervention may be appropriate when the symptoms have failed to respond to aggressive nonsurgical medical management.

With the exception of acoustic tumors, vestibular disorders are a matter of life-style and comfort and are not life-threatening. Therefore, the patient who lives with the symptoms must make the decision whether or not to proceed with surgery. The physician should discuss the likelihood of a successful outcome, as well as the nature of potential complications, and leave the ultimate decision up to the patient. In the author's experience, patients have a broad spectrum of responses to their symptoms of vertigo. Some want immediate intervention, but others will consider surgery only when life becomes unbearable.

ACOUSTIC NEUROMAS (VESTIBULAR SCHWANNOMA)

Acoustic neuromas are nerve sheath tumors occurring in the internal auditory canal or cerebellopontine angle.[1] They are the third most common intracranial tumor and account for 8 to 10 percent of all intracranial tumors. Most patients with acoustic neuromas present with progressive unilateral sensorineural hearing loss. However, some patients first complain of vestibular symptoms or sudden hearing loss.[2]

An acoustic neuroma should be suspected in any patient with an unexplained unilateral sensorineural hearing loss, particularly if the patient has abnormal brain-stem auditory responses or hypoactive (or absent) caloric responses. Magnetic resonance imaging (MRI) with gadolinium contrast has become the gold standard for the diagnosis of these tumors. Although there are rare instances of false-positive scans, usually arachnoiditis or arachnoid cysts, an enhancing mass in the cerebellopontine angle extending into the internal auditory meatus is almost always an acoustic neuroma.

Once the diagnosis is established there are three therapeutic options: watchful waiting, radiosurgery, and surgical removal. Watchful waiting is indicated only for patients with very small intracanalicular tumors in which the diagnosis is inconclusive and for patients who are elderly or in poor medical condition. Scans should be repeated at 6- to 12-month intervals and treatment planned if the lesion grows.

Radiosurgery is a new modality whose role in the treatment of acoustic neuromas is still being investigated.[3,4] A single treatment of high-dose irradiation is administered by stereotactically focusing multiple radiation sources on the tumor. Because the radiation beams come from many different angles, an extremely high radiation dose is delivered to the tumor where the beams intersect. With proper geometric planning, the surrounding neural and vascular structures are spared from the high dose of radiation.

The initial results of radiosurgery are encouraging. Tumor control is achieved in 70 to 80 percent of patients, and the procedure has a low incidence of complications, especially facial paralysis.[3,4] The vascular supply to the cochlea is not spared, however, and approximately 60 percent of patients develop hearing loss.[3] It is an ideal treatment for recurrent tumors and for patients whose medical problems make them a poor surgical risk. Radiosurgery is currently available in a very limited number of centers but no doubt will develop wider use as availability of the devices increases.

Surgical removal of acoustic tumors has been the treatment of choice since it was described by Harvey Cushing in 1917.[5] Three basic approaches are used for removal of acoustic neuromas: (1) middle fossa craniotomy, (2) translabyrinthine approach, and (3) suboccipital craniotomy.[6,7] The choice of the approach is based on the size and location of the tumor and whether any attempt will be made to preserve hearing.[6,7]

Middle Cranial Fossa

The middle cranial fossa approach is used for tumors confined to the internal auditory canal in patients who have usable hearing. A vertical incision is made in the scalp superior to the external auditory canal (Fig. 10–1). The soft tissues are elevated from the bone and a 3- × 4-cm temporal craniotomy is performed. The dura and temporal lobe are elevated from the floor of the middle cranial fossa. The internal auditory canal is identified by drilling the bone overlying it. The facial nerve, mastoid air-cell system, and superior semicircular canal are important landmarks. The bone is thinned over the entire extent of the internal auditory canal, and then the dura of the canal is incised. Care is taken not to damage the facial nerve in the anterior-superior quadrant of the internal auditory canal. The cochlear nerve is anterior-inferior in the canal and is safely out of harm's way.

The advantage of the middle cranial fossa approach is that the inner ear and hearing are not destroyed. Care must be taken to avoid damaging the facial nerve because it is superficial in the internal auditory canal. It is extremely difficult to manage tumors that extend through the porus acusticus into the posterior fossa through the middle cranial fossa approach. This procedure, therefore, is indicated only for tumors limited to the internal auditory canal.

Recovery after middle fossa craniotomy is prompt. Unless the patient has significant

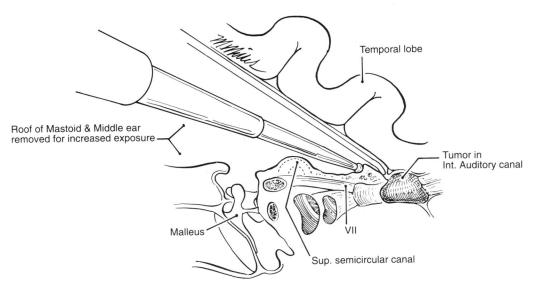

FIGURE 10-1. Middle fossa. This coronal section through the internal auditory canal and middle ear shows the exposure of the internal auditory canal through the middle fossa. A drill is shown passing through a small temporal craniotomy. The temporal lobe is elevated extradurally. The superior semicircular canal is identified and the internal auditory canal exposed by removing the bone over the auditory canal medial to the superior semicircular canal.

vestibular symptoms, he or she should be up and about the next day. Cerebrospinal fluid (CSF) leakage is unlikely, but the patient should be checked for both external leak and a leak down the eustachian tube into the nasopharynx after this and all the other approaches described in this section.

Translabyrinthine Approach

The translabyrinthine approach is the procedure of choice for tumors up to 2.5 cm in diameter when hearing preservation is not a consideration. The tumor is approached similarly to a standard mastoidectomy (Fig. 10-2). The cortical and pneumatized bone of the mastoid are drilled away to expose the sigmoid sinus, posterior fossa dura, and middle fossa dura. The facial nerve is protected by identifying it within the bony canal. A complete labyrinthectomy is performed to expose the internal auditory canal. Once the intracanalicular portion of the tumor is mobilized, the dura of the posterior fossa is incised and the remainder of the tumor is removed.

Recovery after translabyrinthine removal of acoustic tumors is generally prompt, and patients can be out of bed in 2 to 3 days. This rapid recovery is attributable to the lack of pressure or retraction of the cerebellum during the procedure. The disadvantage of the translabyrinthine approach is that it automatically sacrifices hearing. The exposure is excellent for small and medium-sized tumors but is inadequate for tumors larger than 2.5 cm in diameter and those that are adherent to the brain stem. The ideal case for translabyrinthine removal has a clear separation between the tumor and the brain stem on computed tomography or magnetic resonance imaging.

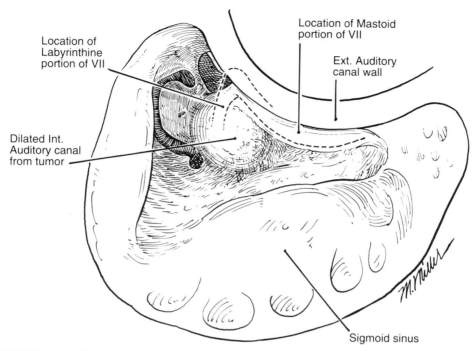

FIGURE 10–2. Translabyrinthine approach for removal of acoustic neuroma. A translabyrinthine approach to the internal auditory canal is shown in surgical position with anterior at the top and superior to the left of the drawing. The tumor is exposed after completion of a labyrinthectomy (see Fig. 10–5). The internal auditory canal has been dilated by the tumor. Removal of the last shell of bone over the tumor as well as the bone from the posterior fossa will allow complete tumor removal.

Suboccipital Craniectomy

Suboccipital craniectomy gives the best exposure when the tumor is large or adherent to the brain stem. In rare cases in which there is good hearing preoperatively, the suboccipital approach offers the possibility of preserving hearing. Maintenance of hearing requires the preservation of both the cochlear nerve and the fragile capillary blood supply of the inner ear. Hearing can be spared in a third to half of the patients in whom it is attempted.[8]

The suboccipital craniectomy differs from the translabyrinthine approach in that the angle of the approach is from behind rather than in front of the sigmoid sinus (Fig. 10–3). The incision is placed 5 to 6 cm behind the ear and a 5-cm piece of the occipital skull is removed. This defect is reconstructed with prosthetic mesh at the end of the procedure. The cerebellum lies between the craniotomy and the cerebellopontine angle; however, the surgery is done in the lateral position and this allows cerebellum to fall away by itself without additional retraction.

After the tumor is identified, the capsule of the tumor is incised and the central core of the tumor is removed with an ultrasonic aspirator or laser. After the tumor has been decompressed, the portion of the tumor within the internal auditory canal is removed by drilling away the posterior surface of the canal. The facial nerve is identified in the fundus of the internal auditory canal where its anatomy is constant. The tumor is

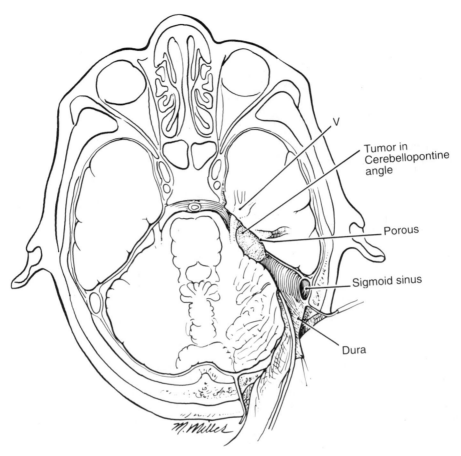

V

Tumor in
Cerebellopontine
angle

Porous

Sigmoid sinus

Dura

FIGURE 10–3. Suboccipital craniectomy. This axial section demonstrates a posterior fossa craniotomy behind the sigmoid sinus. The cerebellum drops away from the posterior surface of the temporal bone. The tumor is exposed in the cerebellopontine angle. The posterior lip of the internal auditory canal must be drilled away to remove the tumor extending into the canal.

mobilized and removed from the brain stem, and the seventh nerve is identified and preserved medial to the tumor.

Recovery time after a suboccipital craniotomy is slower than from the other two approaches because of the magnitude of the procedure, but patients are usually ready for discharge from the hospital within a week. Occasionally, a patient will develop a postcraniotomy headache that requires long-term pain management.

Complications after an acoustic neuroma surgery are relatively uncommon. Hearing loss always occurs in translabyrinthine procedures and is common after suboccipital removal of tumors greater than 1.5 cm. Transient facial paralysis is common with larger tumors. Permanent facial paralysis is seen in fewer than 5 percent of patients. CSF leaks can occur postoperatively. These are usually transient and rarely require secondary surgical correction.

MÉNIÈRE'S DISEASE

Although the underlying cause of Ménière's disease is unknown, a consistent histopathologic finding is hydrops (dilation) of the endolymphatic spaces.[9] The hydrops presumably results from a malfunction of the resorptive function of the endolymphatic sac. The classic constellation of symptoms includes fluctuating hearing loss, episodic vertigo, tinnitus, and a sensation of fullness in the ear.[10] These symptoms, however, do not necessarily develop simultaneously, and many patients do not develop them all. Subcategories of Ménière's disease describe these other conditions, for instance, cochlear hydrops (fluctuating hearing loss alone) or vestibular hydrops (vestibular symptoms without hearing loss).[10]

In most patients, Ménière's disease is ultimately self-limited; over time, the patient suffers deterioration of hearing and a gradual subsiding of the episodic dizzy spells. This evolution, however, may require one or two decades. In the interim, the patient's life-style may be severely impaired.

Medical therapy of Ménière's disease rests on avoiding things known to exacerbate the symptoms: stress, caffeine, alcohol, nicotine, and foods with a high salt content. Diuretics and vestibular suppressant drugs are usually prescribed. This regimen, known as the Furstenberg regimen, can adequately control the symptoms in up to three quarters of patients.[11] A few patients, however, cannot be adequately managed by medical means alone, and surgical intervention must be considered. The surgical procedures for Ménière's disease may be categorized as those designed to improve the function of the endolymphatic sac and those that ablate the vestibular system either with or without preservation of hearing.

Endolymphatic sac procedures attempt to re-establish the function of the sac as the resorptive organ for the endolymph of the inner ear by draining the excess endolymphatic sac into the mastoid cavity.[12] A standard postauricular mastoidectomy is performed, and the sigmoid sinus, mastoid antrum and incus, facial nerve, and lateral and posterior semicircular canals are identified. The endolymphatic sac is found between the posterior surface of the temporal bone and the dura of the posterior fossa. The bone is thinned until the dura and the sac are identifiable through the last layer of bone. This bone is picked away to expose the dura and the overlying endolymphatic sac. The sac is opened, and Silastic sheeting or other shunt device is inserted into the lumen of the endolymphatic sac and allowed to drape into the mastoid cavity. Care must be taken to open the endolymphatic sac without puncturing the underlying dura, which could result in a CSF leak. Any endolymph drained by the shunt is resorbed by the mucous membranes of the mastoid cavity.

It is almost an understatement to say that endolymphatic sac surgery is controversial. The fluid spaces involved are minuscule, and it is doubtful if mechanical means can improve function of the sac. In a clinical trial, similar results were obtained with real and sham operations.[13] Nonetheless, the procedure controls the vertiginous attacks in half to two thirds of patients, and the procedure has the advantage of relative ease and safety.

Although they are more complex procedures, control of vertigo is predictable and reliable in 90 to 95 percent of patients with either vestibular neurectomy or labyrinthectomy. These procedures should completely relieve the vertiginous attacks because vestibular input from that ear is completely eliminated. The loss of all vestibular function on one side can easily be compensated by an intact labyrinth on the opposite side.

When the hearing is worth preserving (ability to detect speech, known as speech reception threshold, is better than 60 dB, and the ability to understand speech, or discrimination score, is better than 50 percent) a vestibular neurectomy through either the middle cranial fossa or retrolabyrinthine space is the procedure of choice.

The middle cranial fossa approach is the same as described above for acoustic tumors. Once the internal auditory canal has been identified and exposed, it can be opened and the superior and inferior vestibular nerves divided.

The vestibular nerve can also be sectioned using either a retrolabyrinthine or retrosigmoid (suboccipital) approach. In the retrolabyrinthine approach, a complete mastoidectomy is performed as described for the endolymphatic sac procedure.[14] In addition, all of the bone medial to the sigmoid sinus is removed to expose the posterior fossa dura. The dura is opened to expose the cerebellopontine angle (Fig. 10–4). The vestibular and auditory branches of the eighth nerve are directly in the field of view, and the vestibular nerve is divided. A disadvantage of this approach is that the auditory and vestibular portions of the eighth nerve are fused as they exit the brain stem and may not have separated before they enter the internal auditory canal. Some surgeons have advocated a retrosigmoid approach in order to drill away the posterior lip of the internal auditory canal. This permits identification of the vestibular nerve after it has separated from the auditory nerve.[15]

If hearing preservation is not a goal, for instance, in cases of unilateral Ménière's disease with severely impaired hearing or discrimination, a labyrinthectomy is the most effective treatment. Labyrinthectomy can be performed either through the external auditory canal or through the mastoid. In the transcanal approach, the tympanic mem-

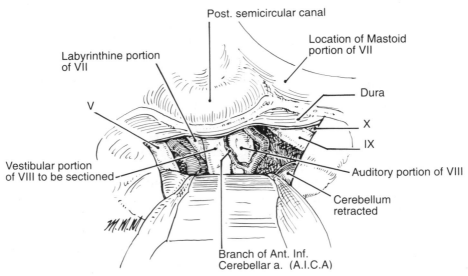

FIGURE 10–4. Retrolabyrinthine vestibular nerve section. This surgeon's view of a right ear in surgical position (anterior — *top;* superior — *left*) shows the exposure for a retrolabyrinthine nerve section. The cerebellopontine angle is exposed by removing the posterior surface of the temporal bone between the sigmoid sinus and the posterior semicircular canal. The dura is opened, and the seventh and eighth nerves are identified. The demarkation between the vestibular and auditory portions of the nerve is usually marked by a small branch of AICA. The vestibular portion of the eighth nerve (superior half) is divided.

brane is elevated to expose the middle ear. The stapes is removed and the vestibule is opened between the oval and round windows. The saccule, utricle, and ampullae of the superior, lateral, and posterior semicircular canals are removed with an angled pick. Reaching the ampulla of the posterior semicircular canal is a blind maneuver and may leave neuroepithelium behind. For this reason, this author prefers the transmastoid approach.

A standard mastoidectomy is performed, and all three semicircular canals are identified. Each one in turn is drilled away and the neuroepithelium identified under direct vision and removed. The three semicircular canals lead to the vestibule where once again the saccule and utricle are removed (Fig. 10–5).

Recently there have been reports of attempts to selectively destroy the vestibular epithelium perfusing the lateral semicircular canal with streptomycin.[16] Although the initial reports were encouraging, subsequent multicenter studies have noted an unacceptably high incidence of sensorineural hearing loss.[17]

It is implicit in all of the procedures described above that the disease is unilateral, or if bilateral, the side producing the majority of symptoms can be determined. Surgical procedures, however, are seldom, if ever, indicated in patients who have active bilateral disease. These patients are extremely difficult to treat, but some hope can be offered these patients with systemically administered streptomycin. Streptomycin is preferentially toxic to the vestibular portion of the inner ear and if given systemically will produce a bilateral chemical labyrinthectomy. Patients are given streptomycin, 1 g twice a day intramuscularly, until the vertigo subsides, usually about 10 days. The patient is left the side effects of bilateral vestibular loss, including difficulty walking in the dark and inability to keep the eyes fixed on a target during head movements (oscillopsia).[18]

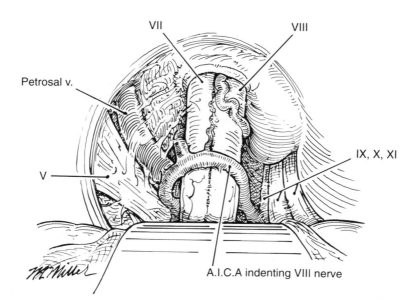

FIGURE 10–5. Labyrinthectomy. A transmastoid labyrinthectomy of the right ear (anterior— *top*; superior—*left*). The three semicircular canals have been identified, and the lateral and posterior canals have been partially opened. The canals will be completely removed, and the vestibule will be opened to remove all neuroepithelium.

POSTTRAUMATIC VERTIGO

Posttraumatic vertigo is managed in an identical manner to Ménière's disease with either a hearing-preserving or hearing-sacrificing form of vestibular ablation. Most authors, however, report less reliable control of recurrent attacks of dizziness.[19] The reasons for these results are unknown.

BENIGN PAROXYSMAL POSITIONAL VERTIGO

Unlike patients with Ménière's disease who develop spontaneous episodes of dizziness, those suffering with benign paroxysmal positional vertigo (BPPV) develop transient symptoms only when they assume certain positions.[10] The most common position is in a lateral or head-hanging position with the diseased ear undermost. The symptoms generally have a few seconds latency before onset, develop in a crescendo-decrescendo pattern, demonstrate torsional nystagmus, and habituate on repeated trials. The site of the pathology is generally thought to be in the posterior semicircular canal. Schuknecht[9] has described debris on the cupula of the posterior semicircular canal, and he has given the condition the name *cupulolithiasis*. It seems probable that the symptoms could arise from dislodged otoconia floating in the posterior semicircular canal as well from those physically attached to the cupula.

BPPV is frequently a self-limiting condition that resolves regardless of what treatment is given.[10] A number of different physical therapy measures have been designed to dislodge the otoconia from the posterior semicircular canal. These measures are effective in the vast majority of patients (see Chapter 16).

Rarely will a patient have persistent symptoms despite physical therapy intervention and the passage of time. In such a case, two surgical procedures can be considered. The first is singular neurectomy; division of the branch of the vestibular nerve to the posterior semicircular canal.[20] This is a technically difficult procedure and has only been described by a few centers. The singular nerve passes just medial to the round window niche before it enters the ampulla of the posterior canal. The lip of the round window is drilled away, but the round window membrane must not be violated. Bone is removed posterior and inferior to the round window membrane with tiny diamond spurs to expose the singular canal. The canal is opened and the nerve avulsed.

Surgical blockade of the flow of endolymph in the posterior semicircular canal has been described recently.[21] In this procedure, the bony posterior semicircular canal is opened without violating the membranous labyrinth. Flow within the membranous labyrinth is blocked by occluding the bony and membranous canals with a bone plug.

Only limited reports of the postoperative course after singular neurectomy and blockage of the posterior semicircular canal appear in the literature. In most cases, it appears that amelioration of symptoms is prompt after these procedures.

PERILYMPH FISTULA

Perilymph fistula is a direct communication between the inner ear and the middle ear, usually through the round or oval windows.[22] Such leaks were initially described in association with barotrauma; however, spontaneous leaks are being described with increasing frequency. The symptoms of perilymph leak include hearing loss, usually sudden or episodic; vertigo associated with the hearing loss; and more recently patients have been described with generalized spacial disorientation and normal hearing. The diagnosis of perilymph fistula, and the indications and timing of surgery, are some of the most controversial subjects in the otologic literature. To date there are no preoperative diagnostic tests that definitively confirm or exclude the presence of a perilymph fistula. Even on surgical exploration there may be disagreements among observers as to the presence or absence of a fluid leak. Biochemical and fluorescent tracer studies as well as protein analyses are being developed as potential markers for the presence or absence of the perilymph fistula.[23]

The middle ear exploration for perilymph fistula is straightforward. The middle ear is approached through the external auditory canal, and the tympanic membrane is elevated (Fig. 10–6). Both the oval and round windows are carefully observed for the repeated accumulation of fluid. The leak may become more obvious with a Valsalva maneuver (increased intrathoracic pressure against a closed glottis). The leak is repaired with autogenous tissue. It is generally believed that the patient should remain at bed rest

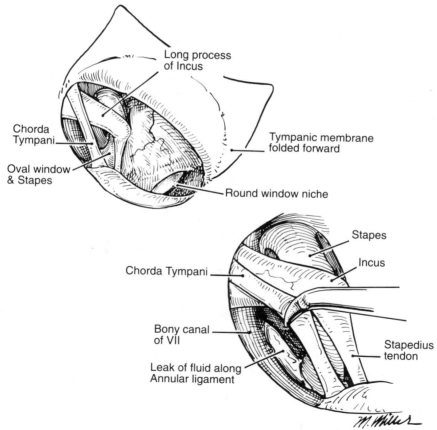

FIGURE 10–6. Perilymphatic fistula. A right middle ear exploration for perilymph fistula is shown in the surgical position (anterior—*top*; superior—*right*). The tympanic membrane has been reflected forward to expose the oval and round windows. Close inspection of the annular ligament of the oval window demonstrates a leak of perilymph. This will be closed with an autologous tissue graft.

for some time after closure of perilymph fistula in order to allow the graft to heal in place.[22]

In most cases, the patient feels better shortly after repair of a perilymph fistula. Patients with persistent symptoms present the physician with the difficult dilemma of deciding if the repair has failed or if the diagnosis was wrong in the first place.

VASCULAR LOOPS

Vascular loops are elongated or tortuous vessels (arteries or veins) within the intracranial cavity that are thought to press on nerve roots as they exit from the brain stem. The first well-described vascular syndrome was hemifacial spasm, an uncontrollable twitching of one side of the face. This was found by Janetta and associates[24] to be caused by an abnormal vessel pressing on the root-entry zone of the facial nerve. This concept has been expanded to include vestibular and auditory disorders.[25] The significance of these vascular loops is difficult to determine because the symptoms overlap over diagnostic categories, including Ménière's disease and perilymph fistula. Furthermore, tortuous vessels are common in the cerebellopontine angle of normal individuals, especially after middle age. Nonetheless, there are documented cases of vessels impinging on nerves causing abnormal stretching or displacement. It has been suggested that radiologic confirmation can be obtained with the combination of high-resolution CT with intravenous and air contrast.

Microvascular loop decompression is performed through a standard posterior craniectomy (Fig. 10–7). The offending artery or vein is carefully dissected from the nerve, and a small piece of muscle or Teflon sponge is interposed to keep the vessel from pressing on the nerve.

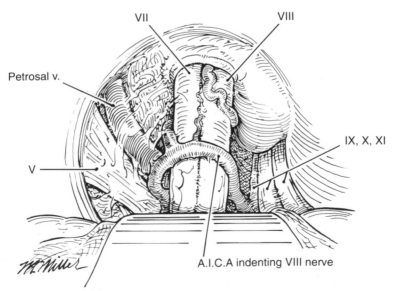

FIGURE 10–7. Retrolabyrinthine exposure of vascular compression. The exposure is the same as shown in Figure 10–4. The AICA is seen compressing the eighth nerve. This is treated by carefully elevating the vessel and interposing muscle or sponge material between the vessel and the nerve.

SUMMARY

The development of surgical intervention for vertigo is a fascinating and challenging branch of neurotology. Unfortunately, at the moment most of the procedures used are ablative rather than restorative. Future developments in this field will be directed toward the rehabilitation and functional restoration of the diseased inner ear.

REFERENCES

1. Nager, GT: Acoustic neurinomas. Acta Otolaryngol (Stockh) 99:245, 1985.
2. Thomsen, J, Terkildsen, K, and Tos, M: Acoustic neuromas: Progression of hearing impairment and function of the eigthth cranial nerve. Am J Otol 5:20, 1983.
3. Yamamoto, M and Noren, G: Stereotactic radiosurgery in acoustic neurinomas. No Shinkei Geka 18:1101, 1990.
4. Flickinger, JC, et al: Radiosurgery of acoustic neurinomas. Cancer 67:345, 1990.
5. Cushing, H: Tumors of the Nervus Acusticus and the Syndrome of the Cerebellopontine Angle. WB Saunders, Philadelphia, 1917.
6. Fisch, U and Mattox, DE: Microsurgery of the Skull Base. Thieme Medical Publishers, New York, 1988.
7. Brackmann, DE: A review of acoustic tumors: 1979–1982. Am J Otol 5:233, 1984.
8. Harner, SG, Laws, ER, and Onofrio, BM: Hearing preservation after removal of acoustic neurinoma. Laryngoscope. 94:1431, 1984.
9. Schuknecht, HR: Pathology of the Ear. Harvard University Press, Cambridge, Mass., 1974.
10. Paparella, MM, et al: Ménière's disease and other labyrinthine diseases. In Paparella, MM, (eds): Otolaryngology. WB Saunders, Philadelphia, 1991, p 1689.
11. Boles, R, et al: Conservative management of Ménière's disease; Furstenberg regimen revisited. Ann Otol 84:513, 1975.
12. Arenerg, IK: The fine points of valve implant surgery for hydrops: An update. Am J Otol 3:359, 1982.
13. Thomsen J, et al: Placebo effect in surgery for Ménière's disease. Arch Otolaryngol 107:271, 1981.
14. Silverstein, H and Norrell, H: Retrolabyrinthine vestibular neurectomy. Otolaryngol Head Neck Surg 90:778, 1982.
15. Silverstein, H, et al: Combined retrolab-retrosigmoid vestibular nerve neurectomy: An evolution in approach. Am J Otol 10:166, 1989.
16. Shea, JJ: Perfusion of the inner ear with streptomycin. Am J Otol 10:150, 1989.
17. Monsell, EM and Shelton, C: Labyrinthotomy with streptomycin infusion: Early results of a multicenter group. The LSI Multicenter Study Group. Am J Otol 13:416–422, 1992.
18. Schuknecht, HF: Ablation therapy in the management of Ménière's disease. Acta Otolaryngol (Stockh) (suppl): 132, 1975.
19. Kemink, JL, et al: Retrolabyrinthine vestibular nerve section: Efficacy in disorders other than Ménière's disease. Laryngoscope. 101:523, 1991.
20. Gacek, RR: Singular neurectomy update. Ann Otol Rhinol Laryngol 91:469, 1982.
21. Parnes, LS and McClure, JA: Posterior semicircular canal occlusion for intractable benign paroxysmal positional vertigo. Ann Otol Rhinol Laryngol 99:330, 1990.
22. Mattox, DE: Perilymph fistulas. In Cummings, CWC, et al (eds): Otolaryngology, Head and Neck Surgery, CV Mosby, St. Louis, 1986, p 3113.
23. Paugh, DR, Telian, SA, and Disher, MJ: Identification of perilymph proteins by two-dimensional gel electrophoresis. Otolaryngol Head Neck Surg 104:517, 1991.
24. Janetta, PJ, et al: Etiology and definitive microsurgical treatment of hemifacial spasm. J. Neurosurg 47:321, 1977.
25. Janetta, PJ: Neurovascular cross-compensation of the eighth cranial nerve in patients with vertigo and tinnitus. In Sammi, M and Janetta, PJ (eds): The Cranial Nerves. Springer-Verlag, New York, 1981, p 552.

CHAPTER 11

Assessment and Management of Central Vestibular Disorders

James A. Sharpe, MD, FRCPC

Damage to central vestibular projections that subserve the vestibulo-ocular reflex (VOR), vestibulospinal reflexes, and vestibular projections to cerebral cortex cause a variety of symptoms ranging from sensations of rotation of oneself or the environment, to oscillopsia, to vague feelings of imbalance. The central VOR refers to the vestibular nuclei and their projections to the ocular motor nuclei, as opposed to the peripheral input to the reflex from the labyrinth and the vestibular nerve. The cardinal symptoms and signs of disorders of the reflex are vertigo and nystagmus. Vestibular nystagmus results from central or peripheral lesions that imbalance the VOR. Slow phases are directed toward the side of the intact VOR pathway, but the direction of nystagmus is named according to the direction of the quick phase, that is, toward the side of the damaged pathway. Because disease processes that involve the brain stem or cerebellum such as infarction, hemorrhage, tumor, or demyelination commonly disrupt the VOR, nystagmus and vertigo are common and important indicators of neurologic disease. Nystagmus and peripheral vestibular disorders are discussed in other chapters in this volume. This chapter reviews the clinical assessment of common central disorders of the VOR and some principles of management.

VERTIGO

Vertigo is an illusion of motion of oneself or the environment. Motion may be horizontal, torsional, vertical, or in the frontal plane. All the symptoms of sea sickness simulate those caused by vestibular disease, since motion sickness arises from vestibular stimulation. Thus, confining the term *vertigo* to a whirling, spinning, or rotating sensation is not useful. Symptoms that the patient complains of are myriad (Table 11–1).[1] Oscillopsia is a category of vertigo, consisting of illusionary to-and-fro movement of the environment. It occurs during head movement in patients with peripheral or central

TABLE 11–1 Symptoms of Vestibular Imbalance

Spinning	Floating
Rotation	Tilting
Off-balance	Seasick
Toppling	Pitching
Staggering	Dizzy
Swaying	Light-headed
Rocking	Unsteady
Falling	Head swimming
Drunken	Ground uneven
Walking on pillow	Foggy head

abnormalities of the VOR, or as a spontaneous symptom, unprovoked by head movement, in patients with nystagmus of central origin. Peripheral vestibular disorders are covered elsewhere in this book. As a general rule, vertigo arising from damage to central vestibular pathways is much less florid than that caused by acute labyrinthine disorders such as Ménière's disease or vestibular neuronitis. However, nystagmus or vertigo of central origin tend to persist, whereas that caused by unilateral peripheral disease usually subsides within weeks; nystagmus may recur when the patient moves his or her head at high accelerations. Resolution of the peripheral disturbance or central adaptation to persisting imbalance of vestibular input explain recovery from labyrinthine or vestibular nerve disorders. In contrast, central lesions often damage cerebellar, vestibular commissural, or other brain-stem connections that are required for altering the gain of the VOR, rebalancing it, canceling it, dumping the storage of its activity, or habituating to its imbalance.

CLINICAL TESTS OF THE VESTIBULO-OCULAR REFLEX

The VOR prevents retinal slip during head movements by moving the eyes at the same velocity as the head but in the opposite direction. In that way, the VOR keeps gaze (the sum of eye position and head position) stable relative to the world. As the head moves to the left, the ampullary nerve of the left horizontal semicircular canal is excited while the ampullary nerve of the right horizontal canal is inhibited. In other words, during head motion in one direction, the VOR is generated by the difference between excitation from the ipsilateral labyrinth and reciprocal inhibition from the contralateral labyrinth. Tests of the VOR by head movement assess the function of both labyrinths. Caloric stimulation (discussed in Chapter 7) is used to test the integrity of one labyrinth at a time.

Inspection of the Eyes During Head Shaking

The function of both labyrinths together and their central projections can be tested in the clinic or at the bedside by having the patient shake his or her head from side to side while viewing a stationary distant point target, such as a Snellen chart letter. At low rates of head motion (under 1 Hz), optokinetic and smooth-pursuit movements add to the VOR and compensate for its malfunction. To assess the VOR without these visual influences, the patient is instructed to shake his or her head rapidly (about 2 to 3 Hz) through an excursion of about 20 to 40 degrees. Guiding the patient's movement with one hand placed on each side of his or her head is expedient to ensure that the patient does not stop moving to see better, and to preserve the desired frequency and amplitude. If the VOR is normal, eye movements will appear smooth, without corrective saccades or nystagmus quick phases, and the patient perceives images to be stable; the eyes move smoothly in the orbit, but they remain stationary with respect to the world, because they move the same amount as the head. If the VOR is abnormal, the patient perceives movements of images in the direction of the nystagmus quick phases, which correct for abnormal vestibular smooth eye movements. If the VOR is hypoactive (eye movements too slow), nystagmus fast phases are directed opposite to head motion. The fixation target appears to move opposite to the direction of head movement. If the VOR is hyperactive (smooth eye movements too fast), nystagmus fast phases appear in the same direction as head motion.[2] Eye movements are more readily seen if the patient wears Frenzel glasses, plus 20-diopter lenses, which magnify and illuminate the eyes; they also blur fixation, impairing visual cancellation of nystagmus, but this advantage is superfluous when the head moves at 2 to 3 Hz.

Nystagmus After Head Shaking

Patients with unilateral peripheral vestibular lesions have nystagmus directed away from the affected side after vigorous head shaking has stopped. The patient is instructed to shake his or her head through 80 degrees of range at about 2 Hz for 20 to 30 seconds.[3,4] Then when the head is stopped, the observer examines the patient's eyes under Frenzel glasses. Recording the eye movements in darkness is preferred, but Frenzel lenses enable the physician to examine this head-shaking-after-nystagmus (HSAN) in the clinic or at the bedside. The nystagmus is conventionally called simply *head-shaking nystagmus*, but the term may be confused with the nystagmus observed during head shaking in patients with abnormal VOR function, as described earlier. Slow phases of HSAN are initially directed toward the impaired ear. HSAN is initially brisk, and lasts less than 20 seconds, but high-resolution oculography reveals that it is often followed by a low-amplitude reversed HSAN with slow phases away from the impaired ear.[3-5]

HSAN can be explained by Ewald's second law of semicircular canal function. Excitation of a canal is a more effective stimulus than inhibition. In other words, stimulation of the left lateral semicircular canal by leftward head movement is a more potent vestibular stimulus than inhibition of input from right lateral semicircular canal by leftward head movement. If a patient with only one remaining labyrinth (say the left side) is rotated to the left (exciting the left labyrinth), a better vestibular response is evoked than from rotation to the right (inhibiting the left labyrinth). Inability of inhibitory stimuli to decrease vestibular nerve-firing rates to less than zero accounts for Ewald's second law. Most fibers in one vestibular nerve can be driven to a firing rate of close to zero during rotation of the head in the opposite direction at only 180 deg/sec. At higher head velocity, the excitatory response from the normal left labyrinth during leftward head rotation overwhelms the inhibitory response. As the head moves from side to side, the imbalance response from the normal left side charges a velocity-storage mechanism[5] in the medial vestibular and prepositus hypoglossi nuclei, resulting in a net predominance of slow phases directed toward the right (nystagmus quick phases beat toward the left). After the head and cupula come to rest, discharge of the velocity-storage mechanism leads to leftward HSAN, beating away from the right-sided lesion.

Central lesions also cause HSAN. Among 60 patients with central disease, HSAN was found in 25 percent.[4] Disorders included stroke and spinocerebellar degeneration, but 65 percent had multiple sclerosis. Central lesions may involve the velocity-storage mechanism by involving the nucleus prepositus hypoglossi and medial vestibular nucleus, precluding the appearance of HSAN.

Visual Acuity During Head Shaking

When a normal person shakes his or her head at 2 to 3 Hz while viewing a Snellen chart 20 feet away, visual acuity should remain the same as that recorded with the head immobile. If acuity falls by several lines, the VOR is overactive or underactive; that is, VOR gain, the ratio of smooth eye movement velocity to head velocity, is above or below the ideal value of 1.0. Its phase might also be abnormal. Normally, the eyes and head are 180 degrees out of phase; by convention, this phase difference is called zero. If the gain of the reflex is too much above or below 1.0, the retinal image remains off the fovea, although it may be transiently stationary on the retina. If there is a phase lead of the eyes before the head or a phase lag of the eyes behind the head, the image is never stationary on the retina. We attribute a drop of three or more lines of Snellen acuity (e.g., 20/20 to 20/60) to an abnormal VOR.

If the patient does not maintain adequate voluntary head motion, the examiner may move the patient's head as described above for inspection of the eyes during head shaking. This passive testing has the advantage of eliminating preprogrammed smooth eye movements that can compensate partially for an impaired VOR when labyrinthine patients move their head actively,[6] but some patients object to having the head moved rapidly in a sinusoidal pattern.

Ophthalmoscopic Assessment of the VOR

One can also assess the VOR during ophthalmoscopy with the pupil dilated. The patient is instructed to shake his or her head from side to side through an excursion of about 20 degrees. The nonvisualized eye is covered. If the VOR functions normally, the optic disc is seen to remain still during head rotation. If the VOR is overactive or underactive, the disc oscillates. If its gain is too high, the optic disc is seen to move in the same direction as the head. If the VOR is underactive, the disc appears to move opposite to the head.[2] Care must be taken that the head does not shift from side to side, because translation of the head causes movement of the optic disc even when the VOR is normal.

During those tests of the VOR, the patient must wear spectacles that are habitually used, because VOR gain (ratio of eye velocity to head velocity) is adapted to the power of corrective lenses.[7] The gain must be adjusted by the magnification power, which is approximated by the relation 40/40-D, where D is the lens power in diopters; thus a 5-diopter myopic patient would have a VOR gain of about 0.89, whereas a 5-diopter hyperopic patient would have a gain of 1.14 during high-frequency head shaking. If the patient did not wear his or her usual glasses, nystagmus would appear. However, spectacles make ophthalmoscopic assessment of the reflex quite difficult.

Oculocephalic Maneuvers

Passive head movements at rather low speeds with the examiner's hand on the patient's head are known as *oculocephalic maneuvers,* and the ocular response is often called the doll's-eye reflex. In unconscious patients, oculocephalic maneuvers assess the VOR in the absence of visual-following reflexes. Nystagmus quick phases are abolished in coma of any cause, so that eye movements appear smooth and excursion of the eyes may be full in range, even if the VOR gain is subnormal. Moreover, in alert patients full ocular excursion does not necessarily indicate that the VOR is normal. If the head is moved at low accelerations, intact smooth pursuit and optokinetic following reflexes may compensate for a defective VOR and elicit full excursion of the eyes despite a subnormal, even absent, VOR. Nonetheless, oculocephalic responses are useful in detecting the range of VOR excursion; in patients with paralysis of saccades and pursuit, the presence of active oculocephalic reflexes indicates sparing of the VOR and signifies that the ophthalmoplegia is caused by supranuclear damage to saccadic and pursuit pathways. Cervico-ocular reflexes are rudimentary or absent in normal humans, but in patients with bilateral loss of labyrinthine function there is an adaptive increase in their gain that compensates, in part, for loss of the VOR.[6] In the rare comatose patient with bilateral labyrinthine damage, intact responses to oculocephalic maneuvers do not specify sparing of the VOR.

Rapid Passive Head Movements to Test Peripheral Function

While the patient fixates a distant target, the head is briskly moved to one side. Normally, the eyes should stay on target, and the examiner should see only a smooth compensatory eye movement. Patients with unilateral vestibular loss make one or more saccades to bring the eyes on target when the head is moved toward the side of the impaired ear. As noted by Gauthier and Robinson,[8] saccades in the same direction as the VOR signify inability of vestibular smooth eye movements to match head velocity. Thus a patient with right vestibular neurectomy will make leftward saccades during rightward head movements but no saccades during leftward head movements.[9,10] Oppositely directed, compensatory, refixation saccades during rapid horizontal head rotations indicate a severe horizontal semicircular canal lesion on the side toward which the head is being rotated. The head must be moved at high velocity because the VOR eventually becomes balanced for low-velocity head movements after unilateral peripheral vestibular damage.

The asymmetry of vestibular smooth eye movements during rapid passive head movements is attributed to Ewald's second law, as invoked to explain HSAN. One semicircular canal responds to head movement in either direction, with excitation occurring in its vestibular nerve during ipsilateral head motion and inhibition in its vestibular nerve during contralateral head motion. Inhibition of canal input (ampullofugal displacement of the cupula away from the utricle) evokes a weaker slow-phase response than excitation of horizontal canal input (ampullopetal displacement of the cupula toward the utricle). This asymmetry should only be evident during high-velocity head movements that are required to drop the firing rate in the normal vestibular nerve to zero. Because this rate cannot drop below zero, the excitatory response from the normal vestibular nerve imbalances the VOR. The ability of the optokinetic tracking reflex to move the eyes smoothly when retinal slip is low contributes to symmetry of smooth eye movements during slow-velocity head movements. In the laboratory, this optokinetic tracking is eliminated by recording the eye movements in darkness and in the clinic by moving the head quickly. The utility of single repeated rapid head movements in demonstrating central lesions has not been established. Both the asymmetric responses to brisk passive head movement and HSAN signify defective high-frequency responses that can occur independently of defective low-frequency VOR responses that are detected by caloric testing.

Visual Cancellation of the VOR

When an object is pursued with the head, the VOR must be cancelled. Otherwise, the VOR would move the eyes opposite to the head motion, away from the target. During cancellation, the head and eyes move simultaneously toward the target. VOR cancellation is tested clinically by rotating the patient to and fro en bloc while he or she fixates an object moving with him or her, such as a finger of an outstretched arm. If cancellation is adequate, the eyes remain stationary in the orbit. Patients with impaired visual cancellation of the VOR exhibit nystagmus during this test. Vestibular smooth eye movements take the eyes off their target, and quick phases (saccades) bring them back to it. Oscillation must be performed at less than 1 Hz; at higher frequencies VOR cancellation is defective in normal subjects. Impaired visual cancellation of the VOR typically corresponds clinically to defective smooth pursuit,[11,12] which is a very sensitive sign of brain disease.[13] Occasionally, smooth pursuit and cancellation are dissociated (see reference 14 for a concise review).

Cancellation is not actually a test of the VOR. Furthermore, if VOR gain is low, cancellation is readily achieved, even if smooth pursuit (or a distinct cancellation system) is impaired. Conversely, if VOR gain is abnormally high, cancellation can be impaired when smooth pursuit (or a cancellation system) is normal.

MIDBRAIN LESIONS AND THE VOR

Vertical gaze palsies are characteristic of damage to the midbrain pretectum, usually caused by infarcts, hemorrhages, or neoplasms arising from the pineal gland. Upward saccades are paralyzed, and smooth pursuit may be spared or paralyzed, but the VOR usually appears intact when assessed by oculocephalic maneuvers. Vertical eye movements have been recorded using electro-oculography in a few studies,[15-17] but this method is imprecise for recording vertical eye motion. A magnetic search coil technique is optimal for measuring vertical gaze. Reduced gain, limited amplitude, and abnormal phase lead of the vertical VOR were measured by the magnetic search coil technique in a patient with a discrete unilateral infarction involving the interstitial nucleus of Cajal (INC) and rostral interstitial nucleus of the medial longitudinal fasciculus (MLF), confirmed by neuropathologic examination.[18] This observation implies that signals mediating the vertical VOR velocity command traverse, and are partially integrated by, the INC.[18] The lesion spared the ocular motor nuclei, indicating that supranuclear lesions of the rostral midbrain can impair the vertical VOR; this concept varies from the prevailing belief that supranuclear lesions spare the vertical VOR.[19,20] The misconception results from the usual method of testing the vertical VOR at the bedside: the oculocephalic maneuver, in which the patient's head is passively flexed and extended while fixating on a target in a well-lit room. As noted earlier, the eye movements that result represent not only the vertical VOR, but visual enhancement of this reflex by smooth-pursuit and optokinetic following mechanisms. Moreover, although the examiner may judge the amplitude of oculocephalic eye movements to be normal, the gain and phase of the vertical VOR cannot be measured at the bedside. Complete assessment of vertical VOR dysfunction requires oculographic recording and quantification of vertical VOR eye movements performed in darkness.

In our laboratory, quantitative study of the vertical VOR, and its control by vision, in patients with focal lesions confined to the rostral midbrain tegmentum,[21] also refuted the clinical aphorism that supranuclear palsies of vertical gaze spare the vertical VOR. In patients with palsy of upward or both upward and downward saccades, we[21] recorded reduced vertical VOR gain, although many patients had full ranges of smooth eye movements to passive oculocephalic maneuvers tested in the clinic. Cervico-ocular reflexes and preprogrammed smooth eye movements may have contributed to the VOR that we measured during active head motion. Moreover, measurement of visual enhancement of the reflex, which simulates oculocephalic (doll's-eye) maneuvers in the clinic, revealed subnormal enhancement of the reflex by a visual target, despite a normal range of excursion. Normality of the vertical VOR and its visual enhancement cannot be assured by gross integrity of oculocephalic reflexes. The combination of vestibulo-ocular hyporeflexia, with poor visual enhancement, and vertical saccade palsy made vision unstable during vertical head motion.

Phase lead of the eyes before the head occurs in patients with midbrain damage.[21] This phase lead contrasts with the phase lag of the vertical VOR that accompanies internuclear ophthalmoplegia[22] (see below). We documented a similar phase lead after a discrete unilateral lesion of the midbrain involving the rostral interstitial nucleus of the medial longitudinal fasciculus (riMLF) and the INC.[18] Abnormal phase lead may be explained by relative preservation of vestibular velocity commands transmitted in the direct VOR pathway with disruption of integrated eye position commands transmitted to motor neurons through the indirect VOR pathway.[23,24] Structures in the rostral midbrain, perhaps the INC, might comprise an element of the velocity to position integrator of the indirect VOR pathway. Damage to the INC or its projections, or to other periaqueductal neurons, might also give rise to phase lead of the VOR, if those neurons participate in the "velocity storage integrator" which prolongs vestibular responses, thereby extending the low-frequency response of the VOR.[25] Our results[18,21] support evidence in animals[24,26] that the INC, or neighboring axons, participate in the integration of vestibular commands from the vertical semicircular canals before they reach vertically acting motor neurons. A positive feedback loop from the vestibular nuclei to the INC, then to the vestibular nucleus and nucleus prepositus hypoglossi in the medulla may comprise the velocity-to-position integrator for vertical eye movements.[24]

Midbrain damage usually spares the horizontal VOR. Acute unilateral lesions of the midbrain tegmentum, however, may paralyze all vestibular smooth eye movements and saccades, in both eyes, contralateral to the lesion. The VOR recovers within hours or days. Loss of the contralateral VOR has been demonstrated in patients with acute infarction or expansive tumor in the midbrain tegmentum,[27,28] and in monkeys with stereotactic lesions in the midbrain reticular formation.[29] The mechanism is uncertain, but acute deprivation of descending[30] collicular or cerebral cortical influences on the vestibular nuclei might account for transient vestibular areflexia[27] in a manner analogous to the diaschisis of spinal shock.

INTERNUCLEAR OPHTHALMOPLEGIA AND THE VOR

Bilateral internuclear ophthalmoplegia (INO), consisting of binocular paresis of adduction and gaze-evoked abducting nystagmus, results from bilateral lesions of the MLF. Multiple sclerosis is the most common cause, but infarction is often responsible, and neoplasms or any other structural lesion of the pontine or midbrain tegmentum may cause INO. Bilateral INO is associated with impairment of the vertical VOR and smooth pursuit and vertical gaze-evoked nystagmus.[22,31,32] We[22] recorded reduced gain and abnormal phase lag of the vertical VOR at frequencies up to 2 Hz in a group of patients with unilateral or bilateral INO. VOR gain increased when the patients viewed a stationary target but remained below the ideal gain of unity, indicating defective visual enhancement of the reflex. Despite a subnormal vertical VOR, patients with INO are unable to adequately cancel this reflex when they pursue a target with combined head and eye motion.[22] Impairment of the vertical VOR and its cancellation in patients with INO indicates that vertical VOR, vertical eye position, and VOR cancellation signals in humans are transmitted from the vestibular nuclei to the third nerve and fourth nerve nuclei, at least in part, in the MLF.

Some neurons in the vestibular nucleus carry a tonic eye position signal during all vertical eye movements and a head velocity and position signal during vertical head movements, and they pause during saccades. These cells transmit the labyrinth-derived head velocity signal, which constitutes an eye velocity command, to vertical ocular motor neurons; this is the direct VOR. A signal of vertical eye position on these vestibular cells is derived by the integration, in the mathematical sense, of eye velocity signals. An integrated velocity signal corrects any phase lead of the eyes and provides an eye position command to motor neurons so that changes in eye position match opposed changes in head position. Structures that perform the neural integration and relay the position commands can be considered the anatomic substrate of the indirect VOR. Single-unit recording studies in the vestibular nucleus and MLF[33,34] reveal that the MLF carries almost all of the eye velocity signal but only about 63 percent of the eye position signal found on motor neurons during vertical head movement. The remaining 37 percent of the vertical eye position signal must reach motor neurons by other routes through the brain stem or brachium conjunctivum, and thus would be spared by MLF lesions. Because this eye position signal is derived from the mathematical integration of VOR eye velocity signals, the eye position signal lags the eye velocity signal by 90 degrees. Because lesions of the MLF can be expected to interrupt the eye velocity command but only 63 percent of the eye position signal, the motor neuron should receive considerable eye position information during vertical head movement. The phase lag of the vertical VOR in INO can be explained by disruption of eye velocity signals of the direct VOR and relative sparing of vertical eye position signals of the indirect VOR.[22]

CEREBELLUM AND LOWER BRAIN STEM

Damage to central vestibular circuits typically lowers or imbalances the gain of the VOR, creating nystagmus. Caloric responses may be reduced or abolished; directional preponderance of caloric nystagmus typically corresponds to the presence of spontaneous nystagmus. Gaze-evoked or primary position vertical nystagmus specifies central disease of the brain stem or cerebellum. An imbalance of vertical smooth pursuit or vestibular tone likely causes upbeat or downbeat nystagmus that occurs in the primary position; however, few quantitative measurements of vertical smooth eye movements have been performed.[35,36] Central vestibular nystagmus is typically not inhibited by fixation. The slow-phase velocity remains the same in darkness. Failure of vision to inhibit the nystagmus can be explained by impairment of smooth pursuit. Indeed, pursuit and vestibular signals traverse the same or neighboring pathways from the vestibular nuclei to ocular motor nuclei. Vestibular imbalance, together with failure of fixation suppression, can account for primary position nystagmus.

Downbeat Nystagmus

Nystagmus that is directed downward while the eyes are in the vertical midposition of the orbit is called downbeat nystagmus and must be distinguished from vertical nystagmus that is evoked only during eccentric gaze, upward or downward. Gaze-evoked vertical nystagmus is directed upward or upward and downward, but rarely downward alone, and is typically accompanied by gaze-evoked horizontal nystagmus. Gaze-evoked vertical nystagmus signifies disease of the vestibulocerebellum or its connections in the brain stem or sedative or anticonvulsant drug intoxication; this form of nystagmus has less specific diagnostic significance than does downbeat nystagmus (in the primary position). Downbeat nystagmus typically increases in intensity during lateral gaze and during downward gaze; it may increase, stop, or reverse direction during convergence. Downbeat nystagmus occurs with dysgenesis of the vestibulocerebellum and medulla in the Chiari malformation,[35,37] hereditary and acquired cerebellar degeneration,[35,38] multiple sclerosis,[37,38] familial periodic ataxia,[39] magnesium depletion,[40] lithium toxicity,[41,42] or anticonvulsant (phenytoin, carbamazapine) toxicity.[43,44] No cause is found in up to 40 percent of patients,[38] many of whom may have cerebellar degeneration.

The pathogenesis of downbeat nystagmus is uncertain but probably involves the selective effect of lesions on projections that mediate the downward VOR[37] or downward smooth pursuit.[35] Upward vestibular bias caused by disruption of posterior semicircular canal projections in the brain-stem tegmentum may be responsible. Each posterior semicircular canal excites the contralateral inferior rectus and the ipsilateral superior oblique muscle via projections in the MLF. Each anterior semicircular canal excites the ipsilateral superior rectus and the contralateral inferior oblique via projections through the brachium conjunctivum. The anterior canals excite the upward VOR, and the posterior canals activate the downward VOR. Disruption of the posterior canal projections in the brain stem might cause the eyes to glide up in downbeat nystagmus—the fast-phase correct orbital position. Excitatory central projections from the posterior, but not anterior, semicircular canals cross in the floor of the fourth ventricle.[45] Midsagittal section in the dorsal midline of the medulla in monkeys causes a loss of downward vestibular tone, resulting in an upward slow-phase drift and downbeat nystagmus.[46] Downbeating is also produced experimentally by ablating the flocculus and nodulus in the monkey.[47,48] Bilateral lesions of the flocculus[47] or nodulus[48] may cause downbeat nystagmus by loss of the inhibitory influence of Purkinje cells on anterior canal or otolithic-ocular relays.

The intensity of downbeat nystagmus often varies with the position of the head in pitch. This nystagmus may stop when the patient is in the supine position or the nystagmus may be precipitated by assuming that position. The asymmetry of the vertical semicircular canal reflexes seem to be modulated by otolith-ocular reflexes.[36] Downbeat nystagmus might also be the effect of a disturbance of the velocity-to-position integrator on vertical smooth eye movements, but this has not been confirmed by measurement of reduced gain and reduced time constant of the downward integrator. Like other forms of vestibular nystagmus, downbeating usually increases in intensity during gaze in the direction of fast phase. This phenomenon is known as *Alexander's law*. A pathologically elevated gain of the neural integrator for upward smooth eye movements was proposed as the cause of downbeat nystagmus with exponentially increasing velocity slow phases in a patient with paraneoplastic cerebellar degeneration.[49] This slow-phase waveform usually signifies congenital nystagmus. The intensity of nystagmus increased during upward gaze, in violation of Alexander's law.[49]

Lithium is an infrequent cause of downbeat nystagmus.[41,42] In one patient who died after lithium overdose, cell death was observed in the medial vestibular nucleus (MVN) and nuclei prepositus hypoglossi (NPH).[41] disruption of horizontal gaze-holding and downbeat nystagmus have been produced by chemically creating lesions in the MVN and NPH in monkeys; these structures comprise the velocity-to-position neural integrator for horizontal eye movements. However, neuropathologic examination of the brain of a second patient with downbeat nystagmus after chronic lithium ingestion failed to show any abnormality of NPH or MVN,[42] suggesting that other factors such as hypoxemia caused the NPH and MVN necrosis.[41]

Suboccipital decompression resolves downbeat nystagmus in some patients with the Chiari malformation and improves it in others.[50] Treatment with base-out prisms can induce convergence and dampen nystagmus and oscillopsia.[51] However, some cases of nystagmus are increased by convergence, and base-in prisms might be more appropriate. Infection of extraocular muscles with botulinum toxin to paralyze them may be effective in stopping horizontal nystagmus, but attempts to stop vertical nystagmus cause disabling ptosis.[51a] Clonazepam reduced or abolished nystagmus and oscillopsia in one series of patients with downbeat, see-saw, or circular nystagmus.[52] Baclofen, a GABA-B agonist, is reported to be effective for both upbeat and downbeat nystagmus.[53] Trihexphenidyl is not more effective than placebo,[54] but benztropine and scopolamine reduced nystagmus slow-phase velocity, improved motion perception, and reduced oscillopsia, as shown by double-blind trial of their intravenous use.[54a]

Upbeat Nystagmus

Upbeat nystagmus also occurs in the vertical midposition of the orbit and should be set apart from gaze-evoked upbeating nystagmus mentioned above. Upbeat nystagmus is likely caused by bilateral disruption of anterior semicircular canal projections that mediate the upward VOR.[55,56] Upbeat nystagmus occurs with lesions in the pontomedullary junction and has also been attributed to lesions of the brachium conjunctivum and superior cerebellar vermis.[55] Drugs are rarely responsible. Nicotine from tobacco smoking can induce upbeat nystagmus in darkness.[57] Primary-position upbeat nystagmus has been associated with lesions in the medullary and pontine tegmentum,[58,60] involving the inferior olive and perihypoglossal nuclei.[59] Upbeat nystagmus in these cases may result from interruption of upward vestibular signals carried by a ventral tegmental pathway,[56] while sparing downward vestibular signals crossing within the more dorsal decussating pathway that includes the MLF.[46] The nystagmus often stops or reverses direction during convergence[60,61] or in supine head position[56,61]; these changes are attributed to an imbalance in the otolithic-ocular reflex when superimposed on an imbalanced canal-driven VOR.[61] Management of upbeat nystagmus is the same as for downbeat nystagmus.

Torsional Nystagmus

Nystagmus with the axis of rotation around the anteroposterior axis of the globe is torsional. Torsional nystagmus accompanies horizontal vectors in peripheral vestibular disease. Purely torsional nystagmus indicates brain-stem damage.[62,63] Torsional jerk nystagmus occurs in medullary disease; the upper poles of the eyes beat contralateral to the side of damage.[62] Involvement of central projections from the anterior and posterior semicircular canals on one side explains the oscillations. Large-amplitude pendular torsion is a component of see-saw nystagmus in patients with diencephalic-midbrain lesions and bitemporal hemianopia. In see-saw nystagmus, the rising eye intorts as the falling eye extorts. Clonazepam has been an effective treatment in a few patients.[52]

Periodic Alternating Nystagmus

Periodic alternating nystagmus (PAN), a type of jerk nystagmus, shifts direction every 90 seconds or so. Between right-beating cycles (about 90 seconds) and left-beating cycles (about 90 seconds), there is a null period of 0 to 10 seconds. PAN occurs with cervicomedullary junction lesions, spinocerebellar degenerations, and anticonvulsant drug (diphenylhydantoin) intoxication. The nystagmus has been modeled by depriving the VOR of visual signals and by increasing the gain of the central velocity storage mechanism of the VOR.[64] Experimental ablation of the nodulus and uvula cause PAN in monkeys when they are in darkness.[65] The nystagmus requires prolongation of the storage mechanism by damage to the nodulus or its connections and deprivation of visual stabilization systems (pursuit or optokinetic) by cerebellar disease or by ocular disease (e.g., cataracts). Baclofen, a GABA analogue, is an effective treatment for acquired PAN;[66] baclofen disengages velocity storage in the VOR; the nodulus and uvula inhibit vestibular rotational responses by using GABA. A congenital form of PAN does not respond to baclofen. A periodic alternating nystagmus with a very short cycle (4 to 9 seconds) was recorded in two patients with infectious mononucleosis.[67] The nystagmus beat right for 3 to 6 seconds, then paused for 1 to 3 seconds, and then beat left for 3 to 6 seconds. Both patients had midline ataxia and dysarthria and recovered. They likely had focal encephalitis involving flocculonodular projections to the vestibular nuclei.

Vestibulo-ocular Hyperreflexia

Elevation of VOR gain is a sign of cerebellar system disease[12,68,69] that has been attributed to loss of inhibitory effects of the vestibulocerebellum on the vestibular nuclei. Flocculectomy increases the gain to 1.17 in the monkey.[47] In humans with cerebellar degeneration, the highest gain recorded for the horizontal VOR is 3[70] (normal < 1). In one reported patient,[70] physostigmine, an acetylcholinesterase inhibitor, reduced the gain and improved visual acuity during head shaking. Reversible chemical lesioning of the olivocerebellar climbing pathway with lidocaine causes reversible increase of VOR gain in cats,[71] suggesting that involvement of this pathway is responsible for vestibulo-ocular hyperreflexia in humans with cerebellar system disease. The dorsal cap of the inferior olivary nucleus is a major visual relay to the flocculus and contains acetylcholinesterase,[72] providing a possible site of action for physostigmine.

CENTRAL POSITIONAL VERTIGO AND NYSTAGMUS: STATIC AND PAROXYSMAL

In contrast to the syndrome of BPPV (see Chapter 16), central positional vertigo is characterized by little dizziness and prominent nystagmus, but the severity of vertigo is not particularly helpful in separating central and peripheral causes. Paroxysmal positional nystagmus that lasts less than 30 seconds or so after assuming a head-hanging position should be distinguished from static positional nystagmus, which persists as long as the head position is maintained (Table 11–2). Both the static and paroxysmal types are usually caused by labyrinthine disorders, but static positional nystagmus more often results from central (brain-stem) disease than does the paroxysmal type. Peripheral static positional nystagmus is probably caused by damage to otolithic receptors, and central static positional nystagmus likely arises from disruption of their projections in the brain stem and cerebellum, because the otolithic organs are sensitive to changes in head position with respect to gravity. Nylen[73] proposed that direction-changing positional nystagmus signifies central disease, whereas direction-fixed positional nystagmus indicates an origin in the labyrinth, but we now know that both direction-fixed and direction-changing positional nystagmus usually arise from the labyrinth, although both can also be manifestations of central disease.[74]

Paroxysmal positional vertigo is the most common cause of vertigo[75] and is typically a benign disorder that may be explained by cupulolithiasis in the posterior semicircular canal.[76] However, transient vertigo and nystagmus may also be evoked in patients with central lesions by rapid changes in head position, such as reaching for an object on a shelf or rolling over in bed, and demonstrated in the clinic by quickly placing the head in the supine or hanging position. In contrast to the benign paroxysmal positional nystagmus (BPPN) of peripheral origin, central paroxysmal positional nystagmus (CPPN) typically begins immediately, does not fatigue after the head-hanging maneuver is repeated several times, and lasts longer than 30 seconds (Table 11–3). Nonetheless, central lesions involving the caudal brain stem or vestibulocerebellum, such as ependymoma, can cause paroxysmal positional nystagmus with features of the peripheral "benign" type.[77] Patients with apparent BPPN should have neurologic examinations and careful follow-up to exclude CPPN. Cranial CT or MRI is advocated only for patients who have atypical features (Table 11–3) that suggest CPPN.

Both static and paroxysmal positional nystagmus are tested in the recumbent position with the head hanging to the right and then to the left. Static and paroxysmal

TABLE 11–2 Central versus Peripheral Static Positional Nystagmus

	Direction	Effect of Fixation	Brain-stem Signs
PERIPHERAL	Torsional, upbeat dysconjugate	Suppression	Absent
CENTRAL	Upbeat or downbeat conjugate	None	Usually present

TABLE 11-3 Central versus Peripheral Paroxysmal Positional Nystagmus

	Direction	Latency (sec)	Duration (sec)	Fatigue	Brain-stem Signs
Peripheral*	Torsional-upbeat, disconjugate	4-10	<30	Typical	Absent
Central	Horizontal or vertical conjugate	<4	>30	Uncommon	Usual

*An uncommon horizontal canal BPPN is purely horizontal, occurs without latency, and lasts more than 30 seconds.[111]

nystagmus of central origin is often evoked with the head supine in the midposition, but BPPN typically requires the head to be accelerated into a head-hanging posture with the affected ear undermost, so as to maximally stimulate a posterior semicircular canal. The nystagmus of BPPN has its slow phase directed in the plane of action of the offending posterior canal; the right posterior canal excites the ocular muscles that act in its plane, the left inferior rectus and the right superior oblique, causing extorting jerk nystagmus in the right eye and upbeating nystagmus in the left eye. CPPN, on the other hand, is typically conjugate and often downward, toward the lower eyelids (Table 11-3).

Nystagmus is inspected with the eyes open and preferably under Frenzel lenses. Accompanying vertigo, if severe, often prompts patients to close their eyes, and prior instructions must be given to keep the eyes open and maintain a steady viewing direction. Fixation inhibits or stops BPPN but has little effect on CPPN because central lesions that affect otolithic or posterior semicircular canal projections also damage brainstem and cerebellar circuits that mediate smooth pursuit and cancellation of the VOR. Patients with cupulolithiasis may experience terrible vertigo but not exhibit nystagmus when examined without Frenzel lenses. Testing with electro-oculography (EOG) and closed eyelids is not appropriate because many normal subjects have positional nystagmus with their eyes closed.[78] Even with the eyes open in darkness, EOG is deficient because it does not record torsional motion of the globe and its misses the vertical component of nystagmus unless electrodes are placed above and below the eye.

Management of central positional vertigo is addressed entirely at treating the brainstem or cerebellar lesions that cause it. There is no rationale for positional exercises or maneuvers that are sometimes employed in BPPN, and they have not received systematic trials. Antivertiginous drugs, such as meclizine or phenergan, can be used to suppress pervasive dizziness that occurs in particular head positions but are not effective in stopping paroxysmal positional vertigo.

OCCLUSIVE VASCULAR DISEASE

Ischemia in the posterior circulation may be diffuse during hypoperfusion caused by cardiac arrhythmia, or focal after thrombosis or embolism of the vertebral or basilar arteries or their paired tributaries—the paramedian arteries, the short circumferential arteries, and the long circumferential arteries: the posterior-inferior cerebellar arteries (PICA), anterior-inferior cerebellar arteries (AICA), and the superior cerebellar arteries (SCA), as shown in Figure 11-1. Transient ischemic attacks (TIAs) in the posterior circulation can be hemodynamic, resulting from generalized poor perfusion, or occlusive from emboli originating in the heart or vertebral artery.

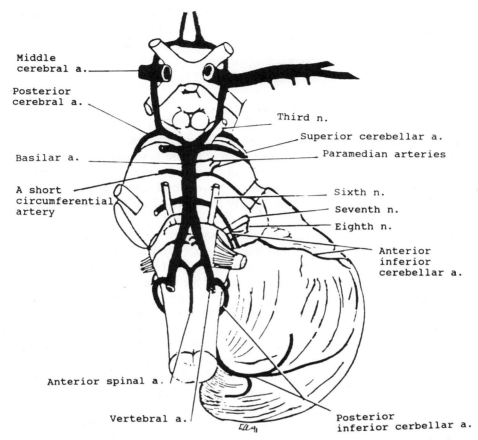

FIGURE 11–1. Basal view of brain stem showing the major branches of the vertebral and basilar arteries.

Patients with vertebral artery disease can be conveniently divided into two groups, those with proximal atherosclerosis affecting the subclavian, innominate, and proximal vertebral arteries, and those with distal disease involving the terminal portion of the extracranial vertebral arteries and intracranial vertebral arteries.

Subclavian Artery Disease

Severe stenosis or occlusion of one subclavian artery proximal to the takeoff of a vertebral artery may lead to reversal of flow down the vertebral artery to nourish the ischemic arm. Blood from the contralateral vertebral artery is "stolen" from the basilar artery to flow down the ipsilateral vertebral artery. This subclavian steal syndrome[79] is occasionally identified by angiography or by noninvasive techniques (Doppler ultrasound or plethysmography) but seldom causes transient CNS symptoms of dizziness, diplopia, visual blurring, facial numbness, and staggering. Ischemic arm symptoms of coldness, cramps, and fatigue and transient brain-stem ischemia are provoked by exercising the arm, but strokes are rare.[80] Coexistent carotid artery disease is a more serious risk of stroke. Surgical correction of left subclavian steal is seldom warranted for relief of neurologic symptoms.

Occlusion or stenosis of the left subclavian artery is more common than disease of the right artery, but right subclavian disease is a greater risk because the carotid artery arises just proximal to it, and clot or atheroma may enter the parent innominate artery and embolize to the right carotid, causing stroke.

Proximal Vertebral Artery Disease

Stenosis within the first few millimeters of the orifice of the vertebral arteries is commonly asymptomatic. Symptoms of transient ischemia (diplopia, staggering, dizziness, blurred vision) are alarming but generally benign because there is a relatively low incidence of stroke in patients with proximal vertebral artery stenosis.[81] The good outcome is explained by rich collateral supply to the distal vertebral arteries from other cervical vessels.

The diagnosis of vertebrobasilar "insufficiency" is employed too loosely to a variety of vestibular symptoms when their mechanism is not known. The terms *vertebrobasilar TIA* or *infarct* should be used if there is sound evidence for a hemodynamic or embolic source and genuine ischemia in the distribution of the vertebral arteries. Chronic hemodynamic insufficiency is rarely, if ever, present after proximal vertebral artery occlusion. Even bilateral occlusion of the origins of the vertebral arteries is typically well tolerated.[82]

Sudden stroke in the posterior circulation is indeed sometimes caused by emoblism from a fresh thrombus in a proximal vertebral artery. Treatment with heparin, then warfarin, anticoagulation for 3 to 4 weeks is justified to prevent further emboli, but long-term anticoagulation is not justified because of the rarity of late embolization once the clot is organized within the vessel wall. Surgical attempts to restore patency to the proximal vertebral artery are not recommended.

Giant cell (temporal) arteritis and Takayasu's disease may also involve the subclavian, innominate, or vertebral arteries in causing brain-stem infarction.[83,84] Temporal arteritis stops where the artery penetrates the dura to enter the cranium. Its external elastic lamina stops at that level, but the relationship between lack of this lamina and absence of arteritis, if any, is unknown.

Extracranial Involvement of the Midartery and Distal Vertebral Artery

An association between cervical vertebral spondylosis and vertebral artery disease was once a popular concept. However, the attribution of vertebrobasilar ischemia to compression of the artery within its bony canal through the transverse foramina of C3 to C6 is seldom well founded. Fewer than 1 percent of patients studied by angiography have occlusive disease within the intravertebral course of the vertebral artery.[85] Spondylitic spurs are usually not positioned to impinge on the transverse foramina, even on turning; they form on the posterior surface of the vertebral body. Moreover, at most sites where arteries contact bone, they erode it, rather than the bone narrowing the artery.

On the other hand, acute cervical trauma or vigorous chiropractic manipulation can cause brain-stem or cerebellar infarcts by occluding the artery or causing intramural dissection, but this typically occurs in the distal part of the vertebral artery after it emerges from the third vertebra, where the artery courses behind the axis and atlas before entering the cranium through the foramen magnum. This distal free segment of the vessel is vulnerable to injury during sports activity or neck manipulation.[86] Spontaneous dissection of the distal artery is increasingly recognized.[87] Neck and head pain are usually accompanied by vertigo and other elements of the lateral medullary syndrome. Clot may enter the lumen through the torn intima and occlude it or embolize or propagate into the intracranial arteries. The dissection usually heals over a few months, and anticoagulation should be used with precaution because the dissection may leak outside the vessel, causing subarachnoid hemorrhage. MRI can be used to identify a clot extending within the wall of the artery inside the cranium, and to select patients at risk for subarachnoid hemorrhage.

Intracranial Disease of the Vertebral Artery

Occlusive disease of the vertebral artery within the skull causes infarction of the lateral medulla that may constitute a typical lateral medullary syndrome (Table 11–4). The infarct is in the distribution of the PICA, which is the largest and the last branch of the vertebral artery before it joins with its fellow from the opposite side to form the basilar artery (see Fig. 11–1). Vertigo is often prominent. Deviation of the limbs and body to the side of the lesion, as if pulled by a strong force, is called *lateropulsion*.[88] Saccades may be driven toward the side of infarction in a phenomenon termed *ipsipulsion*[89]; ipsilateral saccades overshoot their target, contralateral saccades undershoot in a series of hypometric saccades, and vertical saccades are misdirected obliquely toward the side of the medullary infarct. On eyelid closure, the eyes deviate ipsilaterally. The pulsion occurs with medullary damage, but not with damage to the cerebellum alone.[90] *Torsipulsion* is a name used for torsional saccades that are evoked by vertical or horizontal saccades in lateral medullary syndrome patients who have torsional nystagmus;[62] horizontal or vertical saccades may evoke torsional saccades with the upper corneas moving contralateral to the side of the infarct. Contralaterally beating nystagmus is typical, but torsional nystagmus with upward beating is occasionally seen. Pure torsional nystagmus signifies central disruption of input from the anterior and posterior semicircular canals. Discrete lesions of the rostral part of the vestibular nucleus complex can cause torsional and mixed vertical-torsional nystagmus in monkeys,[91] suggesting that this nystagmus pattern signifies infarction that extends rostral to the usual extent of necrosis in the lateral medullary syndrome.

TABLE 11–4 Lateral Medullary Syndrome

Ipsilateral	Contralateral
Dissociated sensory loss (pain and temperature) on face	Nystagmus: horizontal, torsional, hemi-seesaw
Limb ataxia	Dissociated sensory (pain and temperature) loss on body
Lateropulsion of gait	Skew deviation (contralateral hypertropia)
Horner's syndrome	
Vertigo	
Ipsipulsion of saccades	
Torsipulsion of saccades	
Tenth-nerve palsy (dysphagia, dysarthria, vocal cord palsy, palatal and pharyngeal palsy, hiccups)	

Patients may complain of tilting, even inversion, of the visual environment. This complaint is transient and may be a manifestation of the ocular tilt reaction (OTR),[62,92,93] which accompanies some lateral medullary infarcts. The OTR consists of a triad of lateral tilt of the head toward the side of the infarct, torsion of both eyes in the same direction, and skew deviation with the higher eye on the side opposite the infarct (Table 11–4). We[92] were the first to attribute this distinctive triad to projections from one utricle and proposed that they decussate in the caudal brain stem, before ascending to the INC in the midbrain. The torsion and vertical divergence may be oscillatory, comprising hemi-see-saw nystagmus;[62] there is slow-phase depression of the ipsilateral eye, slow-phase elevation of the contralateral eye, and ipsilateral slow torsion of both eyes; nystagmus quick phases are in the opposite direction.

Infarction in its more distal distribution causes only cerebellar infarction, evidenced clinically by ataxia, occipital headache, and dizziness without brain-stem signs. Uncommonly, complete infarction of half of the medulla occurs, causing contralateral hemiparesis and loss of joint position sense in addition to features of the lateral medullary syndrome.

Atheroma in this segment of the vertebral artery, especially if bilateral, is far more ominous than is disease of the proximal artery. Fresh clot may propagate into the basilar artery causing fatal brain-stem infarction, or embolize into its tributaries, usually at its terminal bifurcation into the posterior cerebral arteries. For this reason, four-vessel arterial angiography is warranted in patients with recognized posterior circulation occlusions of major circumferential vessels, if they do not have a cardiac source of embolism. Treatment of initial occlusion is controversial, but heparin for 3 to 4 days followed by warfarin for 4 to 6 weeks may be prudent. If bilateral tight stenosis of the distal vertebral artery or extensive basilar artery stenosis is identified, we use long-term warfarin anticoagulation. If symptoms of ischemia persist, surgical bypass connecting the PICA with the occipital branch of the external carotid may be considered.[94]

Vertigo can be a symptom of cerebellar infarction that spares the brain stem. Ataxia without brain-stem signs and nystagmus evoked by gaze toward the side of the lesion (that is, toward the side of ataxia), imply brain-stem sparing, but MRI is required to confirm it. The following case illustrates this feature.

> A 33-year-old woman bent over to pick up a suitcase and became dizzy with whirling of the environment when she stood up. She had a severe throbbing headache for 3 to 4 hours after onset of vertigo, which lasted about 24 hours. She had a 4-year history of recurrent left hemicranial throbbing headaches lasting about 4 to 36 hours; many were accompanied by blurring vision. Migraine headaches had been diagnosed. Neurologic examination 24 hours after the beginning of symptoms was normal. MRI showed a 2.5-cm lesion in the caudal part of the left side of the cerebellum (Fig. 11–2). Four-vessel angiography revealed occlusion of the distal part of the left PICA. Echocardiograms did not reveal a source of embolism, and tests for anticardiolipin antibody and collagen vascular disease were negative. Cerebellar infarction in the distribution of the distal PICA was diagnosed and attributed to complicated migraine.

Syndromes of the Anterior-Inferior Cerebellar Artery

The anterior-inferior cerebellar artery (AICA) is the source of the internal auditory artery (IAA) in 83 percent of brains; in the remaining cases, the IAA arises from the basilar artery. The IAA nourishes the eighth nerve, then divides into three branches: (1) the anterior vestibular artery supplies the utricle, part of the saccule, the lateral semicir-

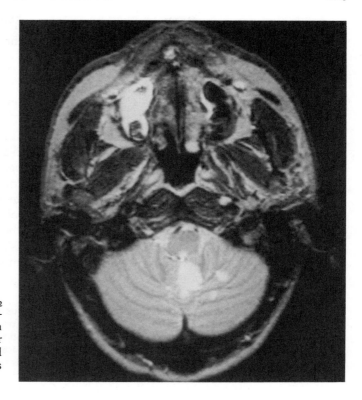

FIGURE 11–2. MRI using T_2 spin echo sequence shows infarct in vestibulocerebellum, in the posterior inferior cerebellar territory, that was associated with vertigo but no other signs (see case description).

cular canal, and the anterior canal; (2) the vestibulocochlear artery feeds the saccule, the utricle, and the posterior canal, and the basal (proximal) turn of the cochlea; and (3) the cochlear artery supplies the rest of the cochlea.[95]

Infarction in the distribution of the AICA affects the dorsolateral pontomedullary region and the inferior cerebellum. As in the lateral medullary syndrome, there is loss of pain and temperature sensation over the ipsilateral face, contralateral trunk and limbs, and ipsilateral ataxia, but distinct features are deafness and tinnitus, which can be attributed to ischemia in the territory of the IAA but might be owing to infarction of the cochlear nuclei or their immediate connections on the lateral edge of the brain stem. Facial palsy is frequent. Vertigo and contralateral nystagmus are prominent. The OTR may occur with occlusion of the AICA.[96] Head tilt occurs toward the side of infarction, as in the lateral medullary syndrome, suggesting that ascending otolithic-ocular fibers that mediate the OTR decussate above the midpontine level.

Vertigo and nystagmus can be isolated manifestations of occlusion of the anterior vestibular artery.[97] After several weeks, recovery occurs by central adaptation and rebalancing of vestibular reflexes (see Chapter 4), but BPPN is said to follow infarction of the labyrinth.[98]

Isolated vertigo may be the only manifestation of TIAs. In one series,[97] 62 percent of patients with vertebrobasilar TIAs had at least one episode of vertigo without other symptoms. Of those with completed stroke in the posterior circulation, 29 percent had isolated vertigo within 2 years of their strokes. This finding conflicts with Fisher's[1] teaching that isolated vertigo is not often caused by vertebrobasilar ischemia. However, Fisher[1] also documented that about 20 percent of basilar artery thrombosis cases have vertigo, unaccompanied by other symptoms, as the first symptom. It typically is a prodromal TIA. Nonetheless, his admonition that isolated vertigo is not vascular in origin until proven so, remains germane, particularly when anticoagulation treatment is contemplated.

Syndrome of the Superior Cerebellar Artery

Infarcts in the distribution of the superior cerebellar artery are also associated with vertigo;[89,99,100] this vertigo might be owing to ischemia to projections from the vestibular nucleus, but imaging may show only lesions in the cerebellar hemisphere in the territory of its distal branches. Ipsilateral limb ataxia and static arm tremor are typical; ipsilateral Horner's syndrome and contralateral spinothalamic (pain and temperature) sensory loss to the face, trunk, and limbs are features of proximal occlusion with infarction of the lateral superior pons. Gaze-evoked or primary position vertical nystagmus can occur, but bilateral or midline ischemia of the midbrain in distal basilar artery perforating branches is probably responsible as vertical nystagmus is absent in most cases.[89,99,100] The following case illustrates the syndrome.

A 17-year-old woman with common migraine headaches had a throbbing headache and spinning vertigo with vomiting and gait instability for 12 hours before admission to hospital. Examination showed a large-amplitude postural and intention tremor of the left arm and left heel-shin ataxia. Other neurologic functions were normal, apart from distinctive saccadic dysmetria: Rightward (contralateral) saccades overshot visual targets; leftward saccades were hypometric; and vertical saccades were directed obliquely away from the side of the ataxic limbs. CT scan (Fig. 11–3) and MRI showed

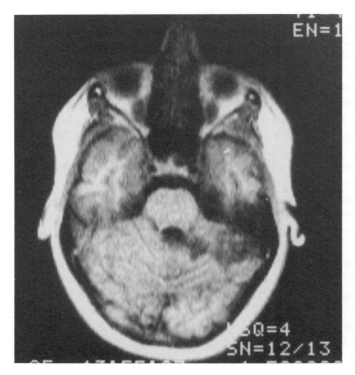

FIGURE 11–3. CT illustrates lucency in rostral part of the left side of the cerebellum involving the anterior lobe and superior peduncle, in the distribution of the superior cerebellar artery.

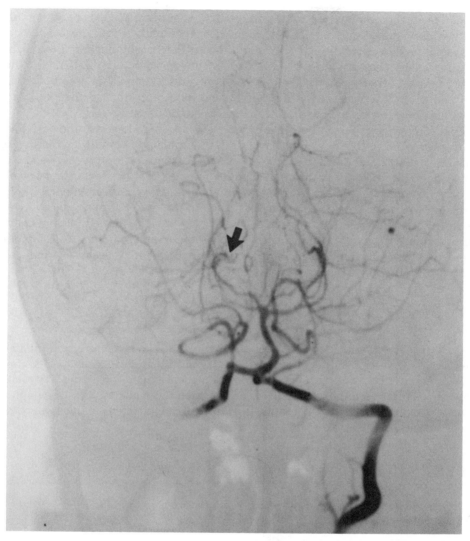

FIGURE 11–4. Posterior-anterior view right vertebral angiogram demonstrates occlusion (*at arrow*) of the distal part of the left superior cerebellar artery in the patient whose CT is shown in Figure 11–3.

an infarct in the rostral part of the left cerebellar hemisphere and vermis, sparing the brain stem. Angiography of the anterior and posterior circulations revealed distal occlusion of the superior cerebellar artery (Fig. 11–4). No evidence of vasculitis or source of embolism were identified by the angiograms or by echocardiography.

The ocular motor triad of hypermetric contralateral saccades, hypometric ipsilateral saccades, and obliquely misdirected vertical saccades is thought to correlate with infarction of the superior cerebellar peduncle or deep nuclei and has been called *contrapulsion*.[89,101] This patient, like the one described above, had vertigo associated with infarction in the territory of a long circumferential branch of the posterior circulation, apparently sparing the brain stem. Vertigo may be caused by disruption of projections from the flocculus or fastigial nucleus to the vestibular nuclei. Both patients had migraine, which is commonly associated with vertigo; as many as 27 percent of migraineurs have vertigo.[102] Moreover, migraine without headache may be responsible for benign paroxysmal vertigo of childhood[103,104] or adulthood.[105] As exemplified by these patients, migraine can be catastrophic with infarction in the posterior circulation.[106] Whether caused by local atherosclerosis, embolism, or migraine, cerebellar infarction must be diagnosed promptly, because swelling of the necrotic cerebellum can rapidly lead to brain-stem compression, coma, and death unless surgically relieved.[107]

Episodic vertigo in patients with known posterior fossa ischemia in the past does not specify recurrent TIAs. They may have BPPN[98] unrelated to vascular disease onset occurring only in certain head postures (see above). Vertigo is often precipitated by rapid head motion and results from incomplete adaptation to a *previous* brain stem or cerebellar infarct or to a labyrinthine disorder when challenged by high-frequency vestibular stimulation. Genuine TIAs can often be stopped and the risk of stroke reduced by about 25 percent with the use of antiplatelet agents: low-dose aspirin (300 mg daily), or sulfinpyrazone, or higher-dose aspirin with or without dipyrimidole.[108] Ticlopidine, a platelet antiaggregant, is an even more promising treatment,[109] because it reduces the risk of stroke 20 percent further than aspirin.[110]

SUMMARY

Disorders affecting the central vestibular pathways, like those affecting the peripheral vestibular system, result in vertigo and nystagmus. Identification of specific changes in VOR and other oculomotor functions and the presence of specific types of nystagmus enable the clinician to localize the site of the lesion along the neuraxis. This chapter has discussed the clinical assessment and the principles of management of the more common brain-stem and cerebellar disorders that affect the VOR.

REFERENCES

1. Fisher, CM: Vertigo in cerebrovascular disease. Arch Otolaryngol 85:529, 1967.
2. Zee, DS: Ophthalmoscopy in evaluation of vestibular disorders. Ann Neurol 3:373, 1978.
3. Hain, TC, Fetter, M, and Zee, DS: Head-shaking nystagmus in patients with unilateral peripheral vestibular lesions. Am J Otolaryngol 8:36, 1987.
4. Kamei, T and Kronhuber, H: Spontaneous and head-shaking nystagmus in normals and in patients with central lesions. Can J Otolaryngol 3:372, 1974.
5. Hain, TC and Spindler, J: Head-shaking nystagmus. In Sharpe, JA and Barber, HO (eds): The Vestibulo-ocular Reflex and Vertigo. Raven Press, New York 1993, p 217.
6. Kasai, T and Zee, DS: Eye-head coordination in labyrinthine-defective human beings. Brain Res 144:123, 1978.
7. Cannon, SC, et al: The effect of rotational magnification of corrective spectacles on the quantitative evaluation of the VOR. Acta Otolaryngol 100:81, 1985.
8. Gauthier, GM and Robinson, DA: Adaptation of the human vestibulo-ocular reflex to magnifying lenses. Brain Res 92:331, 1975.
9. Halmagyi, M and Curthoys, IS: A clinical sign of canal paresis. Arch Neurol 45:737, 1988.
10. Halmagyi, GM, et al: The human horizontal vestibulo-ocular reflex in response to high acceleration stimulation before and after unilateral vestibular neurectomy. Exp Brain Res 81:479, 1990.
11. Zee, DS: Suppression of the vestibulo-ocular reflex. Ann Neurol 1:217, 1977.
12. Sharpe, JA, et al: Visual-vestibular interaction in multiple sclerosis. Neurology 31:427, 1981.
13. Sharpe, JA and Morrow, MJ: Smooth pursuit disorders. In Barber, HO and Sharpe, JA (eds): Vestibular Disorders. Year Book, Chicago, 1988, p 129.
14. Peterson, BW and Leigh, RJ: Modulation and cancellation of the vestibulo-ocular reflex: Physiological and clinical considerations. In Barber, HO and Sharpe, JA: Vestibular Disorders. Year Book, Chicago, 1988, p 24.

15. Buettner-Ennever, JA, et al: Vertical gaze paralysis and the rostral interstitial nucleus of the medial longitudinal fasciculus. Brain 105:125, 1982.
16. Pierrot-Deseilligny, C, et al: Parinaud's syndrome: Electrooculographic and anatomical analyses of six vascular cases with deductions about vertical gaze organization in the premotor structures. Brain 105:667, 1982.
17. Baloh, RW, Furman, JM, and Yee, RD: Dorsal midbrain syndrome: Clinical and oculographic findings. Neurology 35:54, 1985.
18. Ranalli, PJ, Sharpe, JA, and Fletcher, WA: Palsy of upward and downward saccadic, pursuit and vestibular movements with a unilateral midbrain lesion: Pathophysiological correlations. Neurology 38:114, 1988.
19. Bannister, R: Brain's Clinical Neurology. Oxford University Press, London, 1975.
20. Adams, RD and Victor, M.: Principles of Neurology. McGraw-Hill, New York, 1985, p 198.
21. Sharpe, JA and Ranalli, PJ: Vertical vestibulo-ocular reflex control after supranuclear midbrain damage. Acta Otolaryngol (suppl) 481:194, 1991.
22. Ranalli, PJ and Sharpe, JA: Vertical vestibulo-ocular reflex, smooth pursuit, and eye-head tracking dysfunction in internuclear ophthalmoplegia. Brain 111:1299, 1988.
23. Ranalli, PJ and Sharpe, JA: The vertical vestibulo-ocular reflex. In Barber, HO and Sharpe, JA (eds): Vestibular Disorders. Year Book, Chicago, 1988, p 159.
24. Fukushima, K: The interstitial nucleus of Cajal in the midbrain reticular formation and vertical eye movements. Neurosci Res 10:159, 1991.
25. Raphan, T, Matsuo V, and Cohen, B: Velocity storage in the vestibulo-ocular reflex (VOR). Exp Brain Res 35:229, 1979.
26. Crawford, JD, Cadera, W, and Vilis, T: Generation of torsional and vertical eye position signals by the interstitial nucleus of cajal. Science 252:1551, 1991.
27. Zackon, DH and Sharpe, JA: Midbrain paresis of horizontal gaze. Ann Neurol 16:495, 1984.
28. Bril, V, Sharpe, JA, and Ashby, P: Midbrain asterixis. Ann Neurol 6:363, 1979.
29. Shanzer, S and Bender, MB: Oculomotor responses on vestibular stimulation on monkeys with lesions of the brainstem. Brain 82:669, 1959.
30. Pompeiano, O and Walberg, F: Descending connections to the vestibular nuclei. An experimental study in the cat. J Comp Neurol 108:465, 1957.
31. Leigh, RJ, Newman, SA, and King, WM: Vertical gaze disorders. In Lennerstrand, G, Zee, DS, and Keller, EL (eds): Functional Basis of Ocular Motility Disorders. Pergamon Press, Oxford, 1982, p 257.
32. Evinger, LC, Fuchs, AF, and Baker, R: Bilateral lesions of the medial longitudinal fasciculus in monkeys: Effects on the horizontal and vertical components of voluntary and vestibular induced eye movements. Exp Brain Res 28:1, 1977.
33. King, WM, Lisberger, SG, and Fuchs, AF: Response of fibers in medial longitudinal fasciculus (MLF) of alert monkeys during horizontal and vertical conjugate eye movements evoked by vestibular or visual stimuli. J Neurophysiol 39:1135, 1976.
34. Pola, J and Robinson, DA: Oculomotor signals in medial longitudinal fasciculus of monkey. J Neurophysiol 41:245, 1978.
35. Zee, DS, Friendlich, AR, and Robinson, DA: The mechanism of downbeat nystagmus. Arch Neurol 30:227, 1974.
36. Gresty, MA, et al: Analysis of downbeat nystagmus. Otolithic versus semicircular canal influences. Arch Neurol 43:52, 1986.
37. Baloh, RW and Spooner, JW: Downbeat nystagmus: A type of central vestibular nystagmus. Neurology 31:304, 1981.
38. Halmagyi, GM, et al: Downbeating nystagmus. A review of 62 cases. Arch Neurol. 40:777, 1983.
39. Donat, JR and Auger, R: Famililal periodic ataxia. Arch Neurol 36:568, 1979.
40. Saul, R and Selhorst, JB: Downbeat nystagmus with magnesium depletion. Arch Neurol 38:650, 1981.
41. Corbett, JJ, et al: Downbeating nystagmus and other ocular motor defects caused by lithium toxicity. Neurology 39:481, 1989.
42. Halmagyi, GM, et al: Lithium-induced downbeat nystagmus. Am J Ophthalmol 107:664, 1989.
43. Chrousos, GA, et al: Two cases of downbeat nystagmus and oscillopsia associated with carbamazepine. Am J Ophthalmol 103:221, 1987.
44. Alpert, JN: Downbeat nystagmus due to anticonvulsant toxicity. Ann Neurol 4:471, 1978.
45. Carleton, SC and Carpenter, MB: Afferent and efferent connections of the medial, inferior and lateral vestibular nuclei in the cat and monkey. Brain Res 278:29, 1983.
46. Dejong, JMBV, et al: Midsagittal pontomedullary brainstem section: Effects on ocular adduction and nystagmus. Exp Neurol 68:420, 1980.
47. Zee, DS, et al: Effects of ablation of flocculus and paraflocculus on eye movements in primates. J Neurophysiol 446:878, 1981.
48. Fernandez, C, Alzate, R, and Lindsay, JR: Experimental observations on postural nystagmus: II. Lesions of the nodulus. Ann Otol Rhinol Laryngol 69:94, 1960.
49. Zee, DS, Leigh, RJ, and Mathieu-Millaire, F: Cerebellar control of ocular gaze stability. Ann Neurol 7:37, 1980.

50. Spooner, JW and Baloh, RW: Arnold-Chiari malformation. Improvement in eye movements after surgical treatment. Brain 104:51, 1981.
51. Lavin, P, et al: Downbeat nystagmus with a pseudocycloid waveform improvement with base-out prism. Ann Neurol 13:621, 1983.
51a. Leigh, RJ, et al: Effectiveness of botulinumtoxin administered to abolish acquired nystagmus. Ann Neurol 32:633, 1992.
52. Currie, JN and Matuso, V: The use of clonazepam in the treatment of nystagmus-induced oscillopsia. Ophthalmology 93:924, 1986.
53. Dieterich, M, et al: The effects of baclofen and cholinergic drugs on upbeat and downbeat nystagmus. J Neurol Neurosurg Psychiatry 54:627, 1991.
54. Leigh, RJ, et al: Effects of anticholinergic agents upon acquired nystagmus. A double-blind study of triherzyphenidyl and tridihexethyl chloride. Neurology 41:1737, 1991.
54a. Bartar, JJS, Huaman, AG, and Sharpe, JA: Muscarinic antagonists in the treatment of acquired pendular and downbeat nystagmus. Ann Neurol (in press).
55. Nakada, T and Remler, MP: Primary position upbeat nystagmus. Another central vestibular nystagmus? J Clin Neuro-opthalmol 1:185, 1981.
56. Ranalli, PJ and Sharpe, JA: Upbeat nystagmus and the ventral tegmental pathway of the upward vestibulo-ocular reflex. Neurology 38:1329, 1988.
57. Sibony, PA, Evinger, C, and Manning, KA. Tobacco induced primary-position upbeat nystagmus. Ann Neurol 21:53, 1987.
58. Fisher, A, et al: Primary position upbeat nystagmus: A variety of central positional nystagmus. Brain 106:949, 1983.
59. Keane, JR and Itabashi, HH: Upbeat nystagmus: Clinicopathologic study of two patients. Neurology 37:491, 1987.
60. Gilman, N, Baloh, RW, and Tomiyasu, U: Primary position upbeat nystagmus. Neurology 27:294, 1977.
61. Hirose, G, et al: Upbeat nystagmus: Clinicopathological and pathophysiological considerations. J Neurol Sci 105:159, 1991.
62. Morrow, MJ and Sharpe, JA: Torsional nystagmus in the lateral medullary syndrome. Ann Neurol 24:390, 1988.
63. Noseworthy, JH, et al: Torsional nystagmus: Quantitative features and possible pathogenesis. Neurology 38:992, 1988.
64. Leigh, RJ, Robinson, DA, and Zee, DS: A hypothetical explanation for periodic alternating nystagmus: Instability in the optokinetic-vestibular system. Ann New York Acad Sci 374:619, 1981.
65. Waespe, W, Cohen, B, and Raphan, T. Dynamic modification of the vestibulo-ocular reflex by the nodulus and uvula. Science 228:199, 1985.
66. Cohen, B, Helwig, D, and Raphan, T: Baclofen and velocity storage: A model of the effects of the drug on the vestibulo-ocular reflex in the rhesus monkey. J Physiol (Lond) 393:703, 1987.
67. Reis, J, et al: Alternating nystagmus and infectious mononucleosis. Neurophthalmology 9:289, 1989.
68. Zee, DS, et al: Oculomotor abnormalities in hereditary cerebellar ataxia. Brain 99:207, 1976.
69. Baloh, RW, et al: Visual-vestibular interaction and cerebellar atrophy. Neurology 29:116, 1979.
70. Thurston, SE, et al: Hyperactive vestibulo-ocular reflex in cerebellar degeneration: Pathogenesis and treatment. Neurology 37:53, 1987.
71. Demer, JL and Robinson, DA: Effects of reversible lesions and stimulation on olivocerebellar system on vestibulocular reflex plasticity. J Neurophysiol 47:1084, 1982.
72. Marani, E, Voogd, J, and Boekee, A: Acetylcholinesterase staining in subdivisions of the cat's inferior olive. J Comp Neurol 174:209, 1977.
73. Nylen, CO: Positional nystagmus. A review of future prospects. J Laryngol Otol 64:295, 1950.
74. Lin, J, et al: Direction change in positional nystagmus: Incidence and meaning. Am J Otolaryngol 7:306, 1986.
75. Baloh, RW, Honrubia, V, and Jacobson, K: Benign positional vertigo. Clinical and oculographic features in 240 cases. Neurology 37:371, 1987.
76. Schuknecht, H and Ruby, R: Cupulolithiasis. Adv Otorhinolaryngol 20:434, 1973.
77. Watson, P, et al: Positional vertigo and nystagmus of central origin. Can J Neurol Sci 8:133, 1988.
78. Barber, HO and Wright, G: Positional nystagmus in normals. Adv Otolaryngol 19:1973.
79. Reivich, M, et al: Reversal of blood flow through the vertebral artery and its effect on cerebral circulation. N Engl J Med 265:878, 1961.
80. Baker, R, Rosenbaum, A, and Caplan, LR: Subclavian steal syndrome. Comtemp Surg 14:96, 1974.
81. Moufarrij, N, et al: Vertebral artery stenosis: Long term follow up. Stroke 15:260, 1986.
82. Fisher, CM: Occlusion of the vertebral arteries. Arch Neurol 22:13, 1970.
83. Wilkinson, IMS and Russel, RWR: Arteries of the head and neck in giant cell arteritis. Arch Neurol 27:378, 1972.
84. Thomson, GDT, et al: Internuclear ophthalmoplegia in giant cell arteritis. J Rheumatol 16:693, 1989.
85. Radner, S: Vertebral angiography by catheterization. Acta Radiol (suppl) 87:1, 1951.
86. Easton, JD and Sherman, DG: Cervical manipulation and stroke. Stroke 8:594, 1977.
87. Caplan, AR, Zarins, C, and Hemmatti, M: Spontaneous dissection of the extracranial vertebral arteries. Stroke 16:1030, 1985.

88. Bjerver, K and Silfverskiold, BP: Lateropulsion and imbalance in Wallenberg's syndrome. Acta Neurol Scand 44:91, 1968.
89. Ranalli, PJ and Sharpe, JA: Contrapulsion of saccades and ipsilateral ataxia: A unilateral disorder of the rostral cerebellum. Ann Neurol 20:311, 1986.
90. Waespe, W and Wichmann, W: Ocular motor disturbances during visual-vestibular interaction in Wallenberg's lateral medullary syndrome. Brain 113:821, 1990.
91. Uemura, T and Cohen, B: Effects of vestibular nuclei lesions on vestibulo-ocular reflexes and posture in monkeys. Acta Otolaryngol (suppl)315:1, 1973.
92. Rabinovitch, HE, Sharpe, JA, and Sylvester, TO: The ocular tilt reaction. Arch Ophthalmol 95:1395, 1977.
93. Halmagyi, GM, et al: Tonic contraversive ocular tilt reaction due to unilateral meso-diencephalic lesion. Neurology 40:1503, 1990.
94. Ausman, J, Caplan, LR, and Diaz, F: Surgically created posterior circulation vascular shunts. Clin Neurosurg 33:327, 1986.
95. Sunderland, S: The arterial relations of the internal auditory meatus. Brain 68:23, 1945.
96. Keane, JR: Ocular tilt reaction following lateral pontomedullary infarction. Neurology 42:259, 1992.
97. Grad, A and Baloh, RW: Vertigo of vascular origin. Arch Neurol 46:281, 1989.
98. Lindsay, JR and Hemenway, WG: Postural vertigo due to unilateral sudden partial loss of vestibular function. Ann Otol Rhinol Laryngol 65:692, 1956.
99. Davidson, C, Goodhart, SP, and Savitsky, N: The syndrome of the superior cerebellar artery and its branches. Arch Neurol Psychiatry (Chicago) 33:1143, 1935.
100. Kase, CS, et al: Cerebellar infarction in the superior cerebellar artery distribution. Neurology 35:705, 1985.
101. Uno, A, et al: Lateropulsion in Wallenberg's syndrome and contrapulsion in the proximal type of superior cerebellar artery syndrome. Neuro-ophthalmology 975, 1989.
102. Kayan, NA and Hood, JD: Neuro-otological manifestations of migraine. Brain 107:1123, 1984.
103. Watson, P and Steele, JC: Paroxysmal disequilibrium in the migraine syndrome of childhood. Arch Otolaryngol 99:177, 1974.
104. Langzi, G, et al: Benign paroxysmal vertigo in childhood: Longitudinal study. Headache 26:494, 1986.
105. Moretti, G, et al: Benign recurrent vertigo and its connection with migraine. Headache 20:344, 1980.
106. Fisher, CM: Late-life migraine accompaniments as a cause of unexplained transient ischemic attacks. Can J Neurol Sci 7:9, 1980.
107. Tomaszek, DE and Rosner, MJ: Cerebellar infarction: Analysis of 21 cases. Surg Neurol 24:223, 1985.
108. Antiplatelet Trialists' Collaboration. Secondary prevention of vascular disease by prolonged antiplatelet treatment. Br Med J 296:320, 1988.
109. Gent, M, et al: The Canadian American ticlopidine study (CATS) in thromboembolic stroke. Lancet 1:1215, 1989.
110. Hass, WK, Easton, JD, and Adams, HP: A randomized trial comparing ticlopidine hydrochloride with aspirin for the prevention of stroke in high risk patients. N Engl J Med 321:501, 1989.
111. McClure, JA: Functional basis for horizontal canal BPV. In Barber, HO and Sharpe, JA (eds): Vestibular Disorders. Year Book, Chicago, 1988, p 233.

CHAPTER 12

Diagnosis and Management of Neuro-otologic Disorders Due to Migraine

Ronald J. Tusa, MD, PhD

Migraine is a common cause of episodic vertigo and disequilibrium in children and adults. The reported correlation between migraine and vertigo varies according to the type of practice. In a practice treating patients with migraine headaches, 27 to 33 percent out of a population of 700 patients with migraine reported episodic vertigo.[1,2] Thirty-six percent of these patients experienced vertigo during their headache-free period; the others experienced vertigo either just before or during a headache. The occurrence of vertigo during the headache period is much higher in patients with migraine headaches with aura (classic migraine) as opposed to migraine without aura (common migraine).[3] In a practice treating patients with episodic vertigo, 54 percent from a population of 62 patients had a history of migraine.[4] This high percentage may overestimate the prevalence of migraine in this group, because strict criteria for migraine were not used.

This chapter describes recent studies concerning the incidence of migraine, the current classification and criteria used for diagnosing migraine, neuro-otologic syndromes caused by migraine, and the management of migraine.

INCIDENCE OF MIGRAINE

Migraine is an extremely prevalent disorder. An epidemiologic study that involved more than 20,000 individuals between 12 and 80 years of age found 17.6 percent of all females and 5.7 percent of all males had one or more migraine headaches per year.[5] The incidence of migraine in this study is a little lower than previous studies because of the stricter criteria used for the diagnosis. In previous studies, migraine was diagnosed if the individual had an aura, unilateral pain, and nausea, or any two of these symptoms. The study by Stewart and colleagues[5] used the diagnostic criteria recommended by the International Headache Society (IHS),[6] which will be described later. Of those individuals with migraine, approximately 18 percent experienced one or more attacks per month. In both men and women, the prevalence of migraine was highest between the ages of 35 and 45 years.

The type and severity of migraine often varies within the same individual. Migraine with or without aura frequently begins between 12 and 30 years of age. There is often an increased frequency of headache in the mid to late 40s. After the age of 50, migraine is much less common, and it frequently presents as migraine aura without headache.[7]

CLASSIFICATION AND CRITERIA FOR DIAGNOSIS OF MIGRAINE

Migraine disorders are usually subdivided into several types including *common, classic, migraine equivalent, and complicated migraine*. To help standardize terminology and diagnostic criteria, a new classification system for headaches was developed by the IHS.[6] This classification was based on 2 years of discussion among 100 individuals with representatives from seven countries. The classification and criteria for headaches pertinent to neuro-otologic disorders is summarized in Table 12–1. The general features of the relevant types of migraine will be briefly discussed, and then the features of specific neuro-otologic disorders will be presented in more detail.

Migraine without aura, which replaces the classification "common migraine," consists of periodic headaches that are usually throbbing and unilateral, exacerbated by activity, and associated with nausea, photophobia, and phonophobia. These headaches are frequently referred to as "sick" headaches (because of the nausea) or "sinus" headaches (because of their location). Patients usually like to lie down in a quiet dark room during the headache and feel better after sleep. A family history of migraine can usually be obtained in the immediate family.

Migraine with aura, which replaces the classification "classic migraine," is associated with transient neurologic symptoms consisting of sensory, motor, or cognitive disorders. These neurologic disorders usually precede the headache but may develop during or following the headache. The neurologic disorder usually lasts 5 to 20 minutes, but can last up to 1 hour. There are three relevant subtypes. The first is *migraine with prolonged aura*, in which neurologic symptoms can last up to 7 days. The second is called *basilar migraine*, which replaces the classification "basilar artery migraine," and presents with symptoms in the distribution of the basilar artery including vertigo, tinnitus, decreased hearing, and ataxia. The third is called *migraine aura without headache*, which replaces the terms "migraine equivalent spells" and "acephalgic migraine." This presents with the neurologic disorders found in migraine with aura except there is no headache.

Childhood periodic syndromes may be precursors to or associated with migraine. The most important subtype is *benign paroxysmal vertigo of childhood*, which consists of spells of disequilibrium and vertigo in children. These may or may not be associated with headache.

Migrainous infarction, which replaces "complicated migraine," is a migraine with aura associated with an infarct. The infarct can either be documented by neuroimaging or by an aura that does not resolve within 7 days.

Although the IHS classification was a mammoth undertaking, it is still considered preliminary and subject to revision. The classification was primarily developed for research purposes and, therefore, diagnostic criteria were made very specific. Some

TABLE 12–1 IHS Classification of Headache

1.1. *Migraine without aura* (replaces common migraine).
  A. At least five attacks fulfillng B–D.
  B. Headache attacks lasting 4–72 hours untreated. If patient falls asleep and wakes up without migraine, duration of attack is until time of awakening. In children <15 yrs, attack may last 2–48 hrs.
  C. Headache has at least two of the following characteristics:
      1. Unilateral location.
      2. Pulsating quality.
      3. Moderate or severe intensity (inhibits or prohibits daily activities).
      4. Aggravation by walking stairs or similar routine physical activity.
  D. During headache at least one of the following:
      1. Nausea and/or vomiting.
      2. Photophobia and phonophobia.
  E. At least one of the following:
      1. History, physical, and neurologic examinations do not suggest one of the disorders listed in groups 5–11.
      2. History and/or physical and/or neurologic examinations do suggest such disorder, but it is ruled out by appropriate investigations.
      3. Such disorder is present, but migraine attacks do not occur for the first time in close temporal relation to the disorder.
1.2. *Migraine with aura* (replaces classic migraine).
  A. At least two attacks fulfilling B.
  B. At least three of the following:
      1. One or more fully reversible aura symptoms indicating focal cerebral cortical and/or brain stem dysfunction.
      2. At least one aura symptom develops gradually over more than 4 minutes, or two or more symptoms occur in succession.
      3. No aura symptom lasts more than 60 minutes unless more than one aura symptom present.
      4. Headache occurs either before, during, or after aura (but no more than 60 minutes after aura is completed).
  C. Same as E above in criteria 1.1.
1.2.2. *Migraine with prolonged aura* (replaces complicated migraine).
  A. Fulfills criteria for 1.2, but at least one symptom lasts more than 60 minutes and ≤7 days.
1.2.4. *Basilar migraine* (replaces basilar artery migraine).
  A. Fulfills criteria for 1.2.
  B. Two or more aura symptoms of the following types: Visual symptoms in both the temporal and nasal fields of both eyes, dysarthria, vertigo, tinnitus, decreased hearing, double vision, ataxia, bilateral paresthesia, bilateral paresis, decreased level of consciousness.
1.2.5. *Migraine aura without headache* (replaces migraine equivalent or acephalgic migraine). Fulfills criteria for 1.2 but no headache.
1.5. *Childhood periodic syndromes* that may be precursors to or associated with migraine.
1.5.1. *Benign paroxysmal vertigo of childhood*
  A. Multiple, brief, sporadic episodes of disequilibrium, anxiety, and often nystagmus or vomiting.
  B. Normal neurologic examination.
  C. Normal electroencephalogram.
1.6.2. *Migrainous infarction* (replaces complicated migraine).
  A. Patient has previously fulfilled criteria for 1.2.
  B. The present attack is typical of previous attacks, but neurologic deficits are not completely reversible within 7 days and/or neuroimaging demonstrates ischemic infarction in relevant area.
  C. Other causes of infarction ruled out by appropriate investigations.

TABLE 12 – 1 IHS Classification of Headache (*Continued*)

Nonmigraine Headaches

5. Headache associated with head trauma
6. Headache associated with vascular disorders including TIA, hematoma, hemorrhage, arterovenous malformation, arteritis, venous thrombosis, arterial hypertension
7. Headache associated with nonvascular intracranial disorder including high or low cerebrospinal fluid pressure, infection, sarcoid, tumor
8. Headache associated with substances or their withdrawal
9. Headache associated with noncephalic infection
10. Headache associated with metabolic disorder
11. Headache or facial pain associated with disorder of cranium, neck, eyes, ears, nose, sinuses, teeth, mouth or other facial or cranial structures
12. Cranial neuralgias, nerve trunk pain, and deafferentation pain

Adapted from Headache Classification Committee of the International Headache Society.[6]

members on the committee disagree with some of the criteria, such as excluding the bilateral nature of pain in some individuals with migraine.[8] A second edition to the classification is planned for publication in 1993.

NEURO-OTOLOGIC SYNDROMES WITH MIGRAINE

A number of different neuro-otologic syndromes have been described with migraine (Table 12 – 2). These disorders can be divided into those that are due to migraine and those that are associated with migraine.

Disorders Due to Migraine

CHILDHOOD PERIODIC SYNDROMES

There are two neuro-otologic disorders in children due to migraine. Benign paroxysmal vertigo of childhood (1.5.1 by IHS) was first described by Basser.[9] This disorder consists of spells of vertigo and disequilibrium without hearing loss or tinnitus.[10-13] The

TABLE 12 – 2 Neuro-otologic Disorders

Neuro-otologic disorders due to migraine

1. Paroxysmal torticollis of infancy
2. Benign paroxysmal vertigo of childhood
3. Basilar migraine
4. Benign recurrent vertigo of adults
5. Migrainous infarct resulting in vertigo

Neuro-otologic disorders associated with migraine

1. Motion sickness
2. Ménière's disease
3. BPPV

majority of cases occur between 1 and 4 years of age, but they can occur any time during the first decade. Vertigo and disequilibrium typically last for minutes, but they can last up to several hours. Patients may have visual disturbance, flushing, nausea, and vomiting. In the majority of cases, audiograms and caloric tests are normal. These patients also have normal physical examination and normal electroencephalography (EEG). Headache is usually not a major feature of these spells initially. Many of these patients eventually develop migraine with aura, and there is frequently a positive family history for migraine. The differential diagnosis includes Ménière's disease, vestibular epilepsy, perilymphatic fistula, posterior fossa tumors, and psychogenic disorders.

PAROXYSMAL TORTICOLLIS OF INFANCY

This condition was not specifically classified by the IHS but may fit into the same classification as benign paroxysmal vertigo of childhood, because these two disorders frequently occur in the same patient.[12] This disorder was first described by Snyder,[14] and it has now been reported by a number of individuals.[15-17] Paroxysmal torticollis of infancy consists of spells of head tilt and rotation without vertigo, hearing loss, or tinnitus. These spells usually occur in the first 5 years of life and typically last between 10 minutes and several days. They may be associated with nausea, vomiting, pallor, agitation, and ataxia. In the majority of cases, audiograms and caloric tests are normal between the spells. This syndrome is believed to be migraine auras without headache. Some individuals complain of headache when they become older. The differential diagnosis includes posterior fossa tumors and torticollis.

BASILAR MIGRAINE

Basilar migraine (1.2.4 by IHS) was first described by Bickerstaff[18] and has been subsequently reported by a number of individuals.[19,20] This disorder consists of two or more neurologic problems (vertigo, tinnitus, decreased hearing, ataxia, dysarthria, visual symptoms in both hemifields of both eyes, diplopia, bilateral paresthesia or paresis, decreased level of consciousness) followed by a throbbing headache. The majority of these cases occur before 20 years of age, but they can occur up until age 60 years. Vertigo typically lasts between 5 minutes and 1 hour. In the majority of cases, audiograms are normal, but many individuals have abnormal caloric studies. Many of these patients eventually develop migraine headaches with aura, and there is frequently a positive family history for migraine. Transient ischemic attacks (TIAs) need to be considered before basilar migraine is diagnosed. TIAs within the vertebrobasilar circulatory system (vertebrobasilar insufficiency) may cause the same symptoms as basilar migraine, although TIAs usually last less than a few minutes.[21]

BENIGN RECURRENT VERTIGO OF ADULTS

This form of vertigo was not formally classified by the IHS.[6] Based on the symptoms, it may either be referred to as basilar migraine (1.2.4 by IHS), or migraine aura without headache (1.2.5 by IHS). This was first described by Slater[22] and is the most common neuro-otologic syndrome caused by migraine. This disorder consists of spells of vertigo, occasionally with tinnitus but without hearing loss.[23,24] In some individuals, jerk nystagmus may occur during the spell (Case Study 1). Vertigo typically lasts minutes to days, but the majority of instances last less than 1 hour. These spells may occur with or without headache and usually occur between the ages of 20 and 60 years. Peripheral and central vestibular deficits diagnosed by caloric and spontaneous eye movements during electronystagmography have been reported to occur in 5 to 80 percent of individuals with migraine in their headache-free period.[25,26] This variation in abnormality may be due to a difference in criteria used for diagnosing vestibular deficits.[25] Some individuals develop *exercise-induced* spells brought on by a variety of physical activities, including situps, heavy lifting, intercourse, and strenuous aerobic exercises[27] (Case Study 2). In the majority of cases, audiograms and caloric studies are normal. One needs to rule out Ménière's disease, benign paroxysmal positional vertigo (BPPV), TIAs, vestibular epilepsy, and perilymphatic fistula before making a diagnosis of migraine-induced vertigo.

MIGRAINOUS INFARCTION

This migraine with aura is associated with an infarct.[28-30] This IHS classification is 1.6.2. These strokes can be very focal, such as small retinal stroke or infarct within portions of the optic nerve.[31,32] Whether similar focal infarcts can involve the labyrinth and eighth nerve is unclear. Hearing loss, ear fullness, vertigo, and disequilibrium due to a migrainous infarct in the territory of the anterior-inferior cerebellar artery has been described[33] as has vertigo and disequilibrium due to migrainous infarct in the dorsal lateral medulla.[34]

Disorders Associated with Migraine

MOTION SICKNESS

This problem consists of episodic dizziness, tiredness, pallor, diaphoresis, salivation, nausea, and occasional vomiting induced by passive locomotion (e.g., riding in a car) or motion in the visual surround while standing still (e.g., viewing a rotating optokinetic stimulus). One hypothesis is that it is due to a visuovestibular conflict or mismatch.[35] Of patients with migraine, 26 to 60 percent have a history of severe motion sickness compared to 8 to 24 percent in the normal population.[2,3,36] The cause for this relation is not clear.

MÉNIÈRE'S DISEASE

There is considerable confusion between migraine aura without headache and vestibular hydrops (vestibular Ménière's disease). Both can present with transient vertigo, ear fullness, and occasional tinnitus without any decrease in hearing. A history of headaches associated with the spells of vertigo may help to distinguish between these two syndromes, but occasionally the diagnosis is only made following the patient's response to a therapeutic trial (Case Study 3).

Patients with well-documented Ménière's disease may later develop migraine aura without headache. Therefore, they may initially do well with treatment for Ménière's disease for a while and then appear to fail to respond to treatment when in fact they have developed spells of vertigo owing to migraine aura without headache (Case Study 4).

Kayan and Hood[2] and Hinchcliffe[37] have noted a higher-than-expected incidence of both disorders in the same individual. Whether there is a causal link between these two disorders is unclear.

BENIGN PAROXYSMAL POSITIONAL VERTIGO

BPPV and migraine are reported to be associated frequently;[2,38] however, the causal relationship remains obscure. We have occasionally seen patients who had a normal examination but then developed BPPV following a migraine headache (Case Study 5). Whether this occurrence is due to migrainous infarction in the distribution of the superior vestibular artery is unclear.

PATHOPHYSIOLOGY OF MIGRAINE

There are two main hypotheses for the cause of migraine with aura.[39,40] According to the biochemical-vascular hypothesis, the aura is due to ischemia caused by vasoconstriction primarily in specific posterior intracranial vessels; the headache is due to vasodilation, primarily of the extracranial vessels. These vessel changes are thought to be due to abnormal accumulation of vasoactive substances including serotonin, tyramine, and prostaglandin. According to the neurogenic hypothesis, the aura is due to an area of neuronal dysfunction similar to a wave of spreading depression. This neuronal dysfunction may be mediated by neurons containing serotonin. Through autoregulation, blood flow is reduced to this area. Thus, according to this hypothesis, the vascular changes of migraine are epiphenomena secondary to an underlying neurogen mechanism.

Based on these hypotheses, treatment of migraine has included elimination of tyramine from the diet and the use of drugs that change vascular tone or block serotonin and prostaglandin.

MANAGEMENT OF MIGRAINE

Vertigo and disequilibrium secondary to migraine usually respond to the same type of treatment used for migraine headaches. Migraine is triggered by a number of factors, including stress, anxiety, hypoglycemia, fluctuating estrogen, certain foods, and smoking.[41-43] Treatment of migraine can be divided into (1) reduction of risk factors, (2) abortive medical therapy, and (3) prophylactic medical therapy.

Reduction of Risk Factors

All patients with migraine are given a management schedule to follow, which is gone over at the time of their first visit (Table 12–3). There are several triggers for migraine, which are treated by following the schedule:

1. *Stress*: All patients are started on an aerobic exercise program to help reduce stress. This program is gradually increased until the individual is exercising 3 to 5 times per week for at least 30 minutes at the end of the day (jogging, swimming, fast walk, racquetball, tennis, etc.). Several good aerobic exercise programs can be found in a paperback book by Cooper.[44] If patients are reluctant or unable to participate in an exercise program, other stress-reduction programs can be very helpful. These programs include biofeedback and relaxation, which have been shown to significantly reduce the frequency of recurrent migraine disorders in clinical trials.[45] Patients are urged to avoid *hypoglycemia* by eating something at least every 8 hours. Many

TABLE 12–3 Schedule to Treat Migraine Disorders

1. Reduction of stress
   a. Aerobic exercise at end of day (3–4 times/week).
      Get heart rate above 100 and sustain it for at least 20 minutes.
   b. Eat something at least every 8 hours to avoid hypoglycemia. Eat breakfast at same time each morning (breakfast on weekends should be at the same time as on weekdays).
   c. Maintain a regular sleep schedule.
2. Do not smoke or chew any products that contain nicotine.
3. Avoid exogenous estrogen (oral contraceptives, estrogen replacement).
4. Follow diet.
5. Keep a diary.
   a. Time and date of all headaches and/or spells that interfere with daily routine.
   b. Write down any foods that you had that should have been avoided (Table 12–4) during the 24 hours prior to the headache and/or spell.
   c. Bring diary in with you on your next visit!
6. Take medications.

individuals skip breakfast, and so they need to eat breakfast at the same time each morning, including weekends. Finally, they should maintain a regular *sleep schedule* by attempting to go to bed and get up at the same time each day.

2. *Nicotine*: Patients who smoke cigarettes are urged to stop smoking.
3. *Elevated or rapid fluctuations in estrogens*: If female patients are taking estrogen supplements (other then vaginal creams), the doctor should work with the patient's gynecologist to either eliminate the supplement or reduce the estrogen to the lowest level possible for a 3-month trial.
4. *Diet*: All patients are placed on a diet schedule, which is given to them in written form (Table 12–4). This diet is based on the content of tyramine and other substances known to exacerbate migraine.[42,46] Some of these foods cause migraine almost immediately [red wine, monosodium glutamate (MSG)], others cause migraine the next day (chocolate, nuts, cheese).

Finally, all patients are asked to keep a careful *diary*, noting the time and date of all spells or headaches that interrupt their daily activities. They should write down any foods that they had off the diet sheet during the 24 hours prior to the headache or spell. This procedure forces the individual to become more aware of the association of diet to migraine and potentially identifies certain foods from which they should stay away.

Abortive Medical Therapy

The standard drugs used to abort attacks of migraine include aspirin, ibuprofen, isometheptene mucate (Midrin), and ergotamine. These drugs are primarily designed to abort headache; I have not found them effective in aborting migraine auras. Whether their ineffectiveness in aborting auras is due to their delay in absorption (15 to 30 minutes) relative to the average duration of the aura (5 to 20 minutes) or their mode of action is unclear. Drugs such as Sumatriptan, a 5-hydroxytryptamine (HT) agonist that can be delivered subcutaneously, is a very promising drug that may be capable of aborting auras. This drug is now available in the United States and has been found to be very effective in aborting headache in trials outside of the United States.[47]

TABLE 12–4 Diet for Migraine Patients*

	Foods Allowed	Foods to Avoid
Beverages	Decaffeinated coffee, fruit juice, club soda, noncola soda. Limit caffeine sources to 2 cups per day (coffee, tea, cola).	Chocolate, cocoa, certain alcoholic beverages (red wine, port, sherry, scotch, bourbon, gin). Excessive Nutrasweet (no more than 24 oz/day of diet drink).
Meats, fish, poultry	Fresh or frozen turkey, chicken, fish, beef, lamb, veal, pork. Limit eggs to 3 per week. Tuna or tuna salad.	Aged, canned, cured, or processed meats including ham or game, pickled herring, salad and dried fish; chicken liver, bologna; fermented sausage; any food prepared with meat tenderizer, soy souce, or brewer's yeast; any food containing nitrates, nitrites, or tyramine (smoked meats including bacon, sausage, ham, salami, pepperoni, hot dogs).
Dairy products	Milk: Homogenized, 2% or skim. Cheese: American, cottage, farmer, ricotta, cream, Canadian, processed cheese slice. Yogurt (Limit ½ cup per day).	Buttermilk, sour cream, chocolate milk. Cheese: Stilton, bleu, cheddar, mozzarella, cheese spread, roquefort, provolone, gruyere, muenster, feta, parmesan, emmenthal, brie, brick, camembert types, gouda, romano.
Breads, cereals	Commercial bread, English muffins, melba toast crackers, bagels. All hot and dry cereals.	Crackers containing cheese. Fresh yeast-containing bread, coffee cake, doughnuts.
Potato or substitute	White potato, sweet potato, rice, macaroni, spaghetti, noodles.	None.
Vegetables	Any except those to avoid.	Beans such as pole, broad, lima, Italian, fava, navy, pinto, garbanzo. Snow peas, pea pods, sauerkraut, onions (except for flavoring), olives, pickles.
Fruits	Any except those to avoid; Limit citrus fruits to ½ cup per day (1 orange); limit banana to ½ per day.	Avocados, figs, raisins, papaya, passion fruit, red plums.
Soups	Cream soups made from foods allowed in diet, homemade broths.	Canned soup, soup or bouillon cubes, soup base with yeast or MSG (read labels).
Desserts	Any cake or cookies without chocolate, nuts, or yeast. Any pudding or ice cream without nuts or chocolate. Flavored gelatin.	Any products containing chocolate, including ice cream, pudding, cookies, cake, or pies. Mincemeat pie.
Sweets	Sugar, jelly, jam, honey, hard candy.	Chocolate candy or syrup, carob.
Miscellaneous	Salt in moderation, lemon juice, butter or margarine, cooking oil, whipped cream, white vinegar, commercial salad dressings.	Pizza, cheese sauce, MSG in excessive amounts (including Chinese food and Accent), yeast, yeast extract, meat tenderizer, seasoned salt.

TABLE 12–4 Diet for Migraine Patients* (*Continued*)

Foods Allowed	Foods to Avoid
	Mixed dishes (including macaroni and cheese, beef stroganoff, cheese blintzes, lasagna, frozen TV dinners). Chocolate, nuts (including peanut butter). All nonwhite vinegars. Anything fermented, pickled, or marinated.

Modified from Diamond[42] and Shulman et al.[46]

Prophylactic Medical Therapy

When migraine occurs several times a month, prophylactic daily medical therapy designed to prevent migraine should be used. There are a variety of drugs used in this capacity, including beta-blockers, amitriptyline, calcium-channel blockers, lithium carbonate, aspirin, and ibuprofen. All these drugs have been found to be effective in reducing the frequency and severity of headache with or without aura. With the exception of aspirin and ibuprofen, their mode of action may be via their effect on serotonin (5-HT) receptors. There are several types of serotonin receptors. It has been postulated that the abortive drugs are 5-HT1D (or 5-HT1A) agonists, whereas the prophylactic drugs are 5-HT2 antagonists.[48] 5-HT is an intracranial vasoconstrictor, and it rises during aura and falls during the headache. Although calcium channel blockers initially received much attention as a potent drug for migraine, in recent trials they have not been found to be any more effective than placebo,[49,50] and they have minimal effect on serotonin receptors.[48] Their role in preventing migraine auras has not been studied in any controlled manner. Based on personal observations, I have found that propranolol is quite effective in preventing auras, including vertigo; therefore, it is the first drug I use to treat patients with frequent migraine auras. Contraindications include congestive heart disease, cardiac block, asthma, diabetes, or orthostatic hypotension. Patients are started on 40-mg tablets, one table twice daily, increasing in 20-mg increments every 3 to 7 days, depending on patient tolerance of the drug. The effective dose is usually 80 to 200 mg/day, but sometimes as high as 240 mg. As this drug is increased, the heart rate and blood pressure are monitored. Once the therapeutic dose is found, 80-mg tablets three times a day, or long-acting propranolol (80- to 120-mg capsules twice daily) is prescribed. If they remain relatively symptom-free for a few months, then the medication is tapered every 1 to 2 weeks to the lowest effective dose.

Management of Migraine in Children

Treatment of migraine in children has been previously described in the pediatric literature but rarely in the adult literature.[51] Whenever possible, medication should be avoided, and every effort should be used to reduce risk factors. Traditional prophylactic drugs have not been found to be effective in reducing migraine in children in clinical trials.[52]

CASE STUDY 1

A 46-year-old owner of a blacktop paving company was referred for spells of vertigo, nausea, vomiting, oscillopsia, and diaphoresis for the past 2 years, each lasting approximately 30 minutes. He had sustained tinnitus and hearing loss on the right side, which did not fluctuate with his spells of vertigo. In addition, he had a life-long history of sinus pressure discomfort in the forehead, eyes, and behind the nose, for which he took Dristan. His last sinus discomfort was 3 years ago. In addition, he has recently had episodic flashes of light lasting 10 to 15 minutes. He has a history of hypertension and angina, but a normal electrocardiogram (ECG) and coronary angiography. In the last 2 months, the frequency of his spells of vertigo increased to one per week, and the last few spells were associated with left-arm paresthesia and dysarthria. One spell was witnessed, and the patient was found to have a sustained left-beating nystagmus for 20 minutes. The spells became so alarming that a diagnosis of impending basilar artery stroke was made. A four-vessel cerebral arteriogram was normal as was a magnetic resonance imaging (MRI) scan of the head with contrast. In summary, this patient was thought to be having impending brain-stem stroke with possible ischemia to the right brain-stem resulting in vertigo, left-beating nystagmus, and left-arm paresthesia. Of interest was that he also had angina with normal coronary arteries. He had a remote history of "sinus headaches" and recently has been experiencing scintillating scotomas. A diagnosis of migraine aura without headache (1.2.5) was made, and his spells of vertigo stopped after he was placed on a diet and propranolol.

CASE STUDY 2

A 28-year-old real estate developer was referred for thirty, 5- to 10-minute spells of disequilibrium, vertigo, 15-degree tilt of world, and diplopia (vertical and horizontal) over the past 5 years. Many of these spells occurred during a variety of physical activities including running, weight lifting, intercourse, and strenuous aerobic exercises (rowing machine, stair-stepping machine, and stationary bicycle). Because of the exercise-induced nature of these spells, these spells were believed to be due to a perilymphatic fistula, and surgery was recommended. Features more characteristic of migraine included the development of a dull soreness over his left occiput following each spell, the association of certain foods with spells (Chinese food, ice cream, cream cheese), and the frequent omission of breakfast. He had a normal audiogram and no history of barotrauma, ear surgery, or ear infection. A diagnosis of basilar migraine (1.2.4) was made. These spells stopped after he was placed on the antimigraine schedule listed in Table 12–3.

CASE STUDY 3

A 47-year-old medical transcriptionist was referred for a 10-year history of spells of nausea, disequilibrium, occasional vomiting, and ear fullness without hearing loss or tinnitus. Her audiogram was normal. She was diagnosed with probable Ménière's disease and treated with Diuril, Dramamine, Probid, and no caffeine or nicotine. Because she continued to have bad attacks, she was then treated with scopolamine patches. She then began to develop headaches (usually left frontal), and ear pressure with some of the spells, with worsening of symptoms in the summer. She had a history of severe headache with her menses since the age of 30. She had a normal caloric test, computed tomography (CT) scan of the head, and rotary chair test. She was diagnosed with migraine with aura (1.1) and migraine aura without headache (1.2.5). She was placed on an antimigraine schedule and treated with isometheptene at the onset of the spell, which did not help. She was then placed on an increasing dose of amitriptyline and eventually reached a dose of 50 mg each night. For the next year, she continued to get a headache a few days before her menses but no dizzy spells. Because of the complaint of difficulty getting up in the morning and a dry mouth, the amitriptyline was tapered and she was placed on an increasing dose of propranolol. To date, she has had no headaches or spells of vertigo.

CASE STUDY 4

A 35-year-old biochemist was referred for spells of vertigo, nausea, and vomiting lasting for less than 1 hour during the past year. As a teenager, she recalled having occasional bad "sinus headaches." Between the ages of 22 and 32, she had spells of vertigo, nausea, vomiting, fluctuating hearing loss, and tinnitus in the left ear. At that time, she was diagnosed with Ménière's disease and treated with diuretics, antihistamines, and a low-salt diet. Her current spells of vertigo were not associated with fluctuating hearing loss or tinnitus and were not altered by the use of a diuretic and low-salt diet. Two years ago she had a visual scintillation that lasted for a few minutes. She had a normal neurologic examination, normal caloric test, and normal rotary chair test. She had moderate-to-severe low-frequency sensorineural hearing defect and decreased speech discrimination on the left side. Hearing was normal on the right. MRI scan of the head with gadolinium was normal. She was diagnosed with migraine aura without headache (1.2.5). She was placed on an antimigraine schedule. During the next year, her spells of vertigo stopped, hearing in the low frequencies became normal, and she developed normal speech discrimination.

CASE STUDY 5

A 33-year-old professor of history was referred for five spells of vertigo beginning several years ago. These spells usually lasted a few minutes and occurred in the morning around the time of her menses. It was unclear whether they were triggered by head movement. She usually had disequilibrium for up to an hour following the vertigo. She also noted minor right-sided headaches during her menses with queasiness, but denied vomiting, hearing loss, and tinnitus. She recalls having ear infections when she was young. She wondered about anxiety attacks, because she lost her husband 2½ years previously to colon cancer. She had a normal neurologic and neuro-otologic examination. She was reassured that no serious problem was found and was told to come in if she developed another attack. One month later she called and stated that the spells had returned. She stated that she had just finished her menses and had a minor right-sided headache. On examination, she had transient torsional and upbeat nystagmus with the right ear down during the Hallpike-Dix maneuver. A diagnosis of BPPV was made, and she was treated with vestibular exercise. She was also placed on an antimigraine schedule. Her BPPV resolved within 1 week, and she did not have any recurrence of headache or vertigo during the next 6 months she was followed.

SUMMARY

We increasingly recognize that migraine is a common cause of episodic vertigo and disequilibrium in children and adults. Migraine may present as benign paroxysmal vertigo of childhood, paroxysmal torticollis of infancy, and benign recurrent vertigo of adults. In addition, migraine is associated with motion sickness, Ménière's disease, and BPPV. Migraine is triggered by a number of factors, including stress, anxiety, hypoglycemia, fluctuating estrogen, certain foods, and smoking. Episodic vertigo and disequilibrium from migraine should be treated by reducing these risk factors and, if necessary, by medical therapy.

REFERENCES

1. Selby, G and Lance, JW: Observations on 500 cases of migraine and allied vascular headaches. J Neurol Neurosurg Psychiatry 23:23, 1960.
2. Kayan, A and Hood, JD: Neuro-otological manifestations of migraine. Brain 107:1123, 1984.
3. Kuritzky, A, Ziegler, DK, and Hassanein, R: Vertigo, motion sickness and migraine. Headache 21:227, 1981.
4. Eadie, MJ: Some aspects of episodic giddiness. Med J Australia 2:453, 1960.
5. Stewart, WF, et al: Migraine headache: Prevalence in the United States by age, income, race and other sociodemographic factors. JAMA 267:64, 1992.
6. Headache Classification Committee of the International Headache Society: Classification and diagnostic criteria for headache disorders, cranial neuralgias and facial pain. Cephalalgia 8(suppl 7):1, 1988.
7. Fisher, CM: Late-life migraine accompaniments as a cause of unexplained transient ischemic attacks. Can J Neurol Sci 7:9, 1980.
8. Daroff, RB: New headache classification. Neurology 38:1138, 1988.
9. Basser, LS: Benign paroxysmal vertigo of childhood. Brain 87:141, 1964.
10. Fenichel, GM: Migraine as a cause of benign paroxysmal vertigo of childhood. J Pediatr 71:114, 1967.
11. Koenigsberger, MR, et al: Benign paroxysmal vertigo of childhood. Neurology 20:1108, 1970.
12. Parker, W: Migraine and the vestibular system in childhood and adolescence. Am J Otol 10:364, 1989.
13. Watson, P and Steele, JC: Paroxysmal disequilibrium in the migraine syndrome of childhood. Arch Otolaryngol 99:177, 1974.
14. Snyder, CH: Paroxysmal torticollis in infancy. Am J Dis Child 117:458, 1969.
15. Gourley, IM: Paroxysmal torticollis in infancy. Can Med Assoc J 105:504, 1971.
16. Lipson, EH and Robertson, WC: Paroxysmal torticollis of infancy: Familial occurrence. Am J Dis Child 132:422, 1978.
17. Hanukoglu, A, Somekh, F, and Fried, D: Benign paroxysmal torticollis in infancy. Clin Pediatr 23:272, 1984.
18. Bickerstaff, ER: Basilar artery migraine. Lancet 1:15, 1961.
19. Harker, LA and Rassekh, CH: Episodic vertigo in basilar artery migraine. Otolaryngol Head Neck Surg 96:239, 1987.
20. Eviatar, L: Vestibular testing in basilar artery migraine. Ann Neurol 9:126, 1981.
21. Grad, A and Baloh, RW: Vertigo of vascular origin. Clinical and oculographic features. Arch Neurol 46:281, 1989.
22. Slater, R: Benign recurrent vertigo. J Neurol Neurosurg Psychiatry 42:363, 1979.
23. Moretti, G, et al: "Benign recurrent vertigo" and its connection with migraine. Headache 20:344, 1980.
24. Harker, LA and Rassekh, CH: Migraine equivalent as a cause of episodic vertigo. Laryngoscope 98:160, 1988.
25. Schlake, HP, et al: Electronystagmographic investigations in migraine and cluster headache during the pain-free interval. Cephalagia 9:271, 1989.

26. Toglia, JU, Thomas, D, and Kuritzky, A: Common migraine and vestibular function. Electronystagmographic study and pathogenesis. Ann Otol Rhinol Laryngol 90:267, 1981.
27. Imes, RK and Hoyt, W: Exercise-induced transient visual events in young healthy adults. J Clin Neuro-ophthalmol 9:178, 1989.
28. Bartleson, JD: Transient and persistent neurological manifestations of migraine. Stroke 15:383, 1984.
29. Bruyn, GW: Complicated migraine. In Vinken, PJ and Bruyn, GW (eds): Handbook of Clinical Neurology, vol 6, 1968, p 59.
30. Welch, KMA and Levine, SR: Migraine-related stroke in the context of the International Headache Society Classification of Head Pain. Arch Neurol 47:458, 1990.
31. Coppeto, JR, et al: Vascular retinopathy in migraine. Neurology 36:267, 1986.
32. Weintraub, JM and Feman, SS: Ischemic optic neuropathy in migraine. Arch Neurol 100:1097, 1982.
33. Caplan, LR: Migraine and vertebrobasilar ischemia. Neurology 41:55, 1991.
34. Solomon, GD and Spaccavento, LJ: Lateral medullary syndrome after basilar migraine. Headache 22:171, 1982.
35. Brandt, T and Daroff, RB: The multisensory physiological and pathological vertigo syndromes. Ann Neurol 7:195, 1980.
36. Childs, AJ and Sweetnam, MT: A study of 104 cases of migraine. Br Industr Med 18:234, 1961.
37. Hinchcliffe, R: Headache and Meniere's disease. Acta Otolaryngol (Stockh) 63:384, 1967.
38. Schiller, F and Hedberg, WC: An appraisal of positional nystagmus. Arch Neurol 2:309, 1960.
39. Skyhøj Olsen, T, Friberg, L, and Lassen, NA: Ischemia may be the primary cause of neurological deficits in classic migraine. Arch Neurol 44:156, 1987.
40. Olesen, J, Larsen, B, and Lauritzen, M: Focal hyperemia followed by spreading oligemia and impaired activation of rCBF in classic migraine. Ann Neurol 9:344, 1981.
41. Kin, T: Discussion, ideas abound in migraine research; consensus remains elusive. JAMA 257:9, 1987.
42. Diamond, S: Dietary factors in vascular headache. Neurol Forum 2:2, 1991.
43. Silberstein, SD and Merriam, GR: Estrogens, progestins, and headache. Neurology 41:786, 1991.
44. Cooper, KH: The Aerobics Way. Bantam Books, New York, 1977, p 312.
45. Holroyd, KA and Penzien, DB: Pharmacological versus non-pharmacological prophylaxis of recurrent migraine headache: a meta-analytic review of clinical trials. Pain 42:1, 1990.
46. Shulman, KI, et al: Dietary restrictions, tyramine, and the use of monoamine oxidase inhibitors. J Clin Psychopharmacol 9:397, 1989.
47. Ferrari, MD, et al: Treatment of migraine attacks with sumatriptan: The Subcutaneous Sumatriptan International Study Group. N Engl J Med 325:316, 1991.
48. Peroutka, SJ: The pharmacology of current anti-migraine drugs. Headache 30(suppl):5, 1990.
49. Migraine-Nimodipine European Study Group (MINES): European multicenter trial of nimodipine in the prophylaxis of classic migraine (migraine with aura). Headache 29:639, 1989.
50. Albers, GW, et al: Nifedipine versus propranolol for the initial prophylaxis of migraine. Headache 29:214, 1989.
51. Hockaday, JM: Management of migraine. Arch Dis Child 65:1174, 1990.
52. Forsythe, WI and Hockaday, JM: Management of childhood migraine. In Hockaday, JM (ed): Migraine in Childhood. Butterworths, London, 1988, p 63.

Rehabilitation Assessment and Management

CHAPTER **13**

Assessment of Vestibular Hypofunction

Diane F. Borello-France, MS, PT
Susan L. Whitney, PhD, PT, ATC
Susan J. Herdman, PhD, PT

Patients with peripheral vestibular hypofunction differ with respect to the onset and clinical course of their disability and with respect to the final level of recovery, depending on the type and extent of vestibular deficit. Despite these differences, such patients share many of the same symptoms. These symptoms may include dizziness, light-headedness, vertigo, nystagmus, blurred vission, postural instability, gait disturbances, and occasionally falling. In addition, these patients often experience anxiety, depression, and fear related to their disability. As a result of one or more of these symptoms, patients with peripheral vestibular hypofunction often cope with their disability by avoiding certain movements and by decreasing their activity level. This habit, if not treated, will lead to the unfortunate results of physical deconditioning and an alteration of the patient's life-style.

This chapter provides the reader with strategies for the assessment of patients with unilateral peripheral vestibular hypofunction. In order to do so, a brief overview of the functional deficits resulting from unilateral peripheral lesions is provided as a basis for discussing the physical therapy evaluation.

FUNCTIONAL DEFICITS RESULTING FROM UNILATERAL PERIPHERAL LESIONS

Patients with unilateral peripheral vestibular hypofunction may express a multitude of symptoms. These symptoms emerge from functional deficits in vestibulo-ocular and visuo-ocular function, motion perception, postural control, and general physical conditioning.[1]

Vestibulo-ocular and Visuo-ocular Dysfunction

The vestibular system, via the vestibulo-ocular reflex (VOR), plays a major role in gaze stabilization. During movements of the head, the VOR stabilizes gaze (eye position in space) by producing an eye movement of equal velocity and opposite direction to the head movement. The ratio of eye velocity to head velocity is referred to as the gain of the VOR. The ideal gain in a normal subject would equal 1. VOR gain has been shown to be reduced to 25 percent in human beings immediately following unilateral labyrinthine lesions.[2,3]

Normal functioning of the visuo-oculomotor systems is also important. The visuo-oculomotor systems afford an individual the ability to visually pursue a moving object across the visual field (smooth pursuit) without making compensatory head movements. The visuo-ocular system also subserves saccadic eye movements, which are rapid voluntary movements that allow refoveation of stationary targets.

The vestibulo-ocular and visuo-ocular systems work cooperatively to stabilize gaze during head movements and during visually controlled eye movements.[4] Impairment in either or both systems interferes with the patient's ability to maintain gaze during a variety of head movements and situations that are experienced in everyday life. Symptomatic complaints associated with such impairments include dizziness, blurred vision, and occasionally oscillopsia (the illusion that the visual world is moving).

Abnormal Motion Perception

Clinically, the patient experiencing abnormal motion perception may complain of light-headedness, dizziness, or vertigo associated with particular head or body positions and movements. Norre[5] has referred to this condition as "provoked vertigo," which is attributable to the asymmetry in the dynamic vestibular responses following a unilateral vestibular lesion. According to Norre,[5] when movements are signaled, the disturbed vestibular function produces a sensory input different from the one expected in normal conditions. The abnormal vestibular signal is in conflict with normal signals provided by the visual and proprioceptive systems. This "sensory conflict" is thought to produce the symptoms associated with motion misperception.

Postural Dyscontrol

Independent and safe ambulation depends on the ability to perceive successfully the relevant features of one's environment. In addition, information about the orientation of the body with respect to the support surface and gravity is essential to postural control. Information necessary for postural control is derived from an integration of sensory inputs from the visual, somatosensory, and vestibular systems.[6]

Impairment in the function of vestibulospinal reflexes itself is believed to contribute to postural disturbances in patients with peripheral vestibular disorders. Lacour, Roll, and Appaix[7] have shown that producing a unilateral vestibular neurotomy in baboons, induces asymmetric excitability in ipsilateral and contralateral spinal reflexes. Similarly, Allum and Pfaltz,[8] using support surface rotations, reported that tibialis anterior responses in patients with unilateral peripheral vestibular deficits are enhanced contralateral to and reduced ipsilateral to the side of the lesion. These patients also had reduced neck muscle activity and greater-than-normal head angular accelerations during response to the support surface rotations.

Disturbances in vestibulospinal reflex function may account for the locomotor disturbances reported by patients with unilateral peripheral vestibular hypofunction. These patients frequently experience gait instability in situations that require them to walk and move their head, turn, or stop quickly. In addition, clinical observation of their gait frequently reveals deviations such as veering left or right, a widened base of support, decreased gait speed, or decreased head and trunk motion.

Physical Deconditioning

Changes in a patient's overall general physical condition can be considered the most potentially disabling consequence of vestibular dysfunction. Restriction in cervical range of motion is a common clinical finding in patients with vestibular hypofunction. This finding may be associated with a patient's tendency to restrict movements that potentially provoke symptoms. In addition, patients admit to adopting a more sedentary life-style, frequently abandoning premorbid exercise routines or recreational activities. If gone untreated, such changes could possibly lead to more serious physical and psychosocial consequences.

PHYSICAL THERAPY EVALUATION

History

MEDICAL HISTORY

Physical therapy usually is initiated following vestibular laboratory testing and the physician's determination of the patient's diagnosis. The diagnosis, vestibular laboratory test, other diagnostic test results, and the patient's current and past medical histories are important pieces of information that should be obtained by the therapist at the initiation of the physical therapy evaluation. Such information may assist in the identification of problems that could ultimately affect the patient's rehabilitation prognosis and outcome. For example, concurrent disease processes, such as peripheral vascular disease or peripheral neuropathy, could affect and prolong the patient's functional recovery.

Obtaining a complete medication history from the patient is vitally important because there are many medications that can produce or enhance dizziness (see Chapter 9). Certain medications reduce the patient's symptoms by depressing the vestibular system. These medications may also delay or prevent vestibular adaptation and therefore may prolong the recovery period. Consulting with the physician is advisable to determine the possibility of reducing the dose or eliminating the medication completely.

SUBJECTIVE HISTORY

The subjective history of the patient's condition is of critical importance in the evaluation of the patient with a peripheral vestibular problem. Questions that go beyond those usually asked by a physical therapist should be considered (Table 13–1). The use

TABLE 13–1 Questions to Ask a Patient with Vestibular Disease

Have you experienced any dizziness?
What do you mean by "dizzy"?
How would you rate your dizziness?
When did your dizziness first occur?
How often do you become dizzy?
Does dizziness occur in an attack in which you become dizzy and spin?
How long does the attack of vertigo or dizziness last?
During an average day, when do you feel best?
During an average day, when do you feel worst?
Are you completely free of dizziness between attacks?
Does change of position make you dizzy?
Do you become dizzy when you move your head quickly?
Do you become dizzy when you roll over in bed?
Do you become dizzy when you bend your head?
Do you become dizzy when you walk in a busy and crowded place?
Do you take any medications for dizziness?
Have you taken any medications in the past for dizziness?
What makes your dizziness worse or can bring on an attack?

of a questionnaire that the patient can fill out prior to the initial visit is often helpful and saves time (see Appendices A–C). A complete description of the patient's symptoms should be documented so that functional progress can be later assessed. Knowing what positions, movements, or situations aggravate the patient's symptoms may be of importance in treatment planning. In addition, the patient should be asked questions regarding the type, frequency, duration, and intensity of symptoms, and whether or not symptoms are of a fluctuating nature. Intensity of symptoms like vertigo and disequilibrium can be measured using an analog scale similar to that used in the assessment of pain.

Questions related to the patient's perceived disability and psychosocial status should also be included in the initial assessment. Patients may believe they have a psychologic problem rather than a physical one. The patient's condition is one that cannot be seen by their family and friends. Oftentimes, their condition is not well understood and has been misdiagnosed by the medical community.[9] When interacting with these patients, they must be reassured that their disorder is shared by others. This reassurance is essential, because in some cases symptoms are magnified by stress or emotional trauma.

Several attempts have been made to define the patient's subjective symptoms of dizziness in an objective manner.[10] The Dizziness Handicap Inventory (DHI) is a useful clinical tool that can clarify the patient's symptomatic complaints and perceptions of his or her functional abilities (see Appendix B). Items relate to functional, emotional, and physical problems that the patient may have. This inventory can be administered quickly during the initial and discharge visits in an attempt to quantify whether or not the patient thinks he or she has improved. The DHI is consistent with high test-retest reliability ($r = .97$).[10]

Shepard, Telian, and Smith-Wheelock[11] have suggested the use of a disability scale to objectively document the patient's perceived level of disability (Table 13–2). There has been no published study to examine the reliability or validity of this outcome scale. The six-point scale has descriptors that range from the patient having no disability to having long-term disability. Long-term disability was defined as the inability to work for

TABLE 13–2 Scale for Evaluation of Disability

Criterion	Score
No disability—negligible symptoms	0
No disability—bothersome symptoms	1
Mild disability—performing usual duties	2
Moderate disability—disrupts usual duties	3
Recent severe disability—medical leave	4
Established severe disability	5

Adapted from Shepard, NT, Telian, SA, and Smith-Wheelock, M: Habituation and balance retraining: A retrospective review. Neurol Clin 8:459, 1990.

more than 1 year.[11] This scale can be incorporated into the initial and discharge physical therapy evaluation in an attempt to document treatment outcome.

FUNCTIONAL HISTORY

To obtain a complete picture of the patient's functional status, the patient should be questioned about previous and current activity level. A history of the patient's activity level is an important component of the assessment, which often characterizes the extent of the patient's disability. There are patients who have difficulty leaving home because exposure to highly textured visual stimulation causes disequilibrium. This common experience is referred to as the "shopping aisle syndrome." These patients may have a limited ability to interact with their environment, and over time tend to adopt a more sedentary life-style.

PATIENT GOALS

At the beginning of the assessment, the patient should be asked about expectations of physical therapy and functional goals. When the therapist concludes the assessment, determination can be made as to whether these goals are realistic and attainable or whether they need to be modified by the therapist and patient. The final level of recovery for most patients with unilateral vestibular hypofunction, without other complications, should be a return to full activities.

Clinical Examination

The clinical examination of a patient with vertigo and disequilibrium is usually comprehensive (Table 13–3) and therefore time consuming. Discretion should be used as to which portions of the examination need to be performed on each patient. We have described the full examination here and have indicated, where possible, when different portions of the examination would not be necessary.

OCULOMOTOR AND VESTIBULO-OCULAR TESTING

The interaction of the patient's visual and vestibular systems is tested clinically by having the patient perform combinations of head and eye movements. The oculomotor examination is one part of the overall assessment of the "dizzy" patient that may have

TABLE 13–3 Summary of the Clinical Examination of the "Dizzy" Patient

Oculomotor examination

In room light: extraocular movements, diplopia, skew, pursuit, saccades, spontaneous and gaze-evoked nystagmus, VORc, VOR to slow and rapid head thrusts, visual acuity test with head stationary and during gentle oscillation of the head.

With Frenzel lenses: Spontaneous and gaze-evoked nystagmus, head-shaking nystagmus, tragal pressure–induced nystagmus, hyperventilation-induced nystagmus, positional nystagmus.

Sensation

Somatosensory: proprioception, light touch, vibration, kinesthesia, pain; quantified tests: vibration threshold, tuning fork test.

Vision: Visual acuity and field

Coordination: Upper and lower extremities

Optic ataxia/past pointing, rebound, diadokokinesia, heel to shin, postural fixation.

Range of motion: Active and passive ROM

Upper and lower extremity, neck (rotation, extension, flexion, lateral flexion)

Strength (gross)

Grip, upper extremity, lower extremity, trunk

Postural deviations

Scoliosis, kyphosis, lordosis

Positional and movements testing

Hallpike, other positional maneuvers

Sitting balance: Passive or active; anterior-posterior and laterally

Weight shift, head righting, equilibrium reactions upper extremity lower extremity, ability of trunk to recover vertical

Static balance (perform with eyes open and eyes closed)

Romberg, sharpened Romberg, single leg stance, stand on rail, force platform

Balance with altered sensory cues

Eyes open or closed, 'dome', foam

Dynamic balance (self-initiated movements)

Standing reach test (Duncan), Functional (Gabell and Simons), Fukuda's stepping test

Ambulation

Normal gait, tandem walk, walk while turning head, Singleton to right and left

Functional gait assessment

Obstacle course, double-task activities

been performed by a neurologist or otolaryngologist prior to referral for physical therapy and therefore is not always included in the physical therapy assessment.

First the patient is observed for the presence of *spontaneous nystagmus* in room light. In patients with unilateral peripheral vestibular hypofunction, spontaneous nystagmus will be observable in room light during the acute stage after onset of the lesion. Spontaneous nystagmus occurs because of an imbalance in the tonic or resting firing rate of the vestibular neurons. Within a few days, the patient should suppress the nystagmus with visual fixation.

Test smooth pursuit by asking the patient to track a moving object with his or her eyes while the head is stationary. This tracking test should assess the patient's entire visual field. Typically performed in an H-like pattern, this test also assesses the motor function of cranial nerves 3, 4, and 6. Inability to perform down-gaze is not a sign of vestibular deficits but can occur with other neurologic problems (e.g., progressive supranuclear palsy). Patients with this problem may have difficulty seeing objects on the ground as they walk. During the test of smooth-pursuit eye movements, the presence of *gaze-evoked nystagmus* and the quality of the eye movement should be noted. Saccadic pursuit, especially in younger individuals or if asymmetric, should be noted. For the patient with nystagmus, however, determining the quality of pursuit eye movements may be difficult. Care must be taken to distinguish gaze-evoked nystagmus from end-point nystagmus.

Patients can also be tested for *ocular alignment*, particularly for skew deviations that can occur during the acute stage of a unilateral vestibular loss. Skew deviations, in which the eye opposite the side of the lesion is elevated, occur because of the loss of the tonic otolith input from one side. Normally, the tonic input holds the eyes level within the orbit; when there is a unilateral loss, the eye on the side of the lesion drops in the orbit, and the patient complains of vertical diplopia. By convention, the skew is named by the side of the elevated eye (e.g., right hypertropia means the right eye is elevated, but in reality, the left eye has dropped).

Saccadic eye movements are tested by simply asking the patient to look back and forth between two horizontal and two vertical targets. In normal individuals, the target can be reached with a single eye movement or with one small corrective saccade.

The patient can then be asked to voluntarily fixate on a moving target while the head is moved in the same direction. This procedure tests *vestibulo-ocular cancellation* (VORc) and is a function of the parietal lobe. Results should agree with the observations made during the smooth-pursuit test.

Next, the VOR itself is tested. The patient is asked to fixate on a stationary target, and the head is gently turned several times, first horizontally (horizontal canal function) and then vertically (vertical canal function). This procedure should be performed passively, first with slow head movements and then with unpredictable rapid head thrusts. Normal patients will be able to maintain fixation during both slow and rapid head movements. Patients with vestibular deficits often are able to maintain fixation during slow head movements but will make corrective saccades to regain the target with rapid head movements.

Another measure of VOR function is to measure the *degradation of visual acuity* that occurs with head movement. The patient is first asked to read a Snellen wall chart with the head stationary. Then the patient is asked to read the chart while the head is gently oscillated at 1 to 2 Hz. In normal individuals, visual acuity changes at most one line. In patients with unilateral vestibular loss, visual acuity will degrade by three or four lines.

Eye movements can also be observed using Frenzel lenses. These magnifying glasses, with light inside them, enable the clinician to observe eye movements but at the same time greatly decrease the patient's ability to stabilize the eyes with visual fixation. Clinical assessment of oculomotor function using Frenzel lenses should include spontaneous and gaze-evoked nystagmus, head shaking–induced nystagmus, tragal pressure–induced nystagmus, hyperventilation-induced nystagmus, and positional nystagmus (see Chapter 11 for detailed discussion).

During this assessment, the patient is asked to report any symptoms of blurred vision or dizziness. Tests that involve repeated head movements (VOR, head shaking–induced nystagmus) may increase the patient's symptoms. If there is a significant increase in symptoms, the patient may be unable or may refuse to continue with the testing.

SENSORY EVALUATION

Sensation of the extremities and trunk is tested to rule out concurrent pathology and to assist in treatment planning. Kinesthesia and proprioception, vibration sense, light touch, and pain awareness are tested. Probably the most important of these is the assessment of kinesthesia and proprioception, although profound sensory loss affecting touch and pressure sensitivity would obviously affect postural stability.

Proprioception can be assessed by moving the great toes either up or down and asking the patient to identify the position of the toe. Care must be taken to make these relatively small movements or the test becomes too easy. The patient must also be instructed not to guess at the answer. This traditional test of proprioception does not appear to be very sensitive, and patients are quite accurate in perceiving whether the toe is up or down even when other tests indicate sensory deficiencies. *Kinesthesia* can be tested by slowly moving the toe either up or down and asking the patient to state the direction of the movement as soon as he or she first perceives movement. Again, the patient should be instructed not to guess. Perception of the direction of the movement should occur before the toe is moved more than 10 to 15 degrees, although each clinician will have to develop his or her own internal standard for what is normal. *Vibration* can be tested using a tuning fork applied to a bony prominence. One method is to ask the patient to identify when the vibratory sensation stops and then to dampen the tuning fork unexpectedly. Another method is to let the vibration diminish naturally and to time the difference between when the patient and the clinician stop feeling the vibration. Again, each clinician will have to develop his or her own sense of normal. Devices are also available that quantify vibration thresholds. These devices enable the clinician to compare the patient with age-matched normal subjects and to follow changes over time.

Visual acuity should be assessed in the clinic using a Snellen chart. A hand-held Snellen card is not as appropriate because it measures the patient's vision at a distance of only 18 inches. Brandt, Paulus, and Straube[12] suggest that distance acuity of poorer than 20/50 will have a significant effect on postural stability. Additionally, *visual field loss* can also affect balance,[13] and patients with monocular vision may have particular difficulty with depth perception, affecting their ability to walk up and down stairs.

The visual, vestibular, and somatosensory systems all show decrements with age, and the clinician should be familiar with these normal changes to differentiate them from pathologic changes.[14] Furthermore, certain disorders that can affect perception, such as cataract formation, are more likely to occur in the older person. There is some evidence that a decrease in the gain of the VOR occurs with aging, at least at higher frequencies, and there is a more limited adaptive capability.[3,15]

Multisystem involvement can impede the patient's functional progress. A patient with reduced vestibular function and a deficit in somatosensory cues is likely to compensate by using visual mechanisms. This patient will be limited functionally if placed in a situation void of visual information. For example, many patients with reduced somatosensory cues and a peripheral vestibular deficit have difficulty walking in the dark. A treatment plan that does not consider the patient's sensory loss may be ineffective, and the patient's functional independence could suffer.

COORDINATION

An attempt should also be made to rule out any coordination deficits. Vestibular deficits per se do not result in poor coordination or in limb ataxia. Assessment of coordination is especially important, however, as part of the preoperative and postoperative examination of patients with cerebellar angle tumors. Finger to nose, heel to shin, and the ability to perform rapid alternating movements of fingers or feet are gross tests that may be used to subjectively assess the patient's coordination. Other tests of cerebellar function might include truncal stability and tests of tone, such as postural fixation and the rebound phenomenon.

RANGE OF MOTION AND STRENGTH

The patient's range of motion and strength must be assessed in the initial evaluation. Although the neck, trunk, and extremities should be included in this assessment, special attention should be paid to neck range of motion. Patients in whom head movement exacerbates symptoms may have voluntarily restricted active neck motion and may eventually lose range of motion. Furthermore, many of the other assessments involve passive movement of the neck (VOR during rapid head thrusts, head shaking–induced nystagmus, and positional testing), and any limitations in movement or pain associated with neck movement should be identified before attempting those tests. A detailed examination of extremity strength and range of motion is often not necessary; however, a quick screen can indicate if more detailed testing would be appropriate.

POSTURAL EXAMINATION

In addition to assessment of range of motion, the patient's posture should be evaluated. Predisposing orthopedic conditions or postural deviations may complicate the rehabilitation prognosis. Anterior-posterior and medial-lateral views of both the patient's sitting and standing postures should be assessed.

POSITIONAL AND MOVEMENT TESTING

Clinically assessing the positions and movements that provoke the patient's symptoms is important. In this portion of the evaluation, attempts are made to replicate the various positions and movements experienced by the patient throughout the day (Table 13–4). The activities are rated by the patient as to whether they provoke no symptoms or mild, moderate, or severe symptoms. In some situations, the patient may be unable or unwilling to perform the task. This reluctance is especially apparent in the patient who develops severe dizziness early in the evaluation. In addition, a patient may refuse to move into or out of a specific posture because of the fear of eliciting symptoms. Every effort should be made to test the patient using those particular positional changes.

One of the most important positional tests is the *Hallpike maneuver*[16] (Fig. 13–1). This test is most commonly used in patients who complain of vertigo only when they move into certain positions but should be included in almost all assessments. Vertigo and nystagmus occurring when the patient is moved into the Hallpike position are used to diagnose benign paroxysmal positional vertigo (BPPV) (see Chapter 16). In patients with other forms of peripheral vestibulopathy, this maneuver is employed not for diagnostic purposes but as an additional positional and movement test that could potentially

TABLE 13–4 Vestibular Habituation Training: Assessment Guide

Position Changes	Vertigo Type	Intensity	Neuro-veget	Duration
Sitting to supine				
Supine to left side				
Supine to right side				
Supine to sitting				
Standing—turn to right				
Standing—turn to left				
Sitting—put nose to left knee				
Sitting—put nose to right knee				
Sitting turning head counterclockwise				
Sitting turning head clockwise				
Sitting bending forward				
Sitting to standing erect				
Sitting head moves fore-aft				
Sitting to left Hallpike				
Left Hallpike to sitting				
Sitting to right Hallpike				
Right Hallpike to sitting				
Sitting to supine with head hanging				
Supine to sitting				

Adapted from Norre.[5]

provoke symptoms. In the Hallpike maneuver, the patient typically sits with the head turned to one side. The patient then is moved quickly backward so that the head is extended over the end of the table approximately 30 degrees below the horizontal. The maneuver is performed to both the right and left sides. The patient should be cautioned in advance that the maneuver can cause dizziness or vertigo but, nonetheless, it should be performed.

BPPV is a common cause of vertigo. This peripheral vestibular deficit is easily and effectively treated by physical therapy, and therefore it should be distinguished from a vertebral artery problem (see Chapter 16). Although relatively rare, vertebral artery compression can be distinguished from positional vertigo. One way to distinguish between vertebral artery compression and positional vertigo is to perform the vertebral artery test with the patient sitting and leaning forward slightly. In this position, when the head is extended and turned (the head ends up in an upright position), the posterior canal on that side would not be affected by the pull of gravity. Occlusion of blood flow with compression of the vertebral artery produces other neurologic symptoms, such as numbness and weakness, slurred speech, and mental confusion as well as vertigo and nystagmus.

Examples of other movements that can be tested include rolling, supine to sitting, reaching in sitting toward the floor, and sitting to standing. All of these movements should be tested at various speeds and with the eyes open and closed. The speed of the activity will often affect the patient's symptoms. For example, a quickly performed movement could increase the patient's symptoms, while the same movement done at a slower speed may not. Varying the speed and the conditions under which the patient performs the task may affect the patient's functional ability. Positional and movement

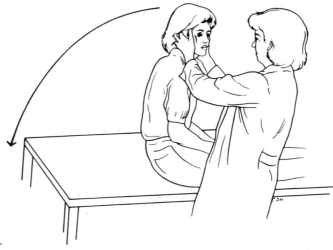

FIGURE 13–1. The Hall-pike-Dix maneuver is used primarily to test for benign paroxysmal positional vertigo. The head is turned to one side, and the patient is moved from sitting into a supine position with the head hanging over the end of the table. The patient is then observed for nystagmus, and complaints of vertigo are noted. The patient is then returned to the upright position. (Adapted with permission from Physical Therapy, 70:381–388, 1990, with permission of the American Physical Therapy Association.)

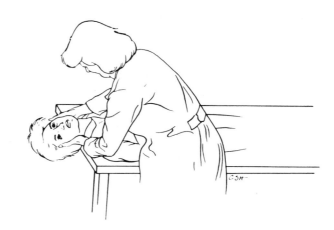

testing is limited only by the imagination of the therapist. In one patient seen in the clinic, the only position that increased her symptoms was the all-fours position, looking under the bed (Fig. 13–2)!

In addition to testing positions and movements that incorporate multiple body segments, the patient is asked to perform head movements. The head movements are typically tested with the patient sitting. These movements are performed at various speeds and with the eyes open and closed. The patient is asked to report if these movements provoke symptoms and whether the symptoms are of a mild, moderate, or severe intensity. If the patient can tolerate further testing, the same movements are tested in the standing position.

BALANCE ASSESSMENT

Sitting Balance

Although many patients with chronic vestibular disorders do not have difficulty with balance in sitting, for some patients including an assessment of sitting balance may

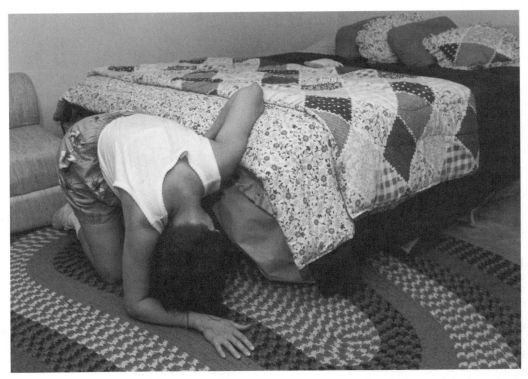

FIGURE 13–2. Patients may experience dizziness or vertigo in positions other than those normally tested. Shown here is the provoking position for one patient who experienced vertigo only when bending over and turning her head.

be appropriate. Patients should be tested while they are leaning anteriorly and posteriorly as well as right and left; tests should be performed both actively and passively. The patient can be observed for weight-shifting ability, head righting, equilibrium reactions in the upper and lower extremities, and the ability to recover to a trunk vertical position.

Static Balance

Static balance tasks have been used clinically in an attempt to document balance function objectively.[17-21] Single-leg stance (SLS), Romberg test, and the sharpened or tandem Romberg test are often included in a static balance test battery and can be performed with eyes open or eyes closed. Traditionally, the variable of interest in this testing has been the time that the patient maintains the position. Normative data for timed tests have been established for SLS, Romberg, and sharpened Romberg tests.[22] The Romberg test has been shown to have low intrasubject variability when measures are repeated over a 5-day period.[23]

We should remember that patients with vestibular deficits may have normal performance on these tests.[24-26] Tests of static balance, such as the Romberg, are fairly easy. Patients may have difficulty with this test only during the acute stage following onset of their vestibular deficit. Of additional importance is remembering that patients with balance disorders other than from vestibular dysfunction may have difficulty with these tests.

Measures of Sway

During performance of static balance tasks, medial-lateral or anterior-posterior stability can be objectively documented using "high-tech" tools such as force platforms or using simple tools such as a sway grid.

When assessing and attempting to replicate standing sway measures, the distance the subject stands from a stable visual target and the foot position of the patient should be standardized. Brandt, Paulus, and Straube[12] hypothesize that one explanation for the variability often found on the Romberg test is the inconsistent positioning of the patient with respect to a target used for visual fixation. The distance that the patient stands from the target should be standardized and should be within 1.5 m. Kirby, Price, and Macleod[27] employed five different foot positions to determine the effect of foot position on sway. They determined that subjects standing in double-limb stance were most stable in the 25 degrees, toe-out position. In addition, they observed that subjects had the greatest medial-lateral sway when their feet closely approximated each other. The standard Romberg position is with heel and toes together.

Postural sway correlates well with measures of the DHI.[28] Of course, both postural sway and the responses to the DHI questionnaire are under "voluntary control," and what is measured is subject to errors according to what the patient wants to convey. Nevertheless, patients who report the greatest disability on the DHI, as a result of their dizziness, also demonstrate the highest measures of sway on posturography.[28] Furthermore, the sway patterns of patients with central pathology differed from that of patients with other vestibular diagnoses. Yoneda and Tokumasu[29] also reported that sway patterns seem to be different between patients with Ménière's disease, BPPV, and vestibular neuronitis, and that these patterns differed from those of a normal comparison group.

ALTERING SENSORY CUES

The Clinical Test for Sensory Interaction in Balance (CTSIB) can be included in the rehabilitation assessment.[30] In some ways, this test is an extension of the Romberg test, which assessed the effect of removing visual cues on postural stability. Referred to as the foam-and-dome test (Fig. 13–3), the CTSIB assesses the influence of vestibular, somatosensory, and visual inputs on postural control. For example, standing on the foam surface and closing the eyes alters somatosensory input and eliminates visual input. In this situation, vestibular input is the most accurate information regarding postural stability. Patients with uncompensated unilateral peripheral vestibular loss may have difficulty maintaining an upright posture when both visual and support surface information are altered.[6] According to Nashner,[6] symmetry and constancy of vestibular information are critical in providing an absolute reference for reorganization of senses in conflicting conditions. The inability of the vestibular system to provide this information may explain why patients with unilateral vestibular lesions often report postural instability when riding on an escalator or when walking on thick carpet across a dimly lit room. If a patient is unstable when both visual and somatosensory cues are altered, a treatment plan might be designed to improve the function of the remaining vestibular system. Depending on the patient, an alternative treatment strategy may focus on altering the patient's environment, such that visual and proprioceptive cues are maximized.

Self-Initiated Movements

In addition to static tests of balance function, self-initiated movements and dynamic tests of balance should be examined. Self-initiated weight shifts, performed in different

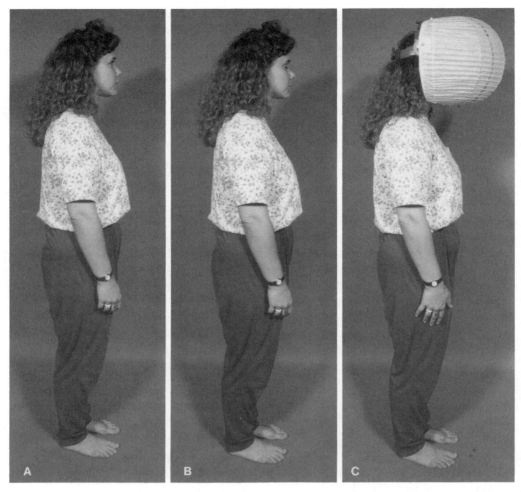

FIGURE 13-3. The Clinical Test of Sensory Integration of Balance. The subject is standing on a level support surface with eyes open (*A*), with eyes closed (*B*), a level surface with the visual conflict dome (*C*),

directions, can be assessed to determine if the patient moves freely and symmetrically. Self-initiated movements should also be tested in functionally relevant contexts, for example, having the patient reach to pick an object from the floor or placing an object on a high shelf.

Duncan and associates[31] have developed the standing reach test. This test functionally and reliably documents performance on a self-initiated task. The subject is asked to reach as far forward as possible. The extent of movement is measured using a simple yardstick (Fig. 13-4). Duncan and colleagues[31] have shown that functional reach, as a measure of a subject's margin of stability, correlates well with center-of-pressure measures obtained from a force platform. This test might be modified so that reaches in different directions are documented (Fig. 13-5).

Gabell and Simons[32] also developed a functional balance test to assess elderly clients at risk for falling. Their assessment examines static positions and rotational and sagittal movements (Table 13-5) and includes criteria for successful performance of each task.

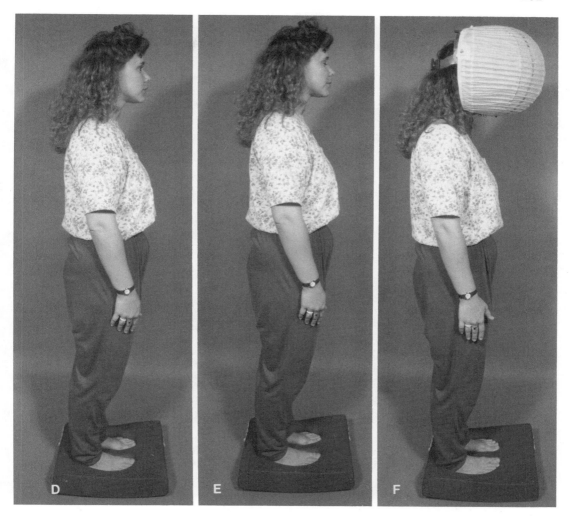

FIGURE 13–3 *Continued.* a compliant surface with eyes open, (*D*), a compliant surface with eyes closed, (*E*) and a compliant surface with the visual conflict dome (*F*). The time the patient performs each task is recorded, and the amount of sway and the patient's movement strategy are documented qualitatively. The results of this test help determine if the patient is dependent on certain sensory cues.

For example, to succeed in one of the rotational stress tasks, the patient must rotate 360 degrees once without staggering or grabbing onto furniture.

Fukuda's stepping test[33] assesses stability during the self-initiated movement of marching, which the patient performs first with eyes open and then with eyes closed. The test is easily administered in the clinic and can be quantified by using a polar coordinate grid placed on the floor (Fig. 13–6). The test is not specific for vestibular dysfunction, but patients with unilateral vestibular deficits often turn excessively when stepping with the eyes closed.[33]

The standing reach test,[31] Gabell and Simon's functional assessment,[32] and Fukuda's stepping test[33] are administered easily and require very little equipment. Such functional measures of balance can easily be used in the clinic or home care setting to document that the patient has made gains in physical therapy.

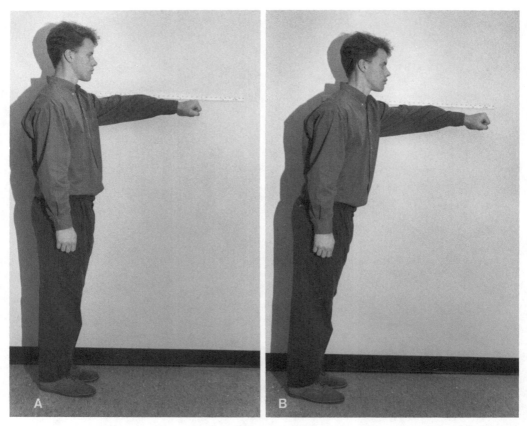

FIGURE 13–4. The distance a patient can reach is one measure of functional balance.[31] (*A*) The patient's acromion is lined up with the yardstick while the patient's arm is held parallel to the yardstick. (*B*) The patient reaches forward as far as possible, while keeping both feet flat on the ground.

Movement Strategy

During the balance assessment, the therapist should observe and document the patient's movement strategy. Three types of movement strategies have been described for controlling anterior-posterior displacements of the center of mass.[34] The *ankle strategy* produces shifts in the center of mass via rotation of the body about the ankle joints. According to Horak and Nashner,[34] the ankle strategy elicits a distal-to-proximal firing pattern of ankle, hip, and trunk musculature. This activation pattern exerts compensatory ankle torques, which are believed to correct for small postural perturbations. The *hip strategy* controls movement of the center of mass by flexing and extending the hips. Unlike the ankle strategy, the muscle activation sequence associated with the hip strategy occurs in a proximal-to-distal fashion. This strategy produces a compensatory horizontal shear force against the support surface. The hip strategy occurs in situations in which the ankle is unable to exert the appropriate torque necessary to restore balance. This situation arises when the task of maintaining balance is more difficult, such as when an individual stands on a small narrow support surface. Finally, a *stepping strategy* is used when the center of mass is displaced outside the base of support. This strategy is employed in response to fast, large postural perturbations.

To function safely and independently throughout the lifespan, humans are required

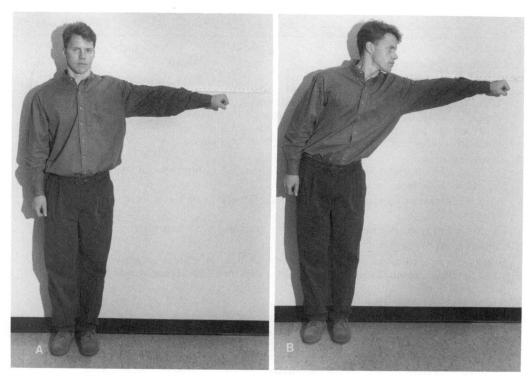

FIGURE 13–5. The distance a patient can reach to the side is another possible functional measure of balance. (A) The patient's acromion is lined up with the edge of the yardstick. (B) The patient reaches to the side as far as possible, while keeping both feet flat on the floor.

to respond, through their movements, to a variety of task situations and environmental contexts. We should logically assume that postural strategies could be task-specific, and therefore categorizing them may prove to be difficult. In addition, individuals vary greatly with respect to body size, proportion, and weight. These considerations, taken together with age-related changes, make the task of categorizing postural strategies difficult. Instead, the physical therapist may be more successful in documenting whether the patient's individual strategy is efficient, safe, and successful with respect to achieving the task goal. With this approach, the clinician's expectations of the patient's responses are not as biased. This notion also has implications for treatment. Current motor learning theory suggests that the learner will be more successful in the task when the learner, not the teacher or therapist, selects the appropriate movement strategy.[35]

Gait Evaluation

Evaluation of the patient's gait provides a dynamic and functional assessment of the patient's postural control mechanism. The gait assessment can be obtained through clinical observation, videotape analysis, or computerized motion analysis. A videotape record of the patient's gait is easily obtained clinically and can be extremely useful for documentation and patient education.

The patient's gait should be assessed in as many situations as are realistically accessible to the therapist. Analysis of the patient walking down a crowded versus

TABLE 13-5 Balance Coding

	Code
1. Static stress	
Unsafe while seated	0
Safe while seated, unsafe standing	1
Steady while standing for 20 sec with aid	2
Steady while standing, 20 sec, no aid, wide base	3
Steady while standing, 20 sec, no aid, narrow base	4
Steady while standing, 20 sec, no aid, long base	5
Steady while standing, 20 sec, no aid, long base, eyes closed	6
2. Rotational stress	
For those who can stand for 20 sec with or without aid. Subject should stand with feet in most stable position.	
Steady while turning head from right to left. (Tested three times, 5 sec of rest between each trial)	a
Can turn 360 degrees without staggering or grabbing onto furniture.	b
3. Sagittal stress	
Subject can arise from chair (with help if necessary), is immediately steady and can stand for 20 sec without help except for aid if uses one. (No code given if cannot perform)	x
4. Directional preponderance	
Coded if subject tends to fall or overbalance in one direction consistently during the above tests.	
Anterior ___ (A) Posterior ___ (P) Right ___ (R) Left ___ (L)	

Adapted from Gabell, A and Simons, MA: Balance coding. Physiotherapy 68:286, 1982.

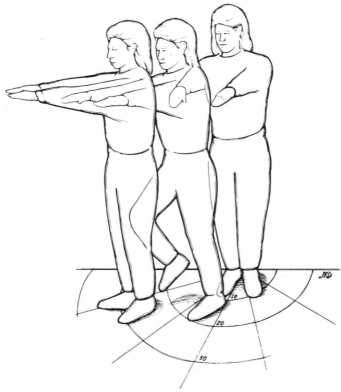

FIGURE 13-6. Fukuda's stepping test assesses balance while the patient marches in place first with eyes open and then with eyes closed. The forward progression of the patient as well as the degree and direction of turning are recorded. Normal subjects will have moved forward less than 50 cm and turned less than 30 degrees at the end of 50 steps. Patients with unilateral vestibular deficits often turn excessively. A polar coordinate grid, placed on the floor, enables easy scoring of the subject's response.

noncrowded hallway may yield very different information about the patient's gait function. Similarly, the patient should be instructed to walk at normal speed, slowly, and quickly. Common clinical observations indicate that patients with vestibular disorders, like other patients, have greater gait instability when asked to walk at a nonpreferred speed.

During the gait assessment, the physical therapist documents the patient's movement strategy, the presence of gait deviations, and whether the patient reports any abnormal sensation of movement. The patient with a peripheral vestibular disorder may select an overall strategy for gait that limits movement of their head and trunk. Clinically, gait is characterized as being stiff or robotlike, and the patient may use excessive visual fixation while walking. Some of the typical gait deviations demonstrated by these patients include inconsistent step lengths, veering to the right or left, a widened base of support, a listing of the head and/or trunk to one side, decreased rotation through the trunk and neck (and decreased arm swing), and "en bloc" and slow turns. In addition to observable gait deviations, patients with a unilateral peripheral vestibulopathy may associate dizziness with their gait instability.

A complete assessment of the patient's gait function should include having the patient perform a variety of tasks while walking. Many of these tasks will cause the patient to lose balance; therefore, during this portion of the gait assessment, the physical therapist may need to guard the patient but without becoming a part of the patient's postural control system. The goal of this assessment is to learn how the patient, not the therapist, solves the problem of postural control.

One of the gait tasks performed by the patient is to walk while moving the head, either to the left and right or up and down. The therapist documents whether the patient experiences symptoms (dizziness, light-headedness, etc.), loss of balance, or an exaggeration of gait deviations. Such a detailed assessment facilitates documentation of the patient's progress.

Many patients with unilateral peripheral vestibular loss experience difficulty when asked to perform gait tasks that require an anticipatory mode of motor control. One such task requires the patient to walk quickly and then to stop immediately on the therapist's command. To enhance task difficulty, the patient may be asked to perform the same task with eyes closed. Another task, the Singleton test, requires the patient to walk quickly and to pivot to the right or left immediately on the therapist's command. To maintain a level of uncertainty, the patient should not be informed ahead of time of the required pivot direction. The speed of the pivot is another factor that must be considered. The patient may slow gait speed as a strategy to avoid disequilibrium during the task. The patient may slow gait speed also to avoid the anticipatory requirements of the task. In such instances, the patient should perform the task at a faster speed, so that the therapist obtains a more complete picture of the patient's gait function.

Observing the ability of the patient to negotiate an obstacle course may also provide the therapist with valuable information about the patient's functional balance (Fig. 13–7). An assessment of the patient's ability to function in an anticipatory mode of control can also be obtained. To assess the patient's ability, the patient self-selects the path to negotiate the obstacle course. In addition, the patient decides whether or not to pick up or step over an object in the course. The patient also decides to negotiate the course quickly or slowly. If, on the other hand, the patient's anticipatory control is of interest, the therapist directs the patient of the path to follow. Task variability and uncertainty is manipulated by the therapist. For example, the therapist decides at which point in the course to throw a ball toward the patient (Fig. 13–8). A temporal constraint may also be added to the task. Asking the patient to negotiate the course as quickly as

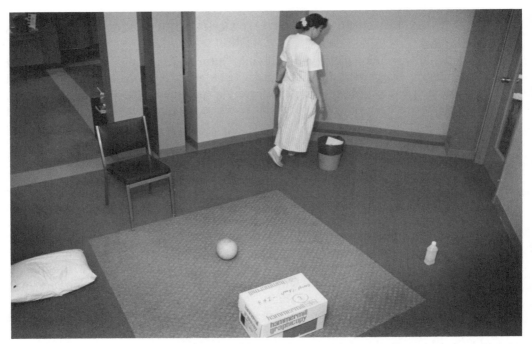

FIGURE 13–7. Patients with vestibular disorders may have difficulty negotiating an obstacle course. The patient selects the path of the course to follow and whether to step over or to pick up objects.

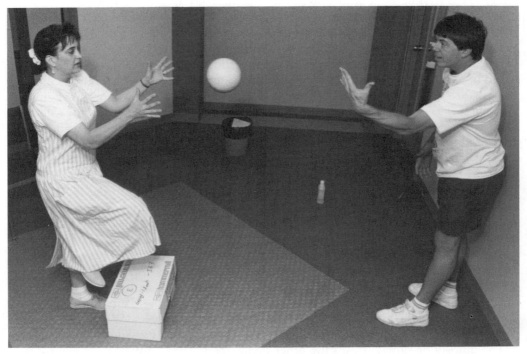

FIGURE 13–8. The obstacle course can also be used to determine how well the patient responds to external perturbations. In this situation, the patient maintains postural control, while simultaneously stepping over a box and catching a ball.

possible enhances task difficulty and provides a means to document the patient's progress subjectively.

The ability of the patient to perform gait tasks while manipulating an object with the hands should also be assessed. Patients with unilateral vestibular loss frequently complain of increased gait instability when carrying a basket of laundry up a flight of stairs or when carrying a bag of groceries. Clinically, the patient's ability to monitor postural control while manipulating an object can be tested in a variety of ways. The patient can be asked to walk, pick up one or more objects off of the floor, and continue walking. Documenting the strategy used by the patient to perform this task is important. Many patients with vestibular loss will bend at the knees and avoid flexing the head or bending at the hips. This strategy may be selected in an attempt to minimize provocation of symptoms or loss of balance. A patient may also be asked to negotiate a flight of stairs while carrying objects of varying weight or size. This task is important to include in the gait assessment, as a patient who demonstrates little difficulty with other gait tasks may express extreme postural instability with this task.

Other gait tasks that can be assessed by the therapist include: sidestepping, backward walking, tandem walking, walking in a figure of eight, and marching or jogging in place. If feasible, the patient should be asked to perform these tasks at various speeds with the eyes open and eyes closed.

THE TRANSITION FROM ASSESSMENT TO TREATMENT

The following points are offered as guidelines in developing a treatment program based on your assessment.

1. *Is there a documented vestibular deficit?:* Review the results of the formal vestibular function tests. If the vestibular function tests are normal, you may *not* be dealing with a vestibular deficit. The results of the vestibular function tests confirm the presence of horizontal canal deficits. Of course, a patient may have a vertical canal lesion without a horizontal canal problem, but that is most likely to occur in BPPV, which is easily recognized. Otolith and central vestibular lesions are more difficult to identify, and we must rely on patient history or on the presence of other deficits that localize the problem to the central nervous system (CNS).

2. *What type of vestibular problem does this patient have?:* The vestibular function tests indicate whether the patient has a peripheral vestibular deficit, a unilateral or a bilateral vestibular deficit, and the degree of the deficit. Some of the exercises for patients with vestibular deficits are designed to improve the remaining vestibular function and therefore are not appropriate for patients with complete vestibular loss. Exercises for BPPV (see Chapter 16) will not help the patient with a unilateral vestibular loss (see Chapter 14).

3. *Not all dizzy patients have a vestibular lesion:* Although nystagmus and complaints of dizziness and vertigo are common in patients with vestibular deficits, these problems can occur in other, nonvestibular, disorders. Nystagmus may be caused by medications, brain-stem or cerebral hemisphere lesions, or may be congenital. Dizziness may occur in patients with peripheral somatosensory deficits (as with patients with peripheral vestibular deficits, these patients feel "dizzy" when they are standing but not when they are sitting), with CNS lesions, with other medical problems such as low blood pressure, or as a side effect of medications. Vertigo, most frequently associated

with peripheral vestibular deficits, can occur with central lesions (often patients with central lesions may not complain of vertigo) and with other medical problems such as presyncope. These patients may have balance problems and may need an individualized exercise program but not necessarily exercises designed to improve vestibular function.

4. *Assess and reassess*: The initial assessment is directed at identifying problems associated with the vestibular deficit, such as increased dizziness or decreased visual acuity with head movements, and with the functional limitations of the patient. The exercise plan, therefore, may include vestibular exercises but must also address the specific problems and level of function of the patient. Developing a problem list will enable the therapist to set goals and devise specific exercises for each of those goals. As the patient responds to the exercises, reassessment is necessary to modify the treatment program.

5. *Quantify the assessment:* Although not all components of the assessment yield quantifiable data, many tests do, such as the patient's subjective complaints, dynamic visual acuity, and some measures of postural stability. Taking the time to objectively measure the patient's performance is important in order to determine the outcome of the patient's treatment, to modify the treatment, to justify further treatment, and to determine when to terminate treatment.

SUMMARY

The physical therapy assessment is multifaceted and is aimed toward identifying the patient's specific functional deficits as well as to establish quantitatively the effects of the vestibular deficit on the patient's vestibulo-ocular and vestibulospinal systems and subjective complaints of disequilibrium and vertigo. The results of the assessment are used to identify specific patient problems and to develop treatment goals for the patient. The results of the assessment also provide the basis for determining whether the treatments used are successful. The use of exercise in the rehabilitation of patients with vestibular disorders is aimed at promoting vestibular compensation and functional recovery.

REFERENCES

1. Shumway-Cook, A and Horak, FB: Rehabilitation strategies for patients with vestibular deficits. Neurol Clin 8:441, 1990.
2. Paige, GD: Nonlinearity and asymmetry in the human vestibulo-ocular reflex. Acta Otolaryngol (Stockh) 108:1, 1989.
3. Allum, JHJ, Yamane, M, and Pfaltz, CR: Long-term modifications of vertical and horizontal vestibulo-ocular reflex dynamics in man. Acta Otolaryngol (Stockh) 105:328, 1988.
4. Baloh, RW: The Essentials of Neurology. FA Davis, Philadelphia, 1984.
5. Norre, ME: Treatment of unilateral vestibular hypofunction. In Oosterveld, WJ (ed): Otoneurology. John Wiley & Sons, New York, 1984, p 23.
6. Nashner, LM: Adaptation of human movement to altered environments. Trends Neurosci 5:358, 1982.
7. Lacour, M, Roll, JP, and Appaix, M: Modifications and development of spinal reflexes in the alert baboon following a unilateral vestibular neurotomy. Brain Res 113:255, 1976.
8. Allum, JHJ and Pfaltz, CR: Influence of bilateral and acute unilateral peripheral vestibular deficits on early sway stabilizing responses in human tibialis anterior muscles. Acta Otolaryngol (Stockh) 406:115, 1984.
9. Reishen, S: A career in the balance. Sports Illustrated, March 18, p 36, 1991.
10. Jacobson, GP and Newman, CW: The development of the dizziness handicap inventory. Arch Otolaryngol Head Neck Surg 116:424, 1990.

11. Shepard, NT, Telian, SA, and Smith-Wheelock, M: Habituation and balance retraining therapy: A retrospective review. Neurol Clin 8:459, 1990.
12. Brandt, T, Paulus, WM, and Straube, A: Visual acuity, visual field and visual scene characteristics affect postural balance. In Igarashi, M and Black, FO (eds): Vestibular and Visual Control on Posture and Locomotor Equilibrium. Karger, Basel, 1985, p 93.
13. Paulus, WM, Straube, A, and Brandt, T: Visual stabilization of posture. Brain 107:1143, 1984.
14. Kenshalo, DR: Age changes in touch, vibration, temperature, kinesthesis and pain sensitivity. In Birren, JE and Schaie, KW (eds): Handbook of the Psychology of Aging. Van Nostrand Reinhold, New York, 1977.
15. Paige, GD: Vestibulo-ocular reflex (VOR) and adaptive plasticity with aging. Soc Neurosci Abstr 15:515, 1989.
16. Brandt, T and Daroff, RB: Physical therapy for benign paroxysmal positional vertigo. Arch Otolaryngol 106:484, 1980.
17. Bohannon, RW, Larkin, PA, and Cook, AC: Decrease in timed balance function and the aging process. Phys Ther 64:1067, 1984.
18. Fregly, AR, Graybiel, A, and Smith, MJ: Walk on floor eyes closed (WOFEC): A new addition to an ataxia battery. Aerospace Med 75:10, 1973.
19. Fregly, AR, Smith, MJ, and Graybiel, A: Revised normative standards of performance of men on a quantitative ataxia test battery. Acta Otolaryngol 75:10, 1973.
20. Fregly, AR and Graybiel, A: An ataxia battery not requiring rails. Aerospace Med 39:277, 1968.
21. Ekdahl, C, Jarnlo, G, and Andersson, S: Standing balance in healthy subjects. Scand J Rehabil Med 21:187, 1989.
22. Black, FO, et al: Normal subject postural sway during the Romberg test. Am J Otolaryngol 3:309, 1982.
23. Thyssen, HH, et al: Normal ranges and reproducibility for the quantitative Romberg's test. Acta Neurol Scand 60:100, 1982.
24. Black, FO, et al: Abnormal postural control associated with peripheral vestibular disorders. Prog Brain Res 76:263, 1988.
25. Horak, FB, Nashner, LM, and Diener, HC: Postural strategies associated with somatosensory and visual loss. Exp Brain Res 82:67, 1990.
26. Nashner, LM, Black, FO, and Wall, C: Adaptation to altered support and visual conditions during stance: Patients with vestibular deficits. J Neurosci 2:536, 1982.
27. Kirby, RL, Price, NA, and Macleod, DA: The influence of foot position on standing balance. Biomechanics 20:423, 1987.
28. Blatchly, CA, Whitney, SL, and Furman, JM: Subjective measures of dizziness and objective measures of balance: Is there a relationship? Neurol Report (Abstr) 14:20, 1990.
29. Yoneda, S and Tokumasu, K: Frequency analysis of body sway in the upright posture. Acta Otolaryngol (Stockh) 102:87, 1986.
30. Shumway-Cook, A and Horak, FB: Assessing the influence of sensory interaction on balance: Suggestion from the field. Phys Ther 66:1548, 1986.
31. Duncan, P, et al: Functional reach: A new clinical measure of balance. J Gerontol 85:529, 1990.
32. Gabell, A and Simons, MA: Balance coding. Physiotherapy 68:286, 1982.
33. Watanabe, T, Hattori, Y, and Fukuda, T: Automated graphical analysis of Fukuda's stepping test. In Igarashi, M and Black, FO (eds): Vestibular and Visual Control on Posture and Locomotor Equilibrium. Karger, Basel, 1985, p 80.
34. Horak, FB and Nashner, L: Central programming of postural movements: Adaptation to altered support-surface configuration. J Neurophysiol 55:1369, 1986.
35. Higgins, S: Motor skill acquisition. Phys Ther 71:123, 1991.

APPENDIX A: DIZZINESS QUESTIONNAIRE*

Name: _____ **Date:** _____

Handedness: _____ **Age:** _____

Name and address of physician(s) to whom you wish our report to be sent:

_____

_____

_____

Please answer these questions to the best of your ability. There is room at the end of each section for additional comments. *Please give necessary details for yes answers.* If you do not have dizziness, answer all questions to the best of your ability.

Exactly when and how did your problem begin?

Was there a specific initial cause?

1. If you have any of these symptoms, please describe them.
   a. Trouble with walking, balance, or falls

   b. Sense of spinning, tumbling, cartwheeling

   c. Sense of being tilted, off balance, or rocking

   d. Moving, tilt, or rotation of the world

   e. Double or blurred or jumping of vision or flashes of light

_____

*Used at Johns Hopkins Hospital, Department of Neurology, Baltimore, MD.

    f. Nausea, vomiting, queasiness

    g. Has anyone observed jerking of your eyes with dizzy spells?

	Yes	No
2. If you have dizziness, vertigo, or imbalance, is it affected or brought on by:		
Changes in position of the head or body (e.g., turning over in bed, bending over, or looking up)	___	___
Standing up	___	___
Rapid head movements	___	___
Walking in a dark room	___	___
Walking on uneven surfaces	___	___
Elevators, escalators	___	___
Climbing stairs or ladders	___	___
Airplane, boat, or car travel	___	___
Loud noises	___	___
Cough, sneeze, strain, laugh, abdominal pressure	___	___
Movement of objects in the environment	___	___
Fluorescent lights	___	___
Shopping malls; narrow or wide open spaces	___	___
Tunnels, bridges, supermarkets	___	___
Exercise (e.g., use of arms, jogging)	___	___
Activity	___	___
Foods, eating or not eating, salt, sugar, monosodium glutamate (MSG)	___	___
Heat, hot showers, or cold	___	___
Time of day	___	___
Swallowing	___	___
Depression, anxiety, nerves, or stress	___	___
Alcohol	___	___
Menstrual periods	___	___

	Yes	No
3. Have you had:		
Infections of ears	___	___
Sinus disease	___	___
Inner-ear disease (e.g., labyrinthitis)	___	___
Migraine or other headaches	___	___
Do or did you have motion sickness (car, boat)	___	___

	Yes	No
Pain, pins/needles, numbness, twitching, or weakness of face	———	———
Ringing in ears, one or both, steady or pulsating, high- or low-pitched	———	———
Difficulty with hearing	———	———
Pain, fullness, popping or pressure in ear	———	———
Trouble chewing, swallowing, speaking	———	———
Tremor or shakiness, stiffness, incoordination	———	———
Sweating, cold feelings	———	———
Palpitations (irregular or fast beating) of the heart	———	———
Crossed eyes, lazy eye, poor vision	———	———
Prescription glasses? What type?	———	———
Coughing, sneezing, straining or laughing that has brought on dizziness, pain, or headache?	———	———
Any problem brought on by airplane travel, underwater diving?	———	———

	Yes	No
4. Recently (within the last year) have you noted:		
Strength or energy change	———	———
Weight or appetite change	———	———
Memory loss (amnesia), change in handwriting	———	———
Skin rash or birthmarks	———	———
Pins and needles, numbness in arms or legs	———	———
Muscle or joint aches	———	———
Diarrhea or constipation	———	———
Fevers or swollen glands	———	———
Bladder problems	———	———
Problems with sexual function	———	———
Problems with sleeping	———	———
Lump in throat	———	———
Burning in body parts	———	———
Shortness of breath	———	———

	Yes	No
5. Questions about your habits		
Do or did you use alcohol? How much?	———	———
Do or did you ever smoke? Caffeine?	———	———
Did you ever use drugs? LSD?	———	———
Your present and prior occupations:	———	———

	Yes	No
6. Injuries		
Ears	_____	_____
Eyes	_____	_____
Head	_____	_____
Neck (e.g., whiplash)	_____	_____
Other	_____	_____

	Yes	No
Surgery		
Ears	_____	_____
Eyes	_____	_____
Head	_____	_____
Neck	_____	_____

	Yes	No
7. Exposures		
Poisons, gases, chemicals	_____	_____
Tropical diseases	_____	_____
Insect or tick bites	_____	_____
Intravenous antibiotics	_____	_____
Military service overseas	_____	_____
Travel to Central or South America, Asia, Africa	_____	_____
AIDS	_____	_____
Blood transfusions within 5 years	_____	_____
Loud noise (guns, machinery, loud music)	_____	_____
Drug therapy for cancer (if yes, what type)	_____	_____
Medications for depression or anxiety or psychiatric disease (if yes, what type and when)	_____	_____
Lithium, Valium, Dilantin, Tegretol, sleeping pills, Xanax, Ativan, phenothiazine, or any other tranquilizers or antidepressants	_____	_____

	Yes	No
8. Infections		
Syphilis or venereal disease	_____	_____
Mononucleosis (Epstein-Barr)	_____	_____
Lyme disease	_____	_____
Meningitis	_____	_____
Other infections	_____	_____

	Yes	No
9. Past or present health has been affected by:		
Heart problems	——	——
Diabetes	——	——
Low sugar (hypoglycemia)	——	——
Thyroid disorders	——	——
Treatment by a psychiatrist or counselor	——	——
Depression, anxiety, severe stress, phobias	——	——
High cholesterol	——	——
High or low blood pressure	——	——
Pain in back of jaw (TMJ), grinding	——	——
Loss of consciousness (faints)	——	——
Seizures or convulsions	——	——
Blood diseases, anemia	——	——
Skin diseases, arthritis	——	——
Neck pain	——	——
List all allergies.		

List other major illnesses, injuries, or other surgery.

	Yes	Specifics
10. Are there any other family members (indicate which one) with:		
Migraine headaches	——	
Ménière's syndrome	——	
Hearing loss	——	
Vertigo or dizziness	——	
Balance problems or tremor	——	
Convulsions or seizures	——	
Diabetes	——	
Cancer or brain tumors	——	
Stroke	——	
Heart disease or high blood pressure	——	
Psychiatric disorders	——	
Health of brothers and sisters?	——	
Are you married?	——	
Health and age of children?	——	
Health of parents?	——	
Any other diseases that run in the family?	——	

If your parents, brothers and sisters, or any children have died, at what age and from what cause?

11a. What are your current medications, include hormones, birth control pills, vitamins, special diet, etc. (name and amount/day)?

11b. What medications have you taken for your dizziness? (What dosage and for how long?)

	Yes	Result	When
12. Have you had a:			
Hearing test	_____		
Evaluation by a neurologist	_____		
Evaluation by an ear doctor	_____		
Caloric test (water or air in ear)	_____		
MRI and/or CT scan of the head or neck	_____		
Arteriogram (blood vessel x-ray)	_____		
BAER (auditory-evoked potentials)	_____		
VER (visual-evoked potentials)	_____		
Sinus x-rays	_____		
Neck x-rays	_____		
Myelogram	_____		
Lumbar puncture (spinal fluid examination)	_____		
EEG (brain wave)	_____		

Additional details:

	Yes	Result	When
Recent general medical checkup? When?	_____		
Blood work	_____		
Urinalysis	_____		
Chest x-ray	_____		
Mammogram	_____		
GYN (pelvic) exam	_____		
Holter monitor for abnormal heart beat	_____		

	Yes	Result	When
Electrocardiogram	———		
Lyme test	———		
Glucose tolerance test (sugar)	———		
B_{12} test	———		
Thyroid test	———		
AIDS test	———		

Additional details:

Any additional comments

APPENDIX B: DIZZINESS INVENTORY

Name: ———————————— **Date:**————————

The purpose of this scale is to identify difficulties that you may be experiencing because of your dizziness or unsteadiness. Please answer "Yes", "No", or "Sometimes" to each question. *Answer each question as it pertains to your dizziness or unsteadiness only.*

	Yes	No	Sometimes
P1. Does looking up increase your problem?	——	——	————
E2. Because of your problem, do you feel frustrated?	——	——	————
F3. Because of your problem, do you restrict your travel for business or recreation?	——	——	————
P4. Does walking down the aisle of a supermarket increase your problem?	——	——	————
F5. Because of your problem, do you have difficulty getting into or out of bed?	——	——	————
F6. Does your problem significantly restrict your participation in social activities such as going out to dinner, the movies, dancing, or to parties?	——	——	————
F7. Because of your problem, do you have difficulty reading?	——	——	————
P8. Does performing more ambitious activities like sports or dancing or household chores such as sweeping or putting dishes away increase your problem?	——	——	————
E9. Because of your problem, are you afraid to leave your home without having someone accompany you?	——	——	————
E10. Because of your problem, are you embarrassed in front of others?	——	——	————
P11. Do quick movements of your head increase your problem?	——	——	————
F12. Because of your problem, do you avoid heights?	——	——	————
P13. Does turning over in bed increase your problem?	——	——	————
F14. Because of your problem, is it difficult for you to do strenuous housework or yardwork?	——	——	————
E15. Because of your problem, are you afraid people may think you are intoxicated?	——	——	————
F16. Because of your problem, is it difficult for you to walk by yourself?	——	——	————
P17. Does walking down a sidewalk increase your problem?	——	——	————
E18. Because of your problem, is it difficult for you to concentrate?	——	——	————
F19. Because of your problem, is it difficult for you to walk around your house in the dark?	——	——	————
E20. Because of your problem, are you afraid to stay home alone?	——	——	————
E21. Because of your problem, do you feel handicapped?	——	——	————

	Yes	No	Sometimes
E22. Has your problem placed stress on your relationships with members of your family or friends?	——	——	————
E23. Because of your problem, are you depressed?	——	——	————
F24. Does your problem interfere with your job or housenold responsibilities?	——	——	————
P25. Does bending over increase your problem?	——	——	————
Total	——	——	————
	(×4)	(×0)	(×2)

Total: ————   F————   E————   P————
              (38)   (36)   (28)

From Jacobson, GP and Newman, CW: The development of the dizziness handicap inventory. Arch Otolaryngol Head Neck Surg 116:424, 1990. Copyright © 1990 The American Medical Association.

APPENDIX C: MULTIDIMENSIONAL DIZZINESS INVENTORY*

Name: _____ Date: _____
     Last   First   Initial

Age (in years): _____ Date of Birth: Month: _____ Day: _____ Year: _____

Sex (check one): _____ Male _____ Female Race: White _____ Black _____ Other _____

When did your dizziness first start? Month: _____ Year: _____

In the last 6 months, what percentage of the time has dizziness interfered with your activities? (Check one) 0%–25% _____; 26%–50% _____; 51%–75% _____; 76%–100% _____

In the last 6 months, on average, how many days per week has dizziness interfered with your activities? _____ number of days per week

Do you have any of the following conditions that have interfered with your activities in the last 6 months?

(check all that apply to you) hearing loss _____; loss of vision _____; pain _____; other _____

Instructions. An important part of your evaluation includes examination of dizziness from your perspective because you know your dizziness better than anyone else. The following questions are designed to help us learn more about your dizziness and how it affects your life. Under each question is a scale to mark your answer. Read each question carefully and then circle a number on the scale under that question to indicate how that specific question applies to you. An example may help you to better understand how you should answer these questions.

Example

How nervous are you when you ride in a car when the traffic is heavy?

0	1	2	3	4	5	6
Not at all nervous						Extremely nervous

If you are not at all nervous when riding in a car in heavy traffic, you would want to circle the number 0. If you are very nervous when riding in a car in heavy traffic, you would then circle the number 6. Lower numbers would be used for less nervousness, and higher numbers for more nervousness.

SECTION I

1. Rate the level of your dizziness at the *present moment*.

0	1	2	3	4	5	6
No dizziness						Very intense dizziness

*Used by R.J. Tusa, MD, Johns Hopkins Hospital, Baltimore, MD.

2. In general, how much does your dizziness interfere with your day-to-day activities?

    0   1   2   3   4   5   6

  No   Extreme

interference   interference

3. Since the time your dizziness began, how much has your dizziness changed your ability to work? (_____ Check here, if you have retired for reasons other than your dizziness.)

    0   1   2   3   4   5   6

  No change   Extreme

                                                change

4. How much has your dizziness changed the amount of satisfaction or enjoyment you get from taking part in social and recreational activities?

    0   1   2   3   4   5   6

  No change   Extreme

                                                change

5. How supportive or helpful is your spouse (significant other) to you in relation to your dizziness?

    0   1   2   3   4   5   6

  Not at all   Extremely

  supportive   supportive

6. Rate your overall mood during the *past week*.

    0   1   2   3   4   5   6

  Extremely   Extremely

    low   high

7. How much has your dizziness interfered with your ability to get enough sleep?

    0   1   2   3   4   5   6

  No   Extreme

interference   interference

8. On the average, how severe has your dizziness been during the *last week*?

    0   1   2   3   4   5   6

  Not at all   Extremely

  severe   severe

9. How able are you to predict when your dizziness will start, get better, or get worse?

    0   1   2   3   4   5   6

  Not at all   Very able to

    able to   predict

    predict

10. How much has your dizziness changed your ability to take part in recreational and other social activities?

    0   1   2   3   4   5   6

  No change   Extreme

                                                change

11. How much do you limit your activities in order to keep your dizziness from getting worse?

    0   1   2   3   4   5   6

  Not at all   Very much

12. How much has your dizziness changed the amount of satisfaction or enjoyment you get from family-related activities?

 0   1   2   3   4   5   6
No change   Extreme
                                                                 change

13. How worried is your spouse (significant other) about you because of your dizziness?

 0   1   2   3   4   5   6
Not at all   Extremely
worried   worried

14. During the past week, how much control do you feel that you have had over your life?

 0   1   2   3   4   5   6
No control   Extreme
                                                                 control

15. On an average day, how much does your dizziness vary (increase or decrease)?

 0   1   2   3   4   5   6
Remains   Changes a lot
the same

16. How much suffering do you experience because of your dizziness?

 0   1   2   3   4   5   6
No   Extreme
suffering   suffering

17. How often are you able to do something that helps to reduce your dizziness?

 0   1   2   3   4   5   6
Never   Very often

18. How much has your dizziness changed your relationship with your spouse, family, or significant others?

 0   1   2   3   4   5   6
No change   Extreme
                                                                 change

19. How much has your dizziness changed the amount of satisfaction or enjoyment you get from work? (_____ Check here, if you are not presently working.)

 0   1   2   3   4   5   6
No change   Extreme
                                                                 change

20. How attentive is your spouse (significant other) to you because of your dizziness?

 0   1   2   3   4   5   6
Not at all   Extremely
attentive   attentive

21. During the *past week* how much do you feel that you've been able to deal with your problems?

 0   1   2   3   4   5   6
Not at all   Extremely
                                                                    well

22. How much control do you feel that you have over your dizziness?

 0   1   2   3   4   5   6
No control   A great deal
at all   of control

23. How much has your dizziness changed your ability to do household chores?

    0   1   2   3   4   5   6
    No change   Extreme
                                                                     change

24. During the *past week,* how successful were you in coping with stressful situations in your life?

    0   1   2   3   4   5   6
    Not at all   Extremely
    successful   successful

25. How much has your dizziness interfered with your ability to plan activities?

    0   1   2   3   4   5   6
    No change   Extreme
                                                                     change

26. During the *past week,* how irritable have you been?

    0   1   2   3   4   5   6
    Not at all   Extremely
    irritable   irritable

27. How much has your dizziness changed or interfered with your friendship with people other than your family?

    0   1   2   3   4   5   6
    No change   Extreme
                                                                     change

28. During the *past week,* how tense or anxious have you been?

    0   1   2   3   4   5   6
    Not at all   Extremely
    tense or   tense and
    anxious   anxious

SECTION II

In this section, we are interested in knowing how your spouse (or significant other) responds to you when he or she knows you are dizzy. On the scale listed below each question, circle a number to indicate how often your spouse (or significant other) responds to you in that particular way when you are dizzy. Please answer all of the 14 questions.

1. Ignores me.

    0   1   2   3   4   5   6
    Never   Very Often

2. Asks me what he/she can do to help.

    0   1   2   3   4   5   6
    Never   Very Often

3. Reads to me.

    0   1   2   3   4   5   6
    Never   Very Often

4. Gets irritated with me.

    0   1   2   3   4   5   6
    Never   Very Often

5. Takes over my jobs or duties.

    0   1   2   3   4   5   6
    Never   Very Often

6. Talks to me about something else to take my mind off the dizziness.

       0   1   2   3   4   5   6

Never   Very Often

7. Gets frustrated with me.

       0   1   2   3   4   5   6

Never   Very Often

8. Tries to get me to rest.

       0   1   2   3   4   5   6

Never   Very Often

9. Tries to involve me in some activity.

       0   1   2   3   4   5   6

Never   Very Often

10. Gets angry with me.

       0   1   2   3   4   5   6

Never   Very Often

11. Gets me medication for my dizziness.

       0   1   2   3   4   5   6

Never   Very Often

12. Encourages me to work on a hobby.

       0   1   2   3   4   5   6

Never   Very Often

13. Gets me something to eat or drink.

       0   1   2   3   4   5   6

Never   Very Often

14. Turns on the T.V. to take my mind off my dizziness.

       0   1   2   3   4   5   6

Never   Very Often

SECTION III

Listed below are 19 daily activities. Please indicate how often you do each of these by circling a number on the scale listed below each activity. Please complete all 19 questions.

1. Wash dishes.

       0   1   2   3   4   5   6

Never   Very Often

2. Mow the lawn. (_____ Check here, if you do not have a lawn to mow.)

       0   1   2   3   4   5   6

Never   Very Often

3. Go out to eat.

       0   1   2   3   4   5   6

Never   Very Often

4. Play cards or other games.

       0   1   2   3   4   5   6

Never   Very Often

5. Go grocery shopping.

       0   1   2   3   4   5   6

Never   Very Often

6. Work in the garden. (_____ Check here, if you do not have a garden.)

       0   1   2   3   4   5   6

Never   Very Often

7. Go to a movie.
   0   1   2   3   4   5   6
   Never   Very Often

8. Visit friends.
   0   1   2   3   4   5   6
   Never   Very Often

9. Help with the house cleaning.
   0   1   2   3   4   5   6
   Never   Very Often

10. Work on the car. (_____ Check here, if you do not have a car.)
    0   1   2   3   4   5   6
    Never   Very Often

11. Take a ride in a car or bus.
    0   1   2   3   4   5   6
    Never   Very Often

12. Visit relatives. (_____ Check here, if you do not have relatives within 100 miles.)
    0   1   2   3   4   5   6
    Never   Very Often

13. Prepare a meal.
    0   1   2   3   4   5   6
    Never   Very Often

14. Wash the car. (_____ Check here, if you do not have a car.)
    0   1   2   3   4   5   6
    Never   Very Often

15. Take a trip.
    0   1   2   3   4   5   6
    Never   Very Often

16. Go to a park or beach.
    0   1   2   3   4   5   6
    Never   Very Often

17. Do the laundry.
    0   1   2   3   4   5   6
    Never   Very Often

18. Work on a needed household repair.
    0   1   2   3   4   5   6
    Never   Very Often

19. Engage in sexual activities.
    0   1   2   3   4   5   6
    Never   Very Often

SECTION IV

Please answer "Yes," "No," or "Sometimes" to each question by circling your response. Answer each question as it pertains to your dizziness or unsteadiness problem only.

	(Circle your answer)		
1. Does looking up increase your problem?	Yes	No	Sometimes
2. Because of your problem, do you feel frustrated?	Yes	No	Sometimes

3. Because of your problem, do you restrict your travel for business or recreation?	Yes	No	Sometimes
4. Does walking down the aisle of a supermarket increase your problem?	Yes	No	Sometimes
5. Because of your problem, do you have difficulty getting into or out of bed?	Yes	No	Sometimes
6. Does your problem significantly restrict your participation in social activities such as going out to dinner, to movies, dancing, or to parties?	Yes	No	Sometimes
7. Because of your problem, do you have difficulty reading?	Yes	No	Sometimes
8. Does performing more ambitious activities like sports, dancing, household chores such as sweeping or putting dishes away increase your problem?	Yes	No	Sometimes
9. Because of your problem are you afraid to leave home without someone to accompany you?	Yes	No	Sometimes
10. Because of your problem, have you been embarrassed in front of others?	Yes	No	Sometimes
11. Do quick movements of your head increase your problem?	Yes	No	Sometimes
12. Because of your problem, do you avoid heights?	Yes	No	Sometimes
13. Does turning over in bed increase your problem?	Yes	No	Sometimes
14. Because of your problem, is it difficult for you to do strenuous housework or yardwork?	Yes	No	Sometimes
15. Because of your problem, are you afraid people may think you are intoxicated?	Yes	No	Sometimes
16. Because of your problem, is it difficult for you to go for a walk by yourself?	Yes	No	Sometimes
17. Does walking down a sidewalk increase your problem?	Yes	No	Sometimes
18. Because of your problem, is it difficult for you to concentrate?	Yes	No	Sometimes
19. Because of your problem, is it difficult for you to walk around your house in the dark?	Yes	No	Sometimes
20. Because of your problem, are you afraid to stay home alone?	Yes	No	Sometimes
21. Because of your problem, do you feel handicapped?	Yes	No	Sometimes
22. Has your problem placed stress on your relationships with your family or friends?	Yes	No	Sometimes
23. Because of your problem, are you depressed?	Yes	No	Sometimes
24. Does your problem interfere with your job or household responsibilities?	Yes	No	Sometimes
25. Does bending over increase your problem?	Yes	No	Sometimes

SECTION V

This scale consists of a number of words that describe different feelings and emotions. Read each item and then mark the appropriate answer in the space next to that word. Indicate to what extent you generally feel this way, that is, how you feel on the average. Use the following scale to record your answers.

1	2	3	4	5
Very slightly or not at all	a little	moderately	quite a bit	extremely

_____interested   _____irritable   _____jittery
_____distressed   _____alert   _____active
_____excited   _____ashamed   _____afraid
_____upset   _____inspired   _____hostile
_____strong   _____nervous   _____enthusiastic
_____guilty   _____determined   _____proud
_____scared   _____attentive

CHAPTER 14

Treatment of Vestibular Hypofunction

Susan J. Herdman, PhD, PT
Diane F. Borello-France, MS, PT
Susan L. Whitney, Phd, PT, ATC

The use of exercise to treat patients with vestibular dysfunction has been advocated since the 1940s. Cawthorne[1] and Cooksey[2] were the first to report an exercise regimen for patients with postconcussion syndrome and other cases of "giddiness." Since that time, much knowledge has been gained that relates to the physiology, pathophysiology, and plasticity of the vestibular system. As this knowledge has grown, so has the use of exercise and physical therapy in the treatment of patients with vestibular disorders.

A clinician who is uncertain about how to manage the patient with unilateral peripheral vestibular hypofunction can draw on a wealth of clinical expertise and knowledge.[3-9] This chapter provides the reader with the background necessary to treat patients with vertigo and disequilibrium. The similarities and differences among the various treatment approaches are examined. Several case studies are presented to illustrate the rehabilitation process of patients with unilateral peripheral vestibular hypofunction. First, the different mechanisms of recovery will be discussed.

MECHANISMS OF RECOVERY FOLLOWING UNILATERAL VESTIBULAR LOSS

Several different mechanisms are involved in the recovery of function following unilateral vestibular loss. These mechanisms include spontaneous recovery, vestibular adaptation or plasticity, and the substitution of other strategies.

Spontaneous Recovery

Disturbances of static vestibular function (nystagmus, skew deviation, and postural asymmetries in stance) recover spontaneously.[10,11] These symptoms and signs are caused by the disruption of *tonic vestibulo-ocular and vestibulospinal responses.*. In the normal individual, when the head is stationary, the tonic firing of the neurons in the vestibular nuclei on each side of the brain stem is balanced. Unilateral loss of the input from the semicircular canals results in a relative imbalance in the inputs between the two sides. For example, loss of the signal from the semicircular canals on one side results in a slow-phase eye movement toward the side of the deficit (away from the intact side). The slow-phase eye movement is interrupted by a quick-phase eye movement in the opposite direction. This quick-phase eye movement resets the eye position, creating a spontaneous nystagmus. Unilateral loss of utricular inputs results in a skew deviation in which the eye on the side of the lesion drops in the orbit. Patients with skew deviations complain of a vertical diplopia.[12] Disruption of the *tonic vestibulospinal responses* produces an asymmetry in the muscle activity in the lower extremities, as measured electromyographically, while the patient is standing,[13] and in a postural asymmetry that can be detected clinically.[14] The timing of the disappearance of these symptoms parallels the recovery of the resting firing rate of the vestibular neurons.[15] Although visual cues can also be used to suppress spontaneous nystagmus and the postural asymmetry, several studies have demonstrated that recovery of spontaneous nystagmus is not dependent on visual inputs per se.[13,16] Nystagmus decreases at the same rate in animals kept in the dark immediately after unilateral labyrinthectomy as in animals kept in a lighted environment.

Vestibular Adaptation

Recovery of the dynamic vestibulo-ocular responses probably is due to the adaptive capability of the vestibular system; that is, the ability of the vestibular system to make long-term changes in the neuronal response to input. Disturbances of the *dynamic vestibulo-ocular response* are distinguished by a decrease in the gain of the response during head movements. The gain of the vestibulo-ocular reflex is decreased by as much as 75 percent for head movements toward the side of the lesion and by 50 percent for head movements away from the side of the lesion in patients with acute unilateral vestibular deficits.[17]

Disturbances of the *dynamic vestibulospinal response* are distinguished by a gait ataxia. Typically, patients ambulate with a widened base of support, frequently side-step, and may drift from one side to another while walking. They decrease trunk and head rotation while walking because these rotations would make them less stable. Head movement would result in an asymmetric vestibular signal that increases their sense of disequilibrium and the ataxia.

The signal for inducing vestibular adaptation is retinal slip, the movement of an image across the retina.[18] This "slip" results in an "error signal" that the brain attempts to minimize by increasing the gain of the vestibular responses. There is a wealth of evidence that recovery from the dynamic disturbances of vestibular function requires both visual inputs and movement of the body and head.[19-21] The gain of the vestibulo-ocular response does not recover when cats or monkeys are kept in the dark following unilateral labyrinthectomy.[16,21] Recovery of vestibulo-ocular gain begins when the animals are returned to a lighted environment. Similarly, if animals are prevented from

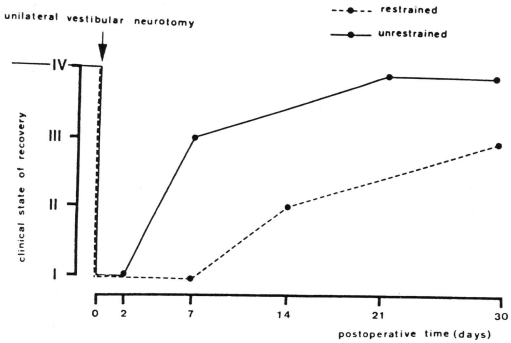

FIGURE 14-1. The effect of restricting mobility on the rate of recovery following unilateral transection of the vestibular nerve. Baboons that were restrained after unilateral vestibular nerve section had a delayed onset of recovery and a more prolonged recovery than animals that were allowed free movement. (From Lacour, Roll, and Appaix,[22] p 265, with permission.)

moving after unilateral vestibular nerve section, there is a delay in the onset of the recovery of postural stability, and the recovery period is prolonged[22] (Fig. 14-1).

Substitution

The third mechanism involved in recovery following vestibular lesions is the substitution of other strategies to replace the lost function. Sensory inputs from muscles and joint facets in the neck produce a slow-phase eye movement, the cervico-ocular reflex, that complements the vestibulo-ocular reflex (VOR) during low-frequency brief head movements.[23,24] Maoli and Precht[25] suggest that neck proprioceptive inputs have increased influence on gaze stability after unilateral vestibular loss. Saccadic eye movements may also be used to regain the visual target, although these eye movements would not be a particularly useful alternative for a poor VOR because patients still would not be able to see the target clearly during head movements.[26]

Recovery of postural stability may be due to the use of visual and somatosensory cues instead of remaining vestibular cues. Although the substitution of visual or somatosensory cues strategy may provide sufficient information for postural stability in many situations, the patient will be at a disadvantage if trying to walk when those cues are inaccurate or even not available, such as in the dark. At an extreme, some patients may modify their behavior to avoid situations where visual or somatosensory cues are diminished, such as going out at night.

Patients may also restrict head movements as a means of seeing clearly or maintaining their balance. This strategy is not particularly desirable because it would result in limited activity and would not provide a mechanism for seeing clearly or for maintaining balance during head movements.

THE ROLE OF EXERCISES IN RECOVERY

Animal studies support the concepts that visuo-motor experience facilitates the rate of recovery and improves the final level of recovery following vestibular dysfunction.[16,20-22] Several animal studies have suggested that exercise may facilitate the process of vestibular compensation. Igarashi and colleagues[27] found that following unilateral labyrinthectomy, squirrel monkeys exercising in a rotating cage had less spontaneous nystagmus than a nonexercise control group. In another similar study, Igarashi and associates[20] found locomotor equilibrium compensation occurred faster (7.3 days as compared to 13.7 days) in a group of squirrel monkeys exercising in a rotating cage compared to a nonexercise group. Similar findings have been observed in cats following unilateral labyrinthectomy.[19]

The use of exercise in the rehabilitation of patients with unilateral peripheral vestibular hypofunction is aimed at promoting vestibular compensation. Rehabilitation approaches recommended by Cawthorne,[1] Cooksey,[2] and by Norre[5] and Norre and De Weerdt[6,7] have focused on achieving compensation through the mechanism of habituation training. Repetition of movements and positions that provoke dizziness and vertigo forms the basic premise of habituation training. Norre[5] and Norre and De Weerdt[7] have compiled numerous case histories and descriptively reported the outcome of their therapeutic approach. Other treatment approaches attempt to achieve compensation through exercises that focus on enhancing the adaptation of the VOR and vestibulospinal reflex.[4,5,8,28]

GOALS OF TREATMENT

The goals of physical therapy intervention are to improve the patient's mobility, overall general physical condition and activity level, functional balance, safety for gait and gait-related activities, and the magnitude of the patient's symptoms (disequilibrium, vertigo, etc.). Patients usually are seen by the physical therapist on an outpatient basis; in some cases, however, the initial treatments occur while the patient is in the hospital. The physical therapist instructs the patient in a home exercise program. The physical therapist must motivate the patient and obtain compliance. To do so, the physical therapist must clarify to the patient the treatment goals and the potential effects of exercise.

Many of the exercises provided to the patient may, at first, enhance the patient's symptoms. This situation may be threatening to patients who are extremely fearful of experiencing their symptoms. Nevertheless, patients should be told that during physical therapy, there may be a period when they may feel worse before they feel better. To assist the patient through this period, the physical therapist should be accessible. For example, the patient should be instructed to telephone the therapist if the symptoms become severe or long-lasting. In such instances, the physical therapist determines if the exercises can be modified or if the exercises should be discontinued until the patient is formally reevaluated.

Excessive exacerbation of the patient's symptoms can also be avoided by conservative exercise prescription. Initially, the patient is provided with only a few key exercises and is instructed to attempt the exercises two to three times per day. The number of repetitions is based on the therapist's assessment of the patient's exercise tolerance. On subsequent visits, the patient is reevaluated and the exercise program expanded, so that all of the initial physical therapy goals are addressed.

TREATMENT APPROACHES

Several different approaches have been advocated in the management of patients with vestibular hypofunction. Four different approaches are presented, although there are elements common to all. Table 14–1 provides a summary and comparison of these different approaches. Two case studies are used to demonstrate the basis for specific exercises used in treatment and the progression of the patient's exercise program.

Cawthorne-Cooksey Exercises

The Cawthorne-Cooksey exercises were developed in the 1940s.[1,2] At the time, Cawthorne was treating patients with unilateral vestibular deficits and postconcussive disorders. In conjunction with Dr. Cooksey, a physiotherapist, Cawthorne developed a series of exercises that addressed their patients' complaints of vertigo and impaired balance. The Cawthorne-Cooksey exercises include movements of the head, tasks requiring coordination of eyes with the head, total body movements, and balance tasks (Table 14–2). Cawthorne and Cooksey recommended that the exercises be performed in various positions and at various speeds of movement. In addition, patients were required to perform the exercises with their eyes open and closed. According to Cawthorne and Cooksey, performing the exercises with the eyes closed decreased the patient's reliance on visual information and possibly forced more effective compensation by the vestibular and proprioceptive mechanisms. They also recommended that patients be trained to

TABLE 14–1 Comparison of Different Exercise Approaches
for the Patient with a Peripheral Vestibular Disorder

Movement	Cawthorne and Cooksey	Norre	Herdman	UPMC
Incorporates head and neck exercises into the treatment approach	X	X	X	X
Uses eye exercises	X		X	X
Uses a functional evaluation to assess the symptoms of the patient	X	X	X	X
Incorporates principles of motor control and learning into designing a treatment program			X	X
Practices mental exercises to increase concentration	X		X	X
Has the patient work in a variety of environments and task contexts	X		X	X

TABLE 14–2 Cawthorne-Cooksey Exercises for Patients
with Vestibular Hypofunction

A. In bed
   1. Eye movements— at first slow, then quick
      a. up and down
      b. from side to side
      c. focusing on finger moving from 3 ft to 1 ft away from face
   2. Head movements at first slow, then quick; later with eyes closed
      a. bending forward and backward
      b. turning from side to side

B. Sitting (in class)
   1. and 2 as above
   3. Shoulder shrugging and circling
   4. Bending forward and picking up objects from the ground

C. Standing (in class)
   1. as A1 and A2 and B3
   2. Changing from sitting to standing position with eyes open and shut.
   3. Throwing a small ball from hand to hand (above eye level).
   4. Throwing ball from hand to hand under knee.
   5. Changing form sitting to standing and turning round in between.

D. Moving about (in class)
   1. Circle round centre person who will throw a large ball and to whom it will be returned.
   2. Walk across room with eyes open and then closed.
   3. Walk up and down slope with eyes open and then closed.
   4. Walk up and down steps with eyes open and then closed.
   5. Any game involving stooping and stretching and aiming such as skittles, bowls, or basket-ball.

   Diligence and perseverance are required but the earlier and more regularly the exercise regimen is carried out, the faster and more complete will be the return to normal activity.

From Dix,[60] with permission.

function in noisy and crowded environments. These situations may be very difficult for patients with vestibular disorders to manage.

To encourage active participation, Cawthorne and Cooksey had patients exercise together in daily group sessions. They believed that a group exercise format would be more economic and more fun for the patient and would make it easier to identify a malingerer.

Hecker, Haug, and Herndon[29] used the Cawthorne-Cooksey exercises to treat a group of patients with vestibular disorders and reported that 84 percent of the patients responded favorably. They also emphasized the importance of performing the exercises regularly. In addition, they noted that emotional stress seemed to affect the patient's progress.

Cooksey[2] stressed that patients should be encouraged to move into positions that provoke symptoms. She believed that with repeated exposure to a stimulus, the patient would eventually tolerate the position without experiencing symptoms. This treatment philosophy is remarkably similar to the philosophy supported by many physical therapists today. Most physical therapy clinics that treat patients with vestibular deficits use some component of the Cawthorne-Cooksey exercises.

Norre's Approach

In 1979, Norre[30] proposed the use of vestibular habituation training for the treatment of patients with unilateral peripheral vestibular loss. According to Norre,[6] an asymmetry in labyrinth function results in a "sensory mismatch." The disturbed vestibular signal produces an input to the brain that conflicts with information received from intact visual and proprioceptive systems. This conflict, Norre believed, produced the symptoms experienced by patients with unilateral peripheral vestibular hypofunction.

Norre expanded on the work of Cawthorne, Cooksey, and Dix[31] and originally developed 34 provoking maneuvers that increased symptoms in patients with unilateral peripheral vestibular loss. Norre later decreased the number of provoking maneuvers to 19 (see Table 13–4). Many of Norre's maneuvers are similar to Cawthorne and Cooksey's original exercises (see Table 14–2).

Norre has used the 19 test maneuvers to obtain an objective measure of his patients' functional condition. In Norre's studies, patients were asked to rate the intensity, type (rotary or atypical), and duration of vertigo produced by each test maneuver. The maneuvers were performed quickly, and each test position was held for 10 seconds prior to returning to the starting position. Norre believed that a 10-second latency period allowed the system enough time to respond to the maneuver.

The 19 test maneuvers were also used by Norre as exercises for patients with provoked vertigo (see Table 13–4). Treatment based on Norre's approach encourages patients to perform the specific movements that increased their symptoms during the functional evaluation. According to Norre and De Weerdt,[32] many of the movements advocated for treatment are not usually incorporated into the patient's normal activities of daily living. These patients avoid such movements in an attempt to decrease their chance of experiencing an episode of vertigo. Thus, Norre and De Weerdt[32] strongly support the use of specific habituation exercises to promote adaptation of the vestibular system.

In addition to the habituation training, Norre and De Weerdt[32] recommended the use of relaxation exercises in the treatment of patients with peripheral vestibular disorders. They also advocated patient education to increase the patient's knowledge about the disability.

Norre has published studies describing the success rate of his therapeutic approach.[6,7,33] Norre's high success rate (70 percent of the subjects report a 75 percent improvement in symptoms after 2 weeks) must be examined cautiously, as subjects were selected from a homogenous diagnostic group. In most physical therapy clinics, patients present with a variety of diagnoses and therefore, the high success rate of Norre and De Weerdt may be impossible to replicate.

More recently, Norre, Forrez, and Beckers[34] have used posturography data to assist in development of a comprehensive rehabilitation program. Norre continues to advocate vestibular habituation training as a key ingredient to the successful rehabilitation of patients with unilateral peripheral vestibular hypofunction.

The Johns Hopkins/University of Miami Program

The exercises used in the Johns Hopkins Hospital vestibular rehabilitation program are based on the mechanisms of vestibular adaptation and on modifications of the Cawthorne-Cooksey regimen.[4,9] Vestibular adaptation is important during development and maturation and also in response to disease and injury. Exercises that facilitate adaptation can be used in patients with vestibular hypofunction as a mechanism to induce recovery.

Guidelines for Developing Exercises

The following points should be considered when developing exercises for the patient with a unilateral peripheral lesion.

1. *The best stimulus to induce adaptation is one producing an error signal:* The central nervous system (CNS) attempts to reduce the error signal by modifying the gain of the vestibular system. The best stimuli appear to be those that incorporate movement of the head and a visual input. Optokinetic stimulation (movement of visual world only) by itself also can increase the gain of the vestibular system, although perhaps not as effectively as head movement combined with a visual stimulus.[18,35-37] Figure 14–2 shows two simple exercises that can be used as the basis for an exercise program for patients with unilateral vestibular lesions. In each, the patient is required to maintain visual fixation on an object while the head is moving.

2. *Adaptation takes time:* The early studies on vestibular adaptation used paradigms in which the stimulus was present for several hours or more.[38-39] This situation would not be appropriate for patients, especially during the acute stage. We now know that vestibular adaptation can be induced with periods of stimulation as brief as 1 to 2 minutes.[40-41] During the time in which the brain is trying to reduce the error signal, the patient may experience an increase in symptoms and must be encouraged to continue to perform the exercise without stopping. Each exercise shown in Figure 14–2, for instance, should be performed for 1 minute without stopping. The time for each exercise can then be gradually increased to 2 minutes.

3. *Adaptation of the vestibulo-ocular system is context specific:* Therefore, for optimal recovery, exercises must stress the system in different ways.[41] For example, adaptation of the vestibular system is frequency-dependent.[42-43] If the system is adapted at a specific frequency, gain will improve most at that frequency. Because normal movement occurs over a wide range of frequencies of head movement, the patient should perform the head movement exercises at many different frequencies for optimal effects. Different head positions can also be used to vary the exercise.

4. *Adaptation is affected by voluntary motor control:*[44,45] VOR gain can be increased even in the dark if the subject simply imagines that he or she is looking at a stationary target on the wall while the head is moving. Although not increasing the gain as much as head movement plus vision combined, these results suggest that mental effort will help improve the gain of the system. Patients should be encouraged to concentrate on the task and should not be distracted by conversation and other activities.

5. *Patients should always work at the limit of their ability:* Although the patient's morale can be lifted through activities that he or she can perform relatively easily, most exercises should stress the patient's ability. For example, with the eye/head exercises, the speed of the head movement should be increased *as long as the patient can keep the visual target in focus.* Balance exercises can be made more difficult by decreasing the base of support, changing head or arm position, manipulating sensory cues, and by moving from static to dynamic activities (Table 14–3).

6. *Other mechanisms are involved in recovery:* These should be included in a well-rounded

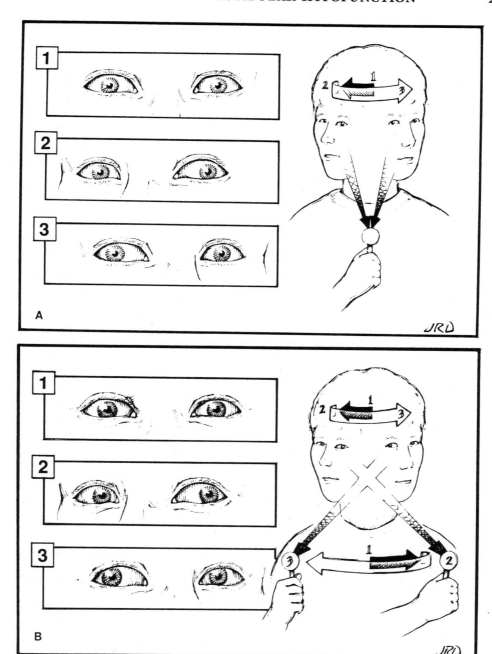

FIGURE 14–2. Exercises to increase the gain of the vestibular system can include (*A*) an X1 viewing paradigm and (*B*) an X2 viewing paradigm. In the X1 paradigm, the visual target is stationary and the subject moves his or her head back and forth while trying to maintain visual fixation on the target. In the X2 paradigm, the target and the head move in opposite directions while the subject tries to keep the target in focus. These exercises can be performed using a small visual target (foveal stimulus) and/or a large visual target (full-field) stimulus, with the head moving either horizontally or vertically. (From Tusa, RJ and Herdman, SJ: Vertigo and disequilibrium. In Johnson, R and Griffin, J (eds): Current Therapy in Neurologic Disease, ed 4. Mosby Year-Book, St. Louis, 1993, p 12, with permission.)

TABLE 14–3 Exercises to Improve Postural Stability

There are many different balance exercises that can be used. These exercises are devised to incorporate head movement (vestibular stimulation) or to foster the use of different sensory cues for balance.

1. The patient stands with his or her feet as close together as possible with both or one hand helping maintain balance by touching a wall if needed. The patient then turns his or her head to the right and to the left horizontally while looking straight ahead at the wall for 1 minute without stopping. The patient takes his or her hand or hands off the wall for longer and longer periods of the time while maintaining balance. The patient then tries moving his or her feet even closer together.
2. The patient walks, with someone for assistance if needed, as often as possible (acute disorders).
3. The patient begins to practice turning his or her head while walking. This will make the patient less stable so the patient should stay near a wall as he or she walks.
4. The patient stands with his or her feet shoulder-width apart with eyes *open*, looking straight ahead at a target on the wall. He or she progressively narrows the base of support from feet apart to feet together to a semi–heel-to-toe position. The exercise is performed first with arms outstretched, then with arms close to the body, and then with arms folded across the chest. Each position is held for 15 sec before the patient does the next-most-difficult exercise. The patient practices for a total of 5 to 15 min.
5. The patient stands with his or her feet shoulder-width apart with eyes open, looking straight ahead at a target on the wall. The patient progressively narrows his or her base of support from feet apart to feet together to a semi–heel-to-toe position. The exercise is performed with eyes *closed*, at first intermittently and then for longer and longer periods of time. The exercise is performed first with arms outstretched, then with arms close to the body, and then with arms folded across the chest. Each position is held for 15 sec, and then the patient tries the next position. The patient practices for a total of 5 to 15 min.
6. A headlamp can be attached to the patient's waist or shoulders, and the patient can practice shifting weight to place the light into targets marked on the wall. This home "biofeedback" exercise can be used with the feet in different positions and with the patient standing on surfaces of different densities.
7. The patient practices standing on a cushioned surface. Progressively more difficult tasks might be hard floor (linoleum, wood), thin carpet, shag carpet, thin pillow, sofa cushion. Graded-density foam can also be purchased.
8. The patient practices walking with a more narrow base of support. The patient can do this first, touching the wall for support or for tactile cues and then gradually touching only intermittently and then not at all.
9. The patient practices turning around while walking, at first making a large circle but gradually making smaller and smaller turns. The patient must be sure to turn in both directions.
10. The patient can practice standing and then walking on ramps, either with a firm surface or with more cushioned surface.
11. The patient can practice maintaining balance while sitting and bouncing on a Swedish ball or while bouncing on a trampoline. This exercise can be incorporated with attempting to maintain visual fixation of a stationary target thus facilitating adaptation of the otolith-ocular reflexes.
12. Out in the community, the patient can practice walking in a mall before it is open and therefore while it is quiet; can practice walking in the mall while walking in the same direction as the flow of traffic; can walk against the flow of traffic.

exercise program. Exercises should synthesize the use of visual and somatosensory cues with the use of vestibular cues, as well as the possibility of central preprogramming to improve gaze and postural stability. For example, balance exercises should "stress" the system by having the patient work with and without visual cues or while altering somatosensory cues by having the patient stand on foam. Removing or altering cues forces the patient to use the remaining cues. Thus if the patient is asked to stand on foam with eyes closed, the use of vestibular cues will be fostered.

Expectations

Recovery from unilateral vestibular lesions is usually quite good, and patients should expect to return to normal activities. Several factors can affect the final level of recovery, and this should be kept in mind when talking to patients about their progress and anticipated recovery.

1. Recovery may be delayed or limited if the patient restricts head movement or if visual inputs are minimized.[16,21,22] Patients with vestibular lesions often prefer to keep their eyes closed and their heads still to minimize symptoms. Another factor that may delay recovery or limit the final level of recovery is the use of medications that suppress vestibular function.[46]
2. Recovery following unilateral vestibular deficits can also be affected by the presence of other disorders affecting the peripheral nervous system or CNS. Deficits of the CNS that affect the vestibular nuclei or the cerebellum may affect vestibular adaptation,[47,48] whereas other lesions can affect structures involved in the substitution of alternative strategies, such as using visual or somatosensory cues for balance. The same is also true for lesions in the peripheral nervous system. To have adequate postural stability, an individual needs two sensory cues. Patients with vestibular deficits plus visual or lower-extremity somatosensory changes generally do not do as well as patients with vestibular deficits alone. Predicting the final level of recovery is even more difficult in patients with combined CNS and vestibular deficits.
3. The rate and final level of recovery can be affected by age-related changes in the vestibular, visual, and somatosensory systems.[49-57] There is evidence that the adaptive capability of the vestibular system itself is reduced in the older person.[53] There is also an increased likelihood that there will be a loss of more than one sensory cue, which would have a significant impact on postural stability. An individual has good stability with eyes closed (loss of one sensory cue) but is less stable if he or she stands with eyes closed and has a vestibular lesion. Third, diminished visual and somatosensory cues may affect the useful substitution of alternative strategies to improve postural stability.

TREATMENT

Acute Vestibular Disorders

Treatment for acute vestibular disorders *should begin early*. When visuomotor experience is prevented during the early stages after unilateral vestibular loss, there is a delay in recovery. In cats and monkeys deprived of vision immediately after labyrinthectomy, the gain of the VOR does not begin to recover until the animals are returned to room light.[16,21] Furthermore, the initiation of the recovery of postural responses is delayed, and the course of recovery is prolonged when motor activity was restricted in baboons after vestibular nerve section compared to unrestrained animals.[22]

There is also evidence that the vestibular system can be modified during the acute stage after unilateral vestibular loss. VOR adaptation can be induced after unilateral labyrinthectomy in cats as early as the third day after surgery.[25] The vestibular system in human beings also can be adapted during the acute stage after unilateral vestibular loss. Pfaltz[40] found an increase in the VOR gain in patients with unilateral vestibular loss stimulated optokinetically compared to untreated patients.

In the beginning of the recovery from the acute stage, *exercise can be for brief periods of time.* Pfaltz's study is also important for showing that even brief periods of stimulation can produce VOR gain changes that would be particularly useful in the treatment of patients during the acute stage of recovery.

During the initial stage following unilateral vestibular loss (UVL), the patient may complain of severe vertigo and may be nauseated and vomiting. Head movement will make these symptoms worse, and the patient usually prefers to lie quietly, often in a darkened room or with eyes closed. At this stage, the patient may also be taking medications to suppress these vegetative responses and may be receiving intravenous fluid replacement. Good visual inputs (bright room lights, curtains open) should be encouraged during the first days after the acute onset of a vestibular deficit.

After 1 to 3 days, the symptoms of nausea and vertigo should resolve, and the spontaneous nystagmus and skew deviation should be decreasing as the resting state of the vestibular neurons recovers. Patients can begin exercises to facilitate adaptation of the vestibular system as early as *2 or 3 days* after the onset of the vestibular loss using gentle, active head movement. Horizontal head movement while fixating a small (foveal), stationary target is performed for only 1 minute followed by a period of rest (X1 viewing, Fig. 14–2, Table 14–4). The exercise is then repeated using vertical head movements. As the patient improves, he or she should try to sustain the head movement for 2 minutes. Although the patient may complain of increased vertigo or disequilibrium

TABLE 14–4 Exercises to Improve Gaze Stability

Acute Stage (Also Used with Chronic, Uncompensated Patients)

1. A business card or other target with words on it (foveal target) is taped on the wall in front of the patient so he or she can read it. The patient moves his or her head gently back and forth horizontally for 1 minute while keeping the words in focus.
2. This is repeated moving the head vertically for 1 minute.
3. Depending on whether this induces any nausea, the exercise is then repeated using a large pattern such as a checkerboard (full-field stimulus), moving the head horizontally.
4. The exercise with the checkerboard is then repeated moving the head vertically.

The patient should repeat each exercise at least 3 times a day.

The duration of each of the exercises is extended gradually from 1 to 2 minutes.

Patients should be cautioned that the exercises may make them feel dizzy or even nauseated but · that they should try to persist for the full 1 to 2 minutes of the exercise, resting between exercises.

Subacute Stage

1. The patient holds a business card in front of him or her so that he or she can read it. The patient moves the card and his or her head back and forth horizontally in *opposite* directions, keeping the words in focus for 1 minute without stopping.
2. This is repeated with vertical head movements and with a large, full-field stimulus.

The duration is gradually extended from 1 to 2 minutes. The patient should repeat each exercise at least 3 times each day.

Chronic Stage

1. The patient fixates on a visual target placed on the wall in front of the patient while gently bouncing up and down on a trampoline (otolith stimulation).

Improve Gaze Stability

with head movements, neither is a reason to stop the exercises. Vomiting, however, is a reason for terminating exercises.

VOR gain in the acute stage after UVL is poor (0.25 to 0.5), and relatively slow head velocities and low frequencies should be used so that the patient can keep the visual target in focus at all times. As the patient improves (within a few days to a week or more), the exercises can be expanded to include use of a full-field stimulus (checkerboard) in addition to the small target they had been using. Within a week or two after the onset, patients can begin the vestibular adaptation exercises that require them to maintain fixation on a visual target that is moving in the opposite direction as their head movement (X2 viewing, Fig. 14–2, Table 14–4). This exercise should be performed with somewhat smaller head movements (and comparably small target movements) because the target cannot be kept in focus while viewing out of the corner of an eye. The head movements may have to be slower as well for the patient to maintain fixation. Both the X1 and the X2 viewing paradigms should be performed at increasing head velocities as the patient improves.

Recovery of postural stability will occur more gradually. Patients can get out of bed with assistance within 1 to 2 days after the onset of the vestibular deficit. They usually, although not always, need assistance with ambulation for a few days. Patients with UVL usually can stand with feet together and their eyes closed within 4 to 5 days after the onset, although they still will have increased sway. Gait will be grossly ataxic for the first week, but patients should be walking independently, albeit with a widened base of support, within 1 week. During this initial stage of recovery, several different balance and gait exercises are appropriate. Goals include increasing the patient's endurance while walking, improving stability while standing with a more narrow base of support (Romberg position) with eyes open and closed, and beginning to turn the head while walking. Exercises to improve balance in sitting or other positions are usually not necessary, and for postoperative patients, bending over must be avoided. Within 2 or 3 days after onset, patients can begin to perform the VOR adaptation exercises while standing as a preparation to walking and turning the head as well.

The exercises used during the chronic stage of recovery are the same as those used with chronic disequilibrium and are discussed below. Recovery from unilateral vestibular neuronitis, labyrinthitis, or from a surgical procedure, such as vestibular nerve section, typically takes 6 weeks although recovery may take up to 6 months in some patients. Patients with vestibular nerve section, for example, are often back at work within 3 weeks. Recovery from resection of acoustic neuroma typically takes longer, although most of the recovery occurs within the first few weeks. After the first 2 or 3 weeks, the main complaints are fatigue, instability when turning quickly, and some increased difficulty walking in the dark. Patients may also complain of greater instability when walking on uneven surfaces or when there is a change in light intensity (opening a door to the outside, walking through intermittent shadows, such as trees). One of the more commonly asked questions is when the patient may begin to drive again. One guideline is that patients should be able to see clearly when making rapid and abrupt head movements.

Chronic Vestibular Deficits

Although patients with chronic vestibular deficits often do not have vertigo or vomiting (the exception being those patients with episodic vestibular disorders such as Ménière's disease), they frequently have limited their movements or at least their head movements in an attempt to avoid precipitating the symptoms of disequilibrium and nausea. Head movements must be encouraged in these patients. The vestibular rehabilitation program may begin with the same adaptation exercises used during the acute stage following UVL. The patients may need to be started slowly, and they often complain that they feel worse rather than better as they perform the exercises because they are stressing the vestibular system by performing head movements that they had been avoiding. Explaining to the patient that this may occur before they begin the exercises is helpful. It is reasonable to expect improved function within 6 weeks in patients who are compliant about doing their exercises but, anecdotally at least, the longer the problem has existed, the longer the time needed to see improved function. Once the patient is able to perform the initial vestibular adaptation exercises, it may be necessary to take the chronic patient through more complex movements in order to habituate the response to movement or at least to make them less fearful that movement will precipitate vertigo. Cawthorne's exercises, such as moving from sitting to standing and turning around in between, and Norre's exercises are very useful at this stage (see Tables 14–2 and 13–4).

Gait exercises can also be more challenging for patients with chronic vestibular disorders, although again, the starting point may be simple static balance exercises with eyes open and closed, on a stable support surface or on foam (Table 14–3). Patients can be taken through a series of exercises that stress their balance by gradually decreasing their base of support. Even if they are unable to maintain the position successfully for the required period of time, practicing will improve their balance. Patients with complete UVL, however, rarely perform the sharpened Romberg with eyes closed at any age. More difficult balance exercises may include walking and turning suddenly or walking in a circle while gradually decreasing the circumference of the circle, first in one direction and then in another. The patient needs the practice of walking in different environments, such as on grass, in malls (walking in an empty mall is easier than in a crowded mall, walking with the crowd is easier than against the crowd), and walking at night. Precautions to prevent falls should always be taken until the patient no longer needs them.

In summary, patients with unilateral vestibular deficits can be expected to recover from the vertigo and/or disequilibrium they first experience. The final level of recovery should be to return to all or most activities (singles tennis may be a problem). Other nervous system disorders can delay or limit the level of recovery. Animal studies and anecdotal evidence in human beings suggest that exercises facilitate recovery of vestibular system function. Early intervention also seems to be important in optimizing recovery. Restricting movement, preventing visual inputs, and the use of vestibular suppressant medications may delay the onset of recovery and may limit the final level of recovery.

University of Pittsburgh Medical Center's Approach

The therapeutic approach employed at the University of Pittsburgh Medical Center (UPMC) is problem-oriented. The physical therapy program prescribed by the physical therapist is based on the problem areas identified during the evaluation and the patient's diagnosis and medical history. For example, the physical therapy program for a patient with Ménière's disease would differ from that provided to a patient with vestibular neuronitis. Specifically, the treatment program for a patient with Ménière's disease would not address the symptom of vertigo. Compensation of vertigo in Ménière's disease is difficult to achieve because of the fluctuating nature of the disease process itself.

Instead, the physical therapy program would focus on improving the patient's balance function in a variety of task and environmental situations, preventing physical deconditioning, and, if indicated, education in environmental modification and safety awareness.

The treatment approach used by physical therapists at the UPMC Jordan Center for Balance Disorders incorporates treatment suggestions offered by Cawthorne and Cooksey, Herdman, Norre, Shumway-Cook, and others. In addition, the UPMC program augments these suggestions by incorporating functional activities and contemporary principles of motor learning and motor control. As with many of the other approaches, the UPMC's general treatment progression includes the following:

1. Increasing and alternating the speed of the exercises
2. Performing exercises in various positions and activities (i.e., head movements performed in sitting, then standing, and finally during walking)
3. Performing exercises in situations of decreasing visual and/or somatosensory input (i.e., eyes open to eyes closed)
4. Exposing the patient to a variety of task and environmental situations and contexts (i.e., walking in the home to walking at a shopping mall)

HEAD MOVEMENT EXERCISES

If a patient experiences exacerbation of symptoms during the head movement assessment, neck exercises are incorporated into the exercise program. The neck exercises developed by Cawthorne[1] and Cooksey,[2] and Norre[5] are employed. If the patient has significant symptoms, these exercises may be performed initially in the supine or sitting position. Later, the patient can perform these exercises in standing or during walking. If straight plane movements of the head produce few symptoms, neck diagonals, with or without a combination of trunk movement, are prescribed. During the head movement exercises, the patient is instructed to hold the position for at least 10 seconds, or until the symptoms dissipate. In addition, the patient is instructed to perform each exercise three to five times. Before instructing the patient to perform neck range of motion exercises, clinical testing of the vertebral artery is advised. The patient lies supine with his or her head over the edge of the table and the therapist passively extends, laterally flexes, and rotates the head. The head is held in this position for approximately 30 sec while the therapist looks for symptoms of arterial compression such as nystagmus, slurred speech, mental confusion, complaints of dizziness, and/or numbness in an extremity. We should recall that nystagmus and dizziness or vertigo would occur in patients with benign paroxysmal positional vertigo (BPPV) in this position (see Chapter 16). The significant characteristics of vertebral artery compression are the other neurologic symptoms that occur during this test. The test is repeated, moving the head to the opposite side. Patients experiencing symptoms should be referred to their physician or to a neurologist. In such cases, neck exercises should be avoided until the physical therapist receives medical clearance from the physician.

Attempts are also made to include neck movements into the patient's daily routine. For example, the patient is instructed to incorporate neck diagonals into the task of loading and unloading the dishwasher. This task requires the patient to focus on the object and move the body, head, and arm synchronously to either pick up or place the object on a high shelf (Fig. 14–3).

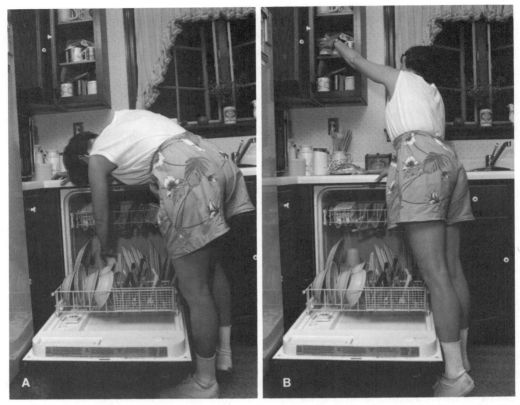

FIGURE 14–3. Neck movements are incorporated into the patient's normal daily routine. In this example, the patient is instructed to perform a neck diagonal exercise while loading and unloading the dishwasher.

EYE AND HEAD EXERCISES

Patients with vestibular disorders often complain of symptoms when performing tasks that require visual tracking or gaze stabilization during head movements. Herdman[3,4] and Toupet[28] have suggested many specific exercises for patients that experience difficulty with tasks requiring visuovestibular interaction. For example, Herdman[3,4] suggests having the patient move the head while reading a business card taped to the wall. These exercises are incorporated into the patient's treatment program if the therapeutic evaluation or subjective complaints of the patient indicate deficits in visuo-ocular or vestibulo-ocular function. At the UPMC, patients with such deficits are also instructed to perform functional tasks or games that require visual tracking or gaze fixation. For example, laser tag requires the patient to move the head while focusing eyes on a moving target. Bouncing and catching a ball may be another appropriate task for some patients. The patient could be advised to bounce the ball off the floor, wall, and/or ceiling in an attempt to vary the task by changing direction of object motion and/or neck position. Using multicolored or highly patterned balls may also enhance task difficulty, because the moving pattern or high color contrast may greatly increase the patient's symptoms. Electronic *Simon Says* requires the patient to watch and remember a sequence of lights that flash in rapid succession in front of the patient. This task incorporates Cawthorne's suggestion to include mental exercises into the exercise regimen.

Exposing the patient to highly textured visual environments may also assist in the remediation of visuovestibular interaction deficits. For example, the patient may be instructed to gradually perform tasks, such as grocery shopping or walking through a shopping mall.

MOVEMENT AND POSITIONAL EXERCISES

During the physical therapy assessment, positions or movements that provoke the patient's symptoms are identified. These positions and movements are then incorporated into the patient's exercise program. Movements, such as rolling, supine to sit, and sit to stand frequently exacerbate the patient's symptoms. Many of the movement and positional exercises used at the UPMC have been adapted from Norre's exercises (see Table 13–4). When initially prescribing these exercises, avoiding those movements or positions that produce severe symptoms is particularly important. Many therapists at the UPMC have experienced that too aggressive an approach initially may lead to patient noncompliance. Instead, UPMC therapists select movements and positions that produce a minimal to moderate level of symptoms. As with the head movement exercises, the patient is instructed to maintain the position for 10 seconds or until the symptoms alleviate. In addition, the patient is told to perform each exercise three to five times.

BALANCE AND GAIT TRAINING

Although many patients with peripheral vestibular hypofunction perform below the norm on static tests of balance, their most common complaint is imbalance during walking. Rarely do these patients report an inability to stand on one leg. Instead, they may complain of difficulty walking on an uphill grade, through a cluttered room, or into a movie theater. Because of the nature of the patient's deficits, balance training should address the dynamic aspects of gait and be task-directed. Balance and gait training are inseparable and are therefore considered together in this discussion.

Based on the evaluation, the therapist identifies the patient's functional balance deficits. Therapeutic exercise prescription should address the patient's specific deficits. For example, a patient may experience disequilibrium when the opportunity to use visual and/or somatosensory input for balance is minimized. In this situation, emphasizing exercises and tasks that require the patient to focus on vestibular instead of visual or somatosensory input is important. Such exercises include walking backward, sidestepping, and braiding performed with the eyes closed, marching in place on foam performed with the eyes open, and later with the eyes closed (Figs. 14–4 and 14–5, Table 14–5), and walking across an exercise mat or mattress in the dark.

Another functional deficit is the instability experienced by patients when faced with situations that require movements of the head during gait. For instance, many patients indicate having difficulty shopping for groceries. To scan the grocery shelves for the desired item, the patient must walk while moving the head left, right, or diagonally. At the same time, the patient must continue to monitor the environment to prevent a collision with another shopper. As a result, this rather ordinary task creates an overwhelming challenge to the patient's postural control system. To overcome this challenge, the patient is first instructed to walk down a corridor while moving the head left and right, up and down, or diagonally. Later, the patient performs the same task while avoiding objects placed in the walking path.

The last deficit to be discussed is the difficulty vestibular patients experience when their gait is unexpectedly disrupted. One seldom walks through a busy shopping mall

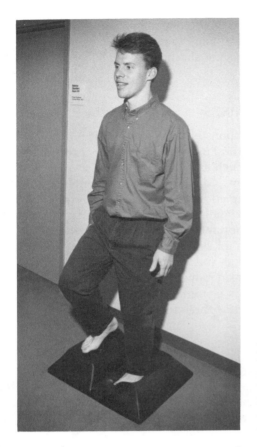

FIGURE 14–4. Activities that promote the use of vestibular information for maintaining balance are frequently included in home exercise programs. In this example, the patient marches in place on a foam cushion, with the eyes open or closed. Closing the eyes maximizes the importance of vestibular information.

without experiencing a sudden head-on encounter with another person. Such tasks require the postural control system to respond quickly. In some cases, the patient may need to improve the ability to anticipate forthcoming events. As indicated in the gait evaluation, an obstacle course can be devised to assess the patient's ability to anticipate or respond quickly to changes in task context. The obstacle course can also be used in treatment. The patient should be instructed to vary the course in as many ways as possible. Having a family member verbally direct the patient on the path to follow is helpful. Commands are given at the moment the patient must encounter or avoid an obstacle, thereby maintaining a level of task uncertainty. Another task that requires the patient to respond quickly to externally imposed constraints is walking and pivoting to the left or right. Again, a family member directs the patient on when and in what direction to pivot.

Patients with vestibular disorders can experience difficulty with many different balance and gait tasks. The above discussion considered only a few. Through a thorough evaluation, the therapist may identify the patient's specific motor control problem. In many instances, this identification is not entirely possible. In such cases, the therapy program should not be limited to specific balance or gait exercises. Instead the therapist should provide the patient with balance and gait activities that challenge the patient's postural control system in a variety of ways.

Trace the Alphabet

A. Stand near a wall or counter in case you need to hold on.

B. Trace the first ten letters of the alphabet on the floor with your foot .

C. Repeat with your other foot.

D. As you get better try and trace the entire alphabet.

E. Do this _____times _____times a day.

F. Do this with your eyes: Open   Closed

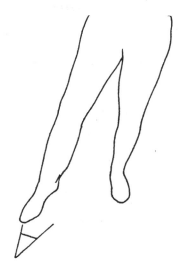

Stepping Forward and Back, Crossing Over

A. Stand near a wall.

B. Cross your foot in front of the other.

C. Bring it back to the starting position.

D. Cross your foot behind the other the foot.

E. Bring it back to the starting position.

F. Repeat the above sequence using the opposite foot.

G. Do this_____times_____times a day.

B

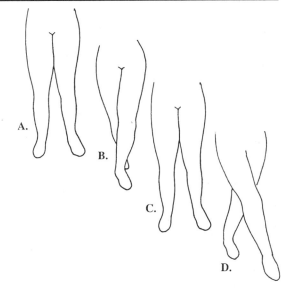

FIGURE 14–5. Balance exercises. Patients receive cards with instructions and diagrams for exercises to perform at home. As the patient progresses, he or she moves on to more difficult and varied exercises.

WALKING PROGRAM

Many patients are advised to begin a regular walking program. The purpose of the walking program is twofold. The first objective is to prevent deconditioning of the patient; the second is to provide realistic challenges to the patient's CNS. Tasks such as walking on uneven terrain, walking through a shopping mall, or crossing the street

TABLE 14–5 Balance and Gait Exercises

1. Do the following exercises in standing. Stand near a kitchen counter, but only hold on if needed.
   a. Walk sideways 15 ft. Repeat in both left and right directions _____ times, twice a day.
   b. Walk backward 15 ft. Repeat _____ times, twice a day.
2. Do the following exercises in standing. Stand with a wall behind you. Have a family member stand nearby if needed. Stand on a pillow or couch cushion, for _____ sec.
   a. Do this with your eyes open. Repeat _____ times, twice a day.
   b. Do this with your eyes closed. Repeat _____ times, twice a day.
   c. Stand on one leg with your eyes open. Repeat _____ times twice a day.
3. Walk down a corridor and practice moving your head left and right. Keep your head turned in each direction for about 3 steps. Walk _____ ft. Repeat _____ times, twice a day. Also repeat by moving your head up and down.
4. Set up an obstacle course. Use chairs, pillows, and furniture as obstacles. Place smaller objects on the floor that you must step over. Change the course each time, so that you do not get used to the same routine.

   You can incorporate stair climbing, sit to stand, or picking up and carrying objects during the obstacle course. Set a timer or clock yourself to see how fast you can finish.

   To add difficulty, have a family member shout out commands (i.e., "Turn left now") or throw a ball toward you unexpectedly.
5. Walk around a darkened room in your house (carpeted preferred) for _____ min.
6. Go grocery shopping, as tolerated.
7. Do your walking program at a shopping mall 1 to 2 times a week.

---

challenge the patient in ways that cannot be stimulated by a therapeutic exercise program (Fig. 14–6). When crossing the street, the patient must conform to the temporal constraints imposed by moving vehicles. Specifically, the patient must determine at what moment to step off of the curb to avoid confronting a vehicle. When crossing the street at a busy intersection, this requirement becomes more difficult to fulfill. In addition, the patient's postural control system must make quick adjustments to offset perturbations caused by changes in terrain or motion of other people.

The initial program requires the patient to walk 15 to 20 minutes, four times per week. Over the subsequent weeks, the patient is instructed to increase to a 30-minute walk. Initially, the patient may be advised to walk in a familiar environment with few challenges. Later, the therapist encourages the patient to expand the walking program to other situations and contexts. Walking in a park and at a shopping mall are frequently recommended. When walking in these situations, patients are advised to experience as many challenges as possible. For example, riding an escalator in a shopping mall may provide an interesting challenge to the patient. The patient must remain balanced while standing on a moving support surface. In addition, the motion of other people toward or to the side of the patient may create a sense of dizziness or imbalance, enhancing the difficulty of the task. Such challenges are necessary to overcome if the patient is to manage safely in a variety of contexts without experiencing an exacerbation of symptoms.

CASE STUDY 1

A 44-year-old woman was referred to Johns Hopkins Hospital for treatment of her acoustic neuroma. For the past year, she has had complaints of disequilibrium and difficulty seeing clearly when walking or riding in a car but was otherwise in

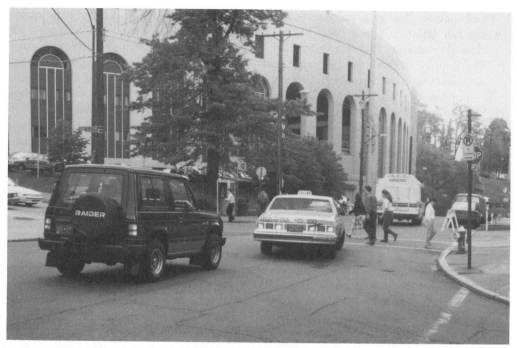

FIGURE 14–6. Patients may have difficulty with walking when they must conform to temporal constraints, for example, when crossing a street before the light changes.

good health. She also complained of a gradual loss of hearing in her left ear. Her audiogram showed a speech-reception threshold (SRT) of 65 and no identifiable speech discrimination. She had normal hearing on the right with 100 percent discrimination. Magnetic resonance imaging (MRI) with gadolinium showed a 4-cm tumor in the left cerebellar-pontine angle that was compressing the lower midbrain, pons, upper medulla, and cerebellum. Facial nerve function appeared to be symmetric and normal. She had decreased light touch sensation on the midportion of the left face to cotton. Corneal reflex was decreased on the left. She had direction-changing gaze-evoked nystagmus. Pursuit, saccades, and VOR cancellation were normal. VOR to slow head movement was normal in both directions. VOR to rapid head thrusts to the right was normal but resulted in corrective saccades with head movements to the left. With Frenzel lenses, gaze-evoked nystagmus was more pronounced to the right than to the left. After head shaking, there was only a single drift of the eyes to the left and a single corrective saccade. No nystagmus was elicited with vertical head shaking. Visual acuity with the head stationary was 20/20 corrected. Quantified visual acuity during active head oscillations at 150 deg/sec degraded to 20/34.

The result of her Romberg test was normal, and the patient could maintain the sharpened Romberg with eyes open for 30 sec. She could not perform the sharpened Romberg tests with eyes closed. Fukuda's stepping test with eyes open resulted in a 22-inch forward progression with no turn. With eyes closed she had a 40-inch forward progression with no turn. The patient ambulated with a normal cadence, stride length, base of support, trunk and neck rotation, and arm swing. She did not appear to use excessive visual fixation to maintain her balance while ambulating. Posturography tests showed that the patient had difficulty maintaining her balance when both visual and somatosensory cues were absent (eyes closed) or altered. She showed mildly increased reliance on visual cues for balance. The latency to force development, gain, and symmetry of her automatic postural responses were within normal limits bilaterally. Short-, middle-, and long-latency responses as measured by electromyography (EMG) were within normal limits bilaterally. Vibration threshold in her left foot was normal but elevated in her right foot [$> \bar{x} + 3$ standard deviations (SD)]. At the time of her initial physical therapy evaluation, the patient was also oriented to the postoperative rehabilitation care.

Comment: This patient is typical of many patients with acoustic neuromas (AN) in that her main complaint was decreased hearing. She additionally had developed some balance problems, but many patients with AN do not notice any changes in balance preoperatively. The absence of vertigo or even disequilibrium in these patients is because of the gradual vestibular loss occurring as the tumor grows rather than an abrupt onset as would occur with vestibular neuronitis. This tumor was quite large and was compressing brain-stem structures and the cerebellum without producing many symptoms or signs other than decreased sensation in the face and a decreased corneal reflex. The direction-changing gaze-evoked nystagmus may have been due to compression of the brain-stem or cerebellum. The patient made corrective saccades with head movements toward the involved side, which indicates an inadequate vestibular system. In addition, her dynamic visual acuity was abnormal (normal is little or no change in acuity with head movement). The fact that she had no head shaking–induced nystagmus, despite having a unilateral vestibular deficit, may be due to poor velocity storage related to the brain-stem compression. Several abnormal findings were noted with assessment of her balance, including inability to perform the sharpened Romberg test with eyes closed, abnormal Fukuda's stepping test with eyes closed, and difficulty maintaining her balance on the posturography tests when both visual and somatosensory cues were altered. We have found that the sharpened Romberg test with eyes closed is sensitive to UVL but not specific for vestibular deficits. Her ability to perform Fukuda's stepping test without turning is a little unusual in a patient with a unilateral deficit; this ability may indicate that compensation is occurring.

Surgical resection of the AN was performed using a suboccipital approach (see Chapter 10). A large tumor, approximately 5 cm in diameter, that filled the posterior fossa and eroded the posterior lip of the internal auditory canal was found. The seventh cranial nerve was monitored throughout the procedure and was intact. The patient did well postoperatively. She had no complaints of vertigo or diplopia. She had a right-beating nystagmus when she looked to the right or upward. She did have a prominent seventh nerve palsy and evidence of involvement of cranial nerves IX and X.

On postoperative day 3, she still had a right-beating nystagmus. Her active neck range of movement was limited by 50 percent due to pain at the surgical site that she described as a pulling sensation. She was beginning to ambulate with contact guarding only. She walked with a widened base of support and minimized rotation through her trunk. Her gait was slow and she occasionally side-stepped. Her balance when turning appeared to be less secure. She appeared to use excessive visual fixation while she walked for balance. She could not turn her head while walking without an increase in her ataxia. She had a negative Romberg test. Sharpened Romberg response was not tested. Posturography showed that she was unable to maintain her balance when both visual and somatosensory cues were altered, and she had increased difficulty when somatosensory inputs alone were altered. Her balance was within normal limits on the other tests. There was no asymmetry in stance. Vestibular adaptation exercises were initiated on postoperative day 3. The initial exercise used was the X1 viewing paradigm, which the patient was to perform both while sitting and while standing. While standing she was to decrease her base of support gradually and bring her feet closer together. The exercise was to be performed using a foveal stimulus with horizontal and vertical head movements. The patient was instructed to perform the exercises three to five times a day for 1 minute each. In addition, she was to practice walking, gradually increasing the distance walked.

Comment: This patient's postural instability and her performance on the various balance tests are typical of patients following resection of AN. Many patients do experience vertigo immediately after the surgery, but this patient probably had lost most of her vestibular function unilaterally because of the size of the tumor. The loss of vestibular function prior to surgery may also account for the minimal nystagmus and the absence of a skew deviation in this patient.

By postoperative day 6, she had a direction-changing gaze-evoked nystagmus, but it had decreased. Her quantitative dynamic visual acuity was 20/60. She had a normal sharpened Romberg response with eyes open, but could not perform it with eyes closed. She was ambulating independently but still had an increased base of support. Her gait was less ataxic, and she no longer used excessive visual fixation to maintain balance. She was independent on stairs with a railing. Her exercise program consisted of the X1 and the X2 viewing paradigms using both a foveal and a full-field stimulus that she was to perform in sitting and in standing positions three times a day. She was to perform each exercise for 2 minutes. She also was instructed to begin practicing turning her head while walking, being careful because it would make her less stable. Each exercise period would take approximately 45 minutes. At this stage, patients are still not allowed to bend over or lift anything more than 5 lb (risk of cerebral spinal fluid leak). The patient was discharged from the hospital on postoperative day 7.

Comment: A rapid recovery of patients with UVL is typical. The effect of the vestibular loss is still obvious (dynamic visual acuity is degraded to 20/60, this patient's gait is still abnormal, especially when she turns her head). Most patients with unilateral vestibular loss are never able to perform the sharpened Romberg test with eyes closed. We typically do not give these patients any kind of assistive device to use when walking. There are 2 or 3 days while they are in the hospital when walking with a cane might be helpful for some patients. Purchasing a cane for these patients is not justifiable because the cane will not be needed at discharge. There are exceptions to this rule, of course, but in the last 200 patients (we see 50 or more AN patients a year), only 3 or 4 have needed an assistive device for walking.

The patient was next seen in the outpatient clinic 3 weeks after surgery. Romberg test was normal and sharpened Romberg test with eyes open was normal, but she could not perform the sharpened Romberg test with her eyes closed. Posturography showed that the patient could maintain her balance within normal limits using vestibular cues. Motor tests showed normal latency, gain, and symmetry of response. The patient ambulated with a normal cadence and a normal base of support. She could turn without loss of balance but did slow down slightly. When asked to turn her head repeatedly while walking, her base of support widened and her gait became slightly ataxic. Her exercise program now included X1 and X2 viewing exercises in stance only, using both a foveal and a full-field stimulus and both horizontal and vertical head movements. She was to perform the exercises with her feet positioned so that her balance was challenged as well (e.g., in a semi-tandem position). She was also to practice standing with and without visual cues while gradually decreasing her base of support (see Table 14–3). She was to continue to practice walking and turning her head, as that was still a problem. She was to begin a walking program to improve her exercise tolerance and was encouraged to walk in different environments such as outdoors, on uneven surfaces, and in a mall.

Comment: The goals for this patient are that she return to full activities, probably within 6 weeks after surgery. Other patients require a longer recovery period and may not return to work for 3 months. The full recovery period following this surgery is 1 year, with fatigue being the main problem. Within 6 months (and usually earlier), patients should be able to participate in sports such as tennis, racquetball, and golf, all of which are good vestibular and balance exercises as well. They may have to change how they play and may have to shift to doubles games rather than singles. Patients will be aware of a sense of imbalance when they turn rapidly toward the side of the deficit but usually do not have any loss of balance. Some patients complain that they have difficulty when balance is stressed, such as when walking in the dark or uneven surfaces or if they have to step backward suddenly. Patients who do not do well should be carefully screened for other problems that would complicate their recovery, such as the coexistence of visual or sensory changes in the feet or of CNS lesions that would prevent vestibular adaptation. Some patients are fearful of moving their heads. These patient may still benefit from vestibular exercises even several months after surgery but will need to be on a more closely supervised program to ensure compliance. This patient also had a facial palsy after surgery. The potential for recovery is good because the nerve was intact after surgery. We do not initiate facial exercises until the patient has more than faint voluntary movements, and then patients are cautioned to practice gentle facial movements rather than forceful movements. In patients with significant synkinesis, we use biofeedback training to improve the quality of the facial movements. Of main concern in patients with facial paresis or palsy is protection of the eye. If lid closure is absent or poor, patients may use either a cellophane moisture chamber or an eye patch to prevent drying of the eye and corneal damage. Patients using either type of patch should be advised to be careful when walking because they have only monocular depth perception cues.

CASE STUDY 2

A 46-year-old woman was referred to UPMC physical therapy with a diagnosis of a right peripheral vestibulopathy. The physician's report indicated that her symptoms appeared suddenly and for no apparent reason. Symptomatic complaints included disequilibrium with rapid head movements, blurred vision, and veering to the right during ambulation. Although somewhat improved, these symptoms had persisted for 2 months. Mrs. M was unable to drive and was on a medical leave from her job. Her past medical history was significant for hypertension and thyroid disease.

Comment: This patient's history is interesting because most patients with unilateral vestibular deficits present with a history of a specific episode of vertigo rather than of disequilibrium. Her complaints of disequilibrium with head movement, blurred vision, and a gait disturbance reflect the disturbance of the dynamic vestibular responses.

The neurologic examination was normal. Her MRI scan and audiogram were unremarkable. Vestibular laboratory testing included an oculomotor screening battery, static positional testing, caloric testing, rotational testing, and posturography. Test results showed a left gaze-evoked nystagmus, a left-beating nystagmus on positional testing, a right vestibular paresis on caloric testing, a left directional preponderance on rotational testing, and abnormal posturography (abnormal response for all six sensory organization conditions and abnormal adaptation to toes-up rotation on movement coordination).

Comment: The left-beating gaze-evoked nystagmus, the left-beating nystagmus on positional testing, and the directional preponderance most likely reflect the right vestibular paresis. The increased difficulty experienced by the patient on all six of the sensory organization tests is unusual but not unheard of during the chronic stage following unilateral vestibular deficits. In some patients, this finding may reflect a functional component to the patient's complaints. Difficulty maintaining balance to sudden toes-up rotations of the support surface may signify a tendency toward retropulsion in some patients but is a nonspecific finding in many patients with balance problems. It may indicate that the patient will have difficulty walking on uneven surfaces.

The patient was assessed in physical therapy 3 days after her neurotologic evaluation. She reported that her symptoms were worsened by looking up, reading, and quick head movements. She reported a decreased activity level and an inability to do grocery shopping or heavy housework. Mrs. M indicated that her symptoms, which occurred several times per day, lasted 2 to 3 minutes.

On clinical evaluation, she reported disequilibrium when moving from the supine to sitting position. Head movements (flexion, extension, left and right rotation, and left and right lateral flexion) tested in the sitting position with eyes open and closed provoked disequilibrium. Disequilibrium and blurred vision occurred when she was asked to track a moving target while keeping her head stationary. In addition, she experienced disequilibrium and blurred vision when asked to move her head while focusing her eyes on an object that was either stationary or moving.

During tests of static balance performance, she maintained single-legged stance (SLS) with her eyes open for 14 seconds on the left foot and 18 seconds on the right foot. With her eyes closed, she could only perform SLS for 3 seconds on either foot. On the Clinical Test for Sensory Interaction in Balance (CTSIB)[58,59] (see Chapter 13), she maintained all conditions for 30 seconds. However, she experienced disequilibrium during the test, especially for the condition requiring her to stand on foam with her eyes closed.

The patient could ambulate independently, but considerable veering to the right and left, decreased trunk rotation, and decreased arm swing were noted during gait. Disequilibrium was produced when the following advanced gait tasks were performed: walking with right and left head movements, walking and stopping quickly, and walking with pivot turns to the right or left. She was able to tandem walk five steps with her eyes open and one step with her eyes closed before losing her balance.

Comment: The patient's complaints of disequilibrium were almost always associated with movement of the head, which reflects the persistent defect in the dynamic vestibulospinal response and VOR. Her complaint of disequilibrium during pursuit eye movements with her head stationary may be related to her nystagmus, although many patients are unaware of nystagmus. The age of the patient must be considered when interpreting whether or not a timed balance test, such as SLS, is normal. In this case, the patient should have been able to maintain SLS with eyes open and closed for at least 28 and 16 seconds, respectively.

The patient was given a home exercise program that consisted of head movements in sitting with eyes open, eye/head exercises (Table 14–6, 1a and 2b), and a walking program. She was told to do the head and eye-head exercises twice a day for 2 weeks. She was advised to walk four times a week. She was seen on two subsequent visits, each 2 weeks apart, upon which she was reevaluated and given a progression in her home exercise program. The following exercises were added to her home program: head movements in sitting with eyes closed, walking with head movements, walking with pivots, and circle walking. She was also given additional eye-head exercises (see Table 14–6, remaining exercises).

After 2 months, the patient was retested in preparation for discharge. She had no symptoms when moving from the supine to sitting position. Head extension and left rotation, performed with the eyes closed, were the only head movements that

---

TABLE 14–6 Eye-Head Exercises

1. Hold an object with printing on it at arm's length, straight out in front of you.
   a. Focus on the words while moving your head as far as you can to the right and left.
      Repeat _____ times, twice a day.
      Also repeat by moving your head up and down.
   b. Focus on the words while moving both your arm and head from left to right.
      Repeat _____ times, twice a day.
   c. Focus on the words while moving both your arm and head up and down.
      Repeat _____ times, twice a day.
2. Hold an object with printing on it in each hand at arm's length, one above and one below eye level.
   a. Alternate looking at each object without moving your head.
      Make sure to focus on the words.
      Repeat _____ times, twice a day.
   b. Alternate looking at each object by moving your head up and down.
      Make sure to focus on the words.
      Repeat _____ times, twice a day.
3. Hold an object in each hand with printing on it at arm's length, one 30 degrees to the right and one 30 degrees to the left of midline.
   a. Alternate looking at each object without moving your head.
      Make sure to focus on the words.
      Repeat _____ times, twice a day.
   b. Alternate looking at each object by moving your head left and right.
      Make sure to focus on the words.
      Repeat _____ times, twice a day.

continued to produce mild disequilibrium. The patient continued to have mild disequilibrium when asked to track a moving object while maintaining a stable head position. Other tasks, which required movement of her head with fixation of her eyes on a stationary or moving object, no longer produced symptoms of disequilibrium and blurred vision.

Timed static balance measures, performed with eyes open, improved to 22 and 29 seconds for left and right SLS, respectively. The same tasks performed with eyes closed were unchanged from the initial physical therapy evaluation. The patient no longer complained of symptoms when performing the CTSIB. Her gait no longer revealed any abnormalities. She was able to tandem walk 15 steps with her eyes open and 3 steps with her eyes closed. In addition, walking and moving the head left and right was the only advanced gait task that continued to produce mild disequilibrium.

At discharge, her activity level had improved. She was walking 25 minutes, four times a week. She was able to drive and perform heavy housework without difficulty. She felt that her symptoms had significantly improved. Her symptoms typically occurred once per week, lasting only 1 minute. At discharge, the patient was instructed in a maintenance home program that consisted of head movements, eye-head movements, and a walking program.

The patient underwent vestibular testing approximately one month after her discharge from physical therapy. At the time of retesting, she indicated that she had returned to work part time. Vestibular testing was much improved as compared to her initial test results. She no longer had a gaze-evoked nystagmus or a left-beating nystagmus on positional testing. Repeated posturography revealed normal adaptation to toes-up rotation on movement coordination testing. On sensory organization testing, only condition 5 continued to reveal an abnormal response. Rotational testing indicated a reduction in the left directional preponderance seen on initial testing.

Comment: Although it is preferable to begin treatment of patients with vestibular deficits as soon as possible after onset of the vestibular deficit, in many cases exercises are not needed, and patients will recover on their own. This patient, however, continued to have disequilibrium and was unable to function at work or around the home. The exercise program, and perhaps time, resulted in improvement in her sense of disequilibrium and in her postural stability that was documented both subjectively and objectively.

SUMMARY

This chapter presents treatment strategies for the physical therapy management of patients with unilateral peripheral vestibular hypofunction. Patients with unilateral peripheral vestibular hypofunction may present with a variety of functional deficits. The physical therapy treatment program should address all of the patient's functional deficits. The use of exercise in the rehabilitation of patients with vestibular disorders is aimed at promoting vestibular compensation. Several case studies are presented to illustrate the rehabilitation management of patients with unilateral peripheral vestibular hypofunction.

REFERENCES

1. Cawthorne, T: The physiological basis for head exercises. J Chartered Soc Physiother 30:106, 1944.
2. Cooksey, FS: Rehabilitation in vestibular injuries. Pro R Soc Med 39:273, 1946.
3. Herdman, SJ: Exercise strategies for vestibular disorders. Ear Nose Throat 68:961, 1989.
4. Herdman, SJ: Assessment and treatment of balance disorders in the vestibular-deficient patient. In Duncan, P (ed): Balance Proceedings of the APTA Forum. American Physical Therapy Association, Nashville, 1990, p 87.
5. Norre, ME: Treatment of unilateral vestibular hypofunction. In Oosterveld, WJ (ed): Otoneurology. John Wiley, New York, 1984, p 23.
6. Norre, ME and De Weerdt, W: Treatment of vertigo based on habituation. I. Physio-pathological basis. J Laryngol Otol 94:689, 1980.
7. Norre, ME and De Weerdt, W: Treatment of vertigo based on habituation. II. Technique and results of habituation training. J Laryngol Otol 94:971, 1980.
8. Shumway-Cook, A and Horak, FB: Rehabilitation Strategies for Patients with Vestibular Deficits. Neurol Clin 8:441, 1990.
9. Zee, D: Vertigo. In Johnson, R (ed): Current Therapy in Neurologic Disease. CV Mosby, St Louis, 1985, p 8.
10. Precht, W: Recovery of some vestibuloocular and vestibulospinal functions following unilateral labyrinthectomy. Prog Brain Res 64:381, 1986.
11. Fetter, M, Zee, DS, and Proctor, LR: Effect of lack of vision and of occipital lobectomy upon recovery from unilateral labyrinthectomy in Rhesus monkey. J Neurophysiol 59:394, 1988.
12. Halmagyi, GM, Curthoys, IS, and Dai, MJ: Diagnosis of unilateral otolith hypofunction. Diagnostic Neurotol 8:313, 1990.
13. Allum, JHJ and Pfaltz, CR: Postural control in man following acute unilateral peripheral vestibular deficit. In Igarashi, M and Black, O (eds): Vestibular and Visual Control on Posture and Locomotor Equilibrium. Karger, Basel, 1985, p 315.
14. Halmagyi, GM, Curthoys, IS, and Gibson, WPR: Vestibular neurectomy and the management of vertigo. Current Opinion Neurol Neurosurg 1:879, 1988.
15. Yagi, T and Markham, CH: Neural correlates of compensation after hemilabyrinthectomy. Exp Neurol 84:98, 1984.
16. Fetter, M and Zee, DS: Recovery from unilateral labyrinthectomy in Rhesus monkeys. J Neurophysiol 59:370, 1988.
17. Allum, JHJ, Yamane M, and Pfaltz CR: Long-term modifications of vertical and horizontal vestibulo-ocular reflex dynamics in man. Acta Otolaryngol (Stockh) 105:328, 1988.
18. Miles, FA and Eighmy, BB: Long-term adaptive changes in primate vestibuloocular reflex. I. Behavioral observations. J Neurophys 43:1406, 1980.
19. Mathog, RH and Peppard, SB: Exercise and recovery from vestibular injury. Am J Otolaryngol 3:397, 1982.
20. Igarashi, M, et al: Further study of physical exercise and locomotor balance compensation after unilateral labyrinthectomy in squirrel monkeys. Acta Otolaryngol 92:101, 1981.
21. Courjon, JH, et al: The role of vision on compensation of vestibulo ocular reflex after hemilabyrinthectomy in the cat. Exp Brain Res 28:235, 1977.
22. Lacour, M, Roll, JP, and Appaix, M: Modifications and development of spinal reflexes in the alert baboon (Papio papio) following unilateral vestibular neurectomy. Brain Res 113:255, 1976.
23. Kasai, T and Zee, DS: Eye-head coordination in labyrinthine-defective human beings. Brain Res 144:123, 1978.
24. Bronstein, AM and Hood, JD: The cervico-ocular reflex in normal subjects and patients with absent vestibular function. Brain Res 373:399, 1986.
25. Maoli, C and Precht, W: On the role of vestibulo-ocular reflex plasticity in recovery after unilateral peripheral vestibular lesions. Exp Brain Res 59:267, 1985.
26. Segal, BN and Katsarkas, A: Long-term deficits of goal-directed vestibulo-ocular function following total unilateral loss of peripheral vestibular function. Acta Otolaryngol (Stockh) 106:102, 1988.
27. Igarashi, M, et al: Effect of physical exercise upon nystagmus and locomotor dysequilibrium after labyrinthectomy in experimental primates. Acta Otolaryngol 79:214, 1975.
28. Toupet, M: Is vestibular neuritis a human model of compensation? In Lacour, M, et al: (eds): Vestibular compensation: Facts, theories, and clinical perspectives. Elsevier, Paris, 1989, p 229.
29. Hecker, HC, Haug, CO, and Herndon, JW: Treatment of the vertiginous patient using Cawthorne's vestibular exercises. Laryngoscope 84:2065, 1974.
30. Norre, ME: The unilateral vestibular hypofunction. Acta Oto-Rhino-Laryng Belg 33:333, 1979.
31. Dix, MR: The physiological basis and practical value of head exercises in the treatment of vertigo. Practitioner 217:919, 1976.
32. Norre, ME and De Weerdt, W: Positional (provoked) vertigo treated by postural training. Agressologie 22:37, 1981.
33. Norre, ME and Beckers, AM: Vestibular habituation training. Arch Otolaryngol Head Neck Surg 114:883, 1988.

34. Norre, ME, Forrez G, and Beckers, A: Vestibulospinal findings in two syndromes with spontaneous vertigo attacks. Ann Otol Rhinol Laryngol 98:191, 1989.
35. Istl-Lenz Y, Hyden, D, and DWF Schwarz: Response of the human vestibulo-ocular reflex following long-term 2X magnified visual input. Exp Brain Res 57:448, 1985.
36. Davies, P and Jones, GM: An adaptive neural model compatible with plastic changes induced in the human vestibulo-ocular reflex by prolonged optical reversal of vision. Brain Res 103:546, 1976.
37. Collewijn, H, Martins, AJ, and Steinman, RM: Compensatory eye movements during active and passive head movements: Fast adaptation to changes in visual magnification. J Physiol 340:259, 1983.
38. Jones, GM, Guitton, D, and Berthoz, A: Changing patterns of eye-head coordination during 6 h of optically reversed vision. Exp Brain Res 69:531, 1988.
39. Demer, JL, et al: Adaptation to telescopic spectacles: Vestibulo-ocular reflex plasticity. Invest Ophthalmol Vis Sci 30:159, 1989.
40. Pfaltz, CR: Vestibular compensation. Acta Otolaryngol 95:402, 1983.
41. Collewijn, H, Martins, AJ, and Steinman, RM: Compensatory eye movements during active and passive head movements: Fast adaptation to changes in visual magnification. J Physiol 340:259, 1983.
42. Lisberger, SG, Miles, FA, and Optican, LM: Frequency-selective adaptation: Evidence for channels in the vestibulo-ocular reflex. J Neurosci 3:1234, 1983.
43. Goodaux, E, Halleux, J, and Gobert, C: Adaptive change of the vestibulo-ocular reflex in the cat: The effects of a long-term frequency-selective procedure. Exp Brain Res 49:28, 1983.
44. Baloh, RW, et al: Voluntary control of the human vestibulo-ocular reflex. Acta Otolaryngol (Stockh) 97:1, 1984.
45. Furst, EJ, Goldberg, J, and Jenkins, HA: Voluntary modification of the rotatory-induced vestibulo-ocular reflex by fixating imaginary targets. Acta Otolaryngol (Stockh) 103:231, 1987.
46. Zee, DS: The management of patients with vestibular disorders. In Barber, HO and Sharpe, JA (eds): Vestibular Disorders. Year Book Medical Publishers, Chicago, 1987, p 254.
47. Lisberger, SG: Role of the cerebellum during motor learning in the vestibulo-ocular reflex. Trends Neurosci 80:437, 1982.
48. Galiana, HL, Flohr, H, and Jones, GM: A reevaluation of intervestibular nuclear coupling: Its role in vestibular compensation. J Neurophys 51:242, 1984.
49. Bergstrom, B: Morphology of the vestibular nerve. II. The number of myelinated vestibular nerve fibers in man at various ages. Acta Otolaryngol 76:173, 1973.
50. Richter, E; Quantitative study of human scarpa's ganglion and vestibular sensory epithelium. Acta Otolaryngol (Stockh) 90:199, 1980.
51. Rosenhall, U: Degenerative patterns in the degenerating human vestibular neuro-epithelia. Acta Otolaryngol (Stockh) 76:208, 1973.
52. Wall, C, Black, FO, and Hunt, AE: Effects of age, sex and stimulus parameters upon vestibulo-ocular responses to sinusoidal rotation. Acta Otolaryngol (Stockh) 98:270, 1984.
53. Paige, GD: Vestibulo-ocular reflex (VOR) and adaptive plasticity with aging. Soc Neurosci Abstr 15:515, 1989.
54. Kosnik, W, et al: Visual changes in daily life throughout adulthood. J Gerontol Psychol Sci 43:63, 1988.
55. MacLennan, S, et al: Vibration sense, proprioception, and ankle reflexes in old age. J Clin Exp Gerontol 2:159, 1980.
56. Perret, E and Regli, F: Age and the perceptual threshold for vibratory stimuli. Eur Neurol 4:65, 1970.
57. Kenshalo, DR: Age changes in touch, vibration, temperature, kinesthesis and pain sensitivity. In Birren, JE and Schaie, KW (eds): Handbook of the Psychology of Aging. Van Nostrand Reinhold, New York, 1977, p 562.
58. Shumway-Cook, A and Horak, FB: Assessing the influence of sensory interaction on balance: Suggestion from the field. Phys Ther 66:1548, 1986.
59. Horak FB: Clinical measurement of postural control in adults. Phys Ther 67:1881, 1987.
60. Dix, MR: The rationale and technique of head exercises in the treatment of vertigo. Acta Oto-Rhino-Laryng Belg 33:370, 1979.

CHAPTER 15

Assessment and Management of Bilateral Vestibular Loss

Susan J. Herdman, PhD, PT

Patients with bilateral peripheral vestibular deficits are unable to see clearly during head movements and have increased difficulty maintaining their balance, especially when walking in the dark or on uneven surfaces. Unlike exercises for patients with unilateral vestibular deficits, exercises for these patients must be aimed at fostering the substitution of visual and somatosensory cues for the lost vestibular function. This chapter presents the assessment and physical therapy treatment of these patients. Case studies are used to illustrate different points.

PRIMARY COMPLAINTS

Patients with bilateral vestibular loss are primarily concerned with their balance and gait problems. During the acute stage, they may feel off balance even when lying down. More typically, however, they complain of disequilibrium only when they are standing or walking. Patients who develop the problem during the course of a long illness usually do not know they have a balance problem until they get out of bed and, even then, the balance problem often is attributed to weakness. Although there are many motor systems involved with postural stability, these systems cannot substitute completely for the loss of vestibular function.

Another problem for patients with bilateral vestibular loss is the visual blurring that occurs during head movements. Often patients say that objects that are far away appear to be jumping or bouncing. As a result, patients may not be able to read street signs or identify people's faces as they walk, or they may have difficulty seeing clearly while in a moving car.

In "Living without a Balance Mechanism,"[1] a physician treated with streptomycin describes what happened to his visual function as he lost his vestibular function. At the worst stage, his eyes moved every time his heart beat. He ended up wedging his head

316

between the bars of his hospital bed to keep his head stable so he could see. After he had undergone some compensation, he found that if he were stationary he could see clearly, but if he were walking he could not identify the faces of people walking toward him.

ASSESSMENT

The assessment of patients with bilateral vestibular loss (BVL) is similar to that for patients with unilateral vestibular deficits; therefore, only certain aspects of the assessment will be described here. Physical therapy assessment of patients with BVL must address both the visual problems and the postural instability. This assessment must also identify other factors that might affect recovery. A summary of the assessment and the usual findings for patients with BVL is presented in Table 15–1.

**TABLE 15–1   Test Results on Patients with
Bilateral Vestibular Loss**

Oculomotor examination: Abnormal findings in room light including poor VOR to slow and rapid head thrusts, visual acuity with head stationary is usually normal, but during gentle oscillation of the head, acuity would change to 20/100 or worse. With Frenzel lenses: No spontaneous, gaze-evoked, head shaking–induced, tragal pressure–induced, hyperventilation-induced, or positional nystagmus.

Sensation: Somatosensory and visual information is critical to functional recovery and must be carefully evaluated.

Coordination: Should be normal.

Range of motion: Should be normal, but patients will voluntarily restrict head movements because head movement makes them less stable and also results in poor vision.

Strength (gross): Should be normal.

Postural deviations: Should be normal.

Positional and movements testing: Should not result in vertigo.

Sitting balance: Patients may have difficulty maintaining their balance during weight-shifting in sitting during the acute stage but should not have difficulty during the compensated stage.

Static balance:
    Romberg test: Abnormal during acute stage in many patients.
    Sharpened Romberg test: Patients with complete or severe bilateral loss will not be able to perform this with eyes closed.
    Single-leg stance: Normal in many patients during compensated stage when performed with eyes open.
    Stand on rail: Usually not tested.
    Standing on foam surface: Difficult to perform with decreasing base of support. Should not be attempted in many patients.
    Force platform: Normal or close to normal AP sway with eyes open or closed during compensated stage on stable surface.

Balance with altered sensory cues: Increased sway when visual *or* somatosensory cues are altered, loss of balance when *both* visual and somatosensory cues are altered.

Dynamic balance (self-initiated movements): Fukuda's stepping test: normal with eyes open during compensated stage; cannot perform with eyes closed (rapid loss of balance).

Ambulation: The patient's gait is usually at least slightly wide-based during compensated stage although may appear normal. There is a tendency to use visual fixation while walking and to turn en bloc.
    Tandem walk: Cannot perform.
    Walk while turning head: Gait slows and becomes ataxic.
    Singleton: Expect loss of balance.

Vestibular Function

One important consideration in designing a treatment program is whether there is any remaining vestibular function. Vestibular function can be documented using tests such as the rotational chair and caloric tests. This information then is used to determine which exercises to give the patient. Patients with remaining vestibular function may benefit from vestibular adaptation exercises to enhance the remaining vestibular function (see Fig. 14–2). If there is no remaining vestibular function, the exercises must be directed at the substitution of visual and somatosensory cues to improve gaze stability and postural stability.

The presence of remaining vestibular function can be used as a guide in predicting the final level of recovery in patients. Patients with incomplete BVL are often able to return to activities such as driving at night and to some sports. Patients with severe BVL may not be able to drive at night, and some patients will not be able to drive at all because of the gaze instability. Activities such as sports and dancing may be limited because of the visual and the postural problems.

Vestibular function tests can also be used to follow the course of the vestibular loss and of any recovery of vestibular function that might occur.[2,3] Ototoxic medications such as gentamicin result in a gradual loss of vestibular function. Frequently the effects of the vestibular loss only become apparent after the medication treatment has been stopped or at the end of the course of the treatment.[1]

Visual System

While taking the patient's history, the clinician should identify the presence of progressive disorders such as macular degeneration and cataracts. These disorders result in a gradual decrease in available visual cues and will have an adverse effect on balance in the future.

Assessment of visual function should include at least a gross test of visual field and a measure of visual acuity when the head is stationary, since both of these can affect postural stability.[4] Measuring visual acuity during head movement is also important. The vestibular-ocular system normally stabilizes the eyes during head movements; when there is no vestibulo-ocular reflex (VOR) to stabilize the eyes during head movement, small amounts of retinal slip (movement of image across the retina) will degrade vision. For instance, 3 deg/sec of retinal slip would cause visual acuity to change from 20/20 to 20/200. The movement of the head that occurs when in a moving car can cause a degradation of visual acuity that would make driving a car unsafe.

Somatosensory System

Particular attention should be made to assess vibration, proprioception, and kinesthesia in the feet. Although mild deficits in sensation in the feet may have no effects on postural stability in otherwise normal individuals, in patients with vestibular loss, somatosensory deficits may have profound effects on balance and on the potential for functional recovery. As with visual system disorders, being aware of potentially progressive disorders affecting somatosensory information is important.

Balance and Gait

Patients with BVL must be given a detailed assessment of balance and gait. Static balance should be assessed first. In the acute stage, patients with bilateral vestibular deficits may have positive Romberg tests. In the compensated stage, the Romberg test is usually normal, but patients will not be able to perform the sharpened Romberg test with eyes closed, although some patients will be able to perform the sharpened Romberg test with eyes open. Patients with bilateral vestibular deficits will also have difficulty performing tests in which both visual and somatosensory cues are altered. An example of this would be Fukuda's stepping test, in which the eyes are closed and the patient is marching in place. Patients may have normal tests with eyes open but will fall with eyes closed. Determining how well patients use different sensory cues to maintain balance and whether they are dependent on particular sensory cues is critical. Bles, Vianney de Jong, and de Wit[5] have shown that patients with BVL initially are more dependent on visual cues than on somatosensory cues for balance. With time, there is an improvement in the ability of patients to use somatosensory cues. This improvement varies from patient to patient, however, and needs to be carefully assessed (Fig. 15–1).

Gait in patients with bilateral vestibular deficits is wide-based and ataxic. Patients decrease their trunk and neck rotation in an effort to improve stability by avoiding head movements. Arm swing is similarly decreased. Usually patients use excessive visual fixation and therefore have increased difficulty if asked to look up while walking. Patients typically turn "en bloc" and may even stop before they turn. Asking patients to turn their heads while walking results in increased ataxia and often loss of balance.

TREATMENT

The treatment approach for patients with complete loss of vestibular function involves the use of exercises that foster the substitution of visual and somatosensory information to improve gaze and postural stability and the development of compensatory strategies that can be used in situations in which balance is stressed maximally. The mechanisms used to stabilize gaze in the absence of vestibular inputs have been well studied (Table 15–2).[6–8] The mechanisms involved in maintaining postural stability are somewhat less well understood, although research is being done in that area.

Gaze Stability

Subjects without vestibular function must develop different mechanisms to keep the image of the target on the fovea during head movements (Table 15–2). One mechanism that many patients use involves an increase in the effectiveness of the cervico-ocular reflex (COR) in producing compensatory eye movements during head movement. In the COR, sensory inputs from neck muscles and facet joints act to produce a slow-phase eye movement that is opposite to the direction of the head movement during low-frequency, brief head movements. The COR, therefore, complements the VOR although in normal subjects it contributes, at most, 15 percent of the compensatory eye movement. In patients with complete BVL, the COR operates at high- and at low-frequency head movements and contributes up to 25 percent of the compensatory eye movement.

A

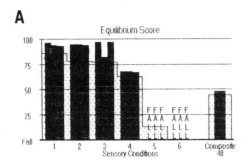

B

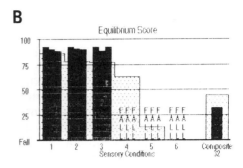

C

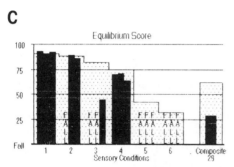

D

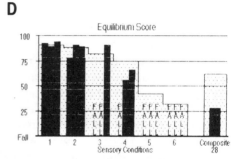

FIGURE 15–1. Posturography test results from patients with bilateral vestibular loss demonstrating the differences in ability to maintain postural stability when different sensory cues are altered or removed. Patients are tested using six different conditions:

	Available Cues	Unavailable or Altered Cues
Test 1:	Vision, vestibular somatosensory	—
Test 2:	Vestibular, somatosensory	No vision
Test 3:	Vestibular, somatosensory	Vision altered
Test 4:	Vision, vestibular	Somatosensory altered
Test 5:	Vestibular	No vision, somatosensory altered
Test 6:	Vestibular	Vision, somatosensory altered

Results show patients who have difficulty when both visual and somatosensory cues are altered (*A*), when somatosensory cues only are altered (*B*), when visual cues only are altered, (*C*) and when either visual *or* somatosensory cues are altered (*D*).

Theoretically, the COR can be potentiated by having the patient perform head movements while maintaining visual fixation on a target (see Fig. 14–2*A*). The exercise, therefore, is exactly the same exercise used to increase VOR gain. This similarity is fortuitous because if there is any remaining vestibular function in these patients, exercises should be designed to increase the gain of the vestibular system as well.

Other mechanisms used to improve gaze stability include modifications in saccadic and pursuit eye movements. Patients with complete BVL may make hypometric saccades toward a visual target. Then, as the head moves toward the target, the eyes would be moved passively into alignment with the target. They may also make accurate saccadic eye movements during combined eye and head movements toward a target and then

TABLE 15-2 Mechanisms to Stabilize Gaze
Enhance the cervico-ocular reflex.
Change amplitude of saccades.
Modify pursuit eye movements.
Use corrective saccades.

make corrective saccades back to the target as the head movement pulls the eyes off the target.

Kasai and Zee[6] found that different patients with complete BVL use different sets of strategies to compensate for the loss of VOR. Therefore, exercises to improve gaze stability should not be designed to emphasize any particular strategy but instead should provide situations in which patients can develop their own strategies to maintain gaze stability (Table 15-3). No mechanism to improve gaze stability fully compensates for the loss of the VOR, however, and patients will continue to have difficulty seeing during rapid head movements.

TABLE 15-3 Exercises to Improve Gaze Stability

Enhance the Cervico-ocular Reflex

Tape a business card on the wall in front of you so that you can read it.

Move your head back and forth sideways, keep the words in focus.

Move your head faster but keep the words in focus. Continue to do this for 1-2 min without stopping.

Repeat the exercise moving your head up and down.

Repeat the exercises using a large pattern such as a checkerboard (full-field stimulus).

Active Eye-Head Movements Between Two Targets

Horizontal targets:

Look directly at one target being sure that your head is also lined up with the target.

Look at the other target with your eyes and then turn your head to the target (saccades should precede head movement). Be sure to keep the target in focus during the head movement.

Repeat in the opposite direction.

Vary the speed of the head movement but always keep the targets in focus.

Note: Place the two targets close enough together that when you are looking directly at one, you can see the other with your peripheral vision. Practice for 5 min resting if necessary. This exercise can also be performed with two vertically placed targets.

Imaginary Targets

Look at a target directly in front of you.

Close your eyes and turn your head slightly, imagining that you are still looking directly at the target.

Open your eyes and check to see if you have been able to keep your eyes on the target.

Repeat in the opposite direction. Be as accurate as possible.

Vary the speed on the head movement.

Practice for up to 5 min, resting if necessary.

Postural Stability

In patients with complete loss of vestibular function, postural stability can be improved by fostering the use of visual and proprioceptive cues. This approach is also used in the treatment of patients with vestibular hypofunction (Table 15–4).

A study on the course of recovery of patients with complete bilateral vestibular deficits over a 2-year period has shown that patients switch the sensory cues on which they rely.[5] Initially, they rely on visual cues as a substitute for the loss of vestibular cues, but over time they become more reliant on proprioceptive cues to maintain balance. In this study, patients were required to maintain balance when facing a moving visual surround. Over the 2-year study, patients recovered the ability to maintain their balance to within normal limits in the testing paradigm except at high frequencies. The vestibular system functions at higher frequencies than do the visual or somatosensory systems, which would account for why neither visual nor somatosensory cues can substitute completely for loss of vestibular cues.

TABLE 15–4   Exercises to Improve Performance of Daily Activities

---

The purpose of these exercises is to force you to develop strategies of performing daily activities even when deprived of vision, proprioception, or normal vestibular inputs. The activities are supposed to help you develop confidence and establish your functional limits. *On all of these exercises, you should take extra precautions so you do not fall.*

1. _____ Stand with your feet as close together as possible with both hands helping you maintain your balance by touching a wall. Take your hand or hands off the wall for longer and longer periods while maintaining your balance. Try moving your feet even closer together. Repeat this for ____ minutes twice each day.

_____ Repeat exercise 1 with eyes closed, at first intermittently and then continuously, all the while making a special effort to mentally visualize your surroundings.

2. _____ Stand with your feet shoulder width apart with eyes open, looking straight ahead at a target on the wall. Progressively narrow your base of support from:

    feet apart to
    feet together to
    a semi–heel-to-toe position to
    heel to toe (one foot in front of the other)
    change your foot position 1 inch at a time

Do the exercise first ____ with arms outstretched and then
                ____ with arms close to your body and then
                ____ with arms folded across your chest.
Hold each position for 15 sec and then move on to the next-most-difficult exercise.

_____ Repeat exercise 2 with eyes closed, at first intermittently and then continuously, all the while making a special effort to mentally visualize your surroundings.

3. _____ Repeat ____ above but while standing on a foam pillow.

4. _____ Walk close to a wall with your hand braced available for balancing. Walk with a more narrow base of support. Finally, walk heel to toe. Do this with eyes _____ (open/closed). Practice for ____ minutes.

5. _____ Walk close to a wall and turn your head to the right and to the left as you walk. Try to focus on different objects as you walk. Gradually turn your head more often and faster. Practice for ____ minutes.

6. _____ Practice turning around while you walk. At first, turn in a large circle but gradually make smaller and smaller turns. Be sure to turn in both directions.

The contribution of proprioceptive inputs from the cervical region to postural stability in patients with complete vestibular loss is not clearly understood. Bles and associates[9] found that changes in the neck position did not affect postural stability in patients with complete BVL. They concluded that proprioceptive signals from the neck do not contribute to postural stability. We do not know, however, if kinesthetic signals from the neck, which would occur during head *movement*, would affect postural stability. Certainly patients with bilateral vestibular dysfunction become less stable when asked to turn their heads while walking. This observation may indicate that kinesthetic cues do not contribute significantly to *dynamic* postural stability and/or that these patients are more reliant on visual cues to maintain postural stability and thus, when the head moves and visual cues are degraded, their balance becomes worse.

The loss of either visual or somatosensory cues in addition to vestibular cues has a devastating effect on postural stability. Such losses also limit the strategies that can be used in rehabilitation. Paulus, Straube, and Brandt[10] reported a case in which the patient had a complete BVL plus a loss of lower-extremity proprioception. This patient relied on visual cues to maintain balance. When the effectiveness of the visual cues was degraded (i.e., by fixating on a visual target more than 1 M away), his postural stability deteriorated significantly.

Compensatory Strategies

Patients can be taught, and often develop on their own, strategies to use when in situations in which their balance will be stressed. For example, they learn to turn on lights at night if they have to get out of bed. They may also wait, sitting at the edge of the bed, before getting up in the dark to allow themselves to waken more fully and for their eyes to adjust to the darkened room. They should be advised to use lights that come on automatically and to have emergency lighting in and outside the house in case of a power failure. Patients may need to learn how to plan to move around environments with busy visual environments such as shopping malls and grocery stores. For some patients, moving in busy environments may require the use of some type of assistive device, such as a shopping cart or a cane, but for many patients with BVL no assistive devices are needed after the patient becomes comfortable walking in that environment.

Guidelines to Treatment and Prognosis

There are several factors to remember when working with patients with bilateral vestibular deficits:

1. Recovery following bilateral deficits is slower than for unilateral lesions and can continue to occur over a 2-year period.
2. Recovery is easily upset by other medical problems such as having a cold or receiving chemotherapy.
3. To maintain recovered function, patients may always need to be doing some exercises, at least intermittently.

4. Postural stability will never be completely normal. The patient may have a negative Romberg test and may be able to maintain the sharpened Romberg position with eyes open but not with eyes closed.

5. Initially, the patient may need to use a cane or a walker while ambulating. Some patients, especially older patients, need to use a cane at least some of the time. Most younger patients, however, are eventually able to walk without any assistive devices. Ambulation during the acute stage will be wide-based and ataxic with shortened stride length and side-stepping to the right and left. The patient will turn en bloc, and turning the head will cause increased instability. Ambulation will improve but, again, it will not be normal.

6. Patients will be at increased risk for falls when walking in low-vision situations, over uneven surfaces, or when they are fatigued.

EVIDENCE THAT EXERCISE FACILITATES RECOVERY

There is some evidence that experience facilitates recovery following bilateral ablation of the labyrinth. Igarashi and co-workers[11] trained monkeys to run along a straight platform. Their performance was scored by counting the number of times they moved off the straight line. A two-stage ablation of the labyrinth was then performed. After the unilateral ablation, animals given specific exercises recovered faster than nonexercised animals, but all animals eventually achieved preoperative functional levels. After ablation of the second labyrinth, all monkeys had difficulty with the platform run task. The control group reached preoperative balance performance levels in 81 days, whereas the exercise group reached preoperative levels in 62 days. This result actually was not significantly different because of the large variation in individual animals. Igarashi and colleagues also looked at how long the animals took to have eight consecutive trial days in a row in which they could keep their balance at preoperative levels. The exercise group achieved this criterion in 118 days. The control group took longer. One animal took 126 days, another took 168 days, and one animal had not achieved that criterion at 300 days. The conclusions that can be made from this study are that (1) recovery from bilateral deficits occurs more slowly than does recovery from unilateral lesions, (2) exercise impacts that rate of recovery in bilateral and unilateral lesions, and (3) the final level of function may be improved if exercises are given after bilateral lesions.

Telian and associates[12] studied the effectiveness of vestibular rehabilitation for patients with bilateral vestibular deficits using balance exercises, vestibular habituation exercises, and general conditioning exercises. They were unable to demonstrate a significant change in functional activity in these patients following treatment. There are several confounding aspects to their study, however. There is evidence that the strategies used by patients with BVL to maintain balance change with time. Whether time was a factor, and therefore some patients may have already compensated for the loss of vestibular function, is unclear. Vestibular rehabilitation may not affect the final level of recovery but may only affect the rate of recovery. Vestibular adaptation exercises may not be appropriate for these patients. Vestibular habituation exercises are designed to decreased unwanted responses to vestibular signals. Based on the results of their study, the authors now use exercises designed to enhance remaining vestibular function and to facilitate the COR as well as using balance exercises. A more recent perspective, controlled study by Krebs and co-workers[13] shows that vestibular rehabilitation exercises improve functional, dynamic stability during locomotion in patients with BVL.

CASE STUDY 1

The patient is a 34-year-old woman with a history of diabetes and renal failure who had been on peritoneal dialysis for $1\frac{1}{2}$ years. She had been treated with gentamicin 9 and 6 months earlier for peritonitis. She had no complaints of disequilibrium after either of those drug courses. Two months later she again developed peritonitis and again received intravenous gentamicin. After a few days, she complained of vertigo and tinnitus, developed disequilibrium, and could not walk unassisted. She also complained that she was not able to see clearly when her head was moving. She was admitted to the hospital for a workup of her vertigo and disequilibrium.

Significant findings on clinical examination included a spontaneous nystagmus with fast phases to the left, poor VOR to slow head movements, and large corrective saccades with rapid head movements bilaterally, worse with head movements to the right than to the left. The test for head-shaking nystagmus was not performed because the patient complained of severe nausea following even gentle head movements and vomited. She also had a positive Romberg test. Sharpened Romberg and Fukuda's stepping tests were not performed. The patient could not ambulate without the assistance of two people.

Comment: This patient's signs and symptoms (vertigo, disequilibrium, oscillopsia, spontaneous nystagmus, and poor VOR) were suggestive of a vestibular disorder. Furthermore, her history included multiple treatment with gentamicin, an ototoxic medication. With bilateral dysfunction due to treatment with an ototoxic drug, the symptoms of oscillopsia and disequilibrium develop over time and may not appear until after the drug treatment is finished. Once the symptoms appear, they may continue to become worse for several weeks. With some patients, there is a partial reversal of the symptoms with time. Often the vestibular symptoms are accompanied by hearing loss. Typically, however, the vestibular loss is symmetric and patients do not develop vertigo or spontaneous nystagmus, both of which are associated with unilateral vestibular loss or with asymmetric bilateral vestibular deficits. Although gentamicin usually results in a BVL, symptoms of asymmetric effects on the vestibular and auditory systems have been reported.[3] Her poor VOR to slow head movements and the presence of corrective saccades during rapid head thrusts bilaterally suggested a bilateral vestibular deficit that was confirmed by the rotational test results. This patient's gait disturbance appeared to be unusually severe and further testing showed a moderate loss of proprioceptive and kinesthetic perception in her feet that would contribute significantly to her problem. This sensory loss was probably due to her diabetes. This finding was particularly important in developing her exercise program and in predicting her final level of recovery.

Computerized tomography (CT) and magnetic resonance imaging (MRI) tests were normal. Audiogram showed an asymmetric sensory-neural hearing loss, right worse than left (Fig. 15–2). Caloric tests showed a poor response bilaterally to warm or cool water, although ice water in the left ear did result in a weak but appropriate response. There was a directional preponderance to the right. Rotational chair test showed a severe bilateral vestibular deficit (Fig. 15–3). There was little optokinetic after-nystagmus, and the VOR time constant (Tc) was 2.4 to 60 deg/sec step rotations. At 240 deg/sec step rotation, some vestibular response was evident. The gain of the response was 0.15, and the Tc was 2.4.

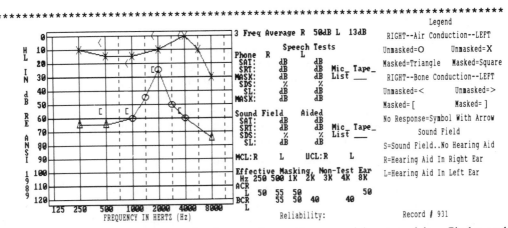

FIGURE 15–2. Hearing test results from patient with gentamicin ototoxicity. Circles and triangles indicate right ear, and X and squares indicate left ear, respectively. Note asymmetry in hearing loss for this patient.

TREATMENT

At this point, the patient was started on a vestibular rehabilitation program. She performed the X1 viewing paradigm exercise (see Fig. 14–2, A), first with horizontal head movements for 1 minute and then vertical head movements for 1 minute. Because head movement exacerbated her nausea, she rested for 10 minutes or more between each of these exercises. Initially, she performed these exercises while sitting, up to five times a day. She also practiced standing unsupported, first with her feet apart and her eyes open and then gradually moving her feet together and briefly closing her eyes. She was instructed on how to use a walker, and an emphasis was placed on increasing her endurance. Initially, she needed contact guarding while using the walker and would occasionally lose her balance, espe-

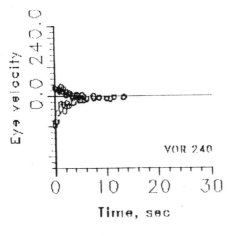

FIGURE 15–3. Plot of the decay in slow-phase eye velocity with time during VOR after-nystagmus. Patient is first rotated in a chair in complete darkness for 2 minutes, and then the chair is stopped. The slow-phase eye movements that occur are due to the discharge of the velocity storage system and represent the function of the vestibular system. These results show the poor peak slow-phase eye velocity (35 degrees sec) and the short time constant (< 2 seconds) in a patient with bilateral vestibular loss. A step rotation at 240 deg/sec was used. Eye movements were recorded using electro-oculography.

cially when trying to turn or if she moved her head too quickly. After 4 days, she was able to walk independently with the walker and was discharged from the hospital. At that time, she no longer had nausea with gentle head movements.

Comment: Although this patient had a bilateral vestibular deficit, the caloric and rotary chair tests showed that she had remaining vestibular function (response to ice water caloric on the left and a Tc of 2.4 sec at 60 deg/sec rotations). Her initial exercise program, therefore, consisted of vestibular adaptation exercises, because she had remaining vestibular function, and of ambulation training. Her balance exercises were designed to gradually increase the difficulty of maintaining balance by slowly decreasing her base of support, changing her arm positions (arms out, arms at side, arms across the chest), and then altering her use of visual cues. Although she had decreased sensation in her feet, subtracting visual cues was used as a treatment approach in order to facilitate her ability to use the remaining somatosensory and vestibular cues.

FOLLOW-UP

The patient continued to be followed as an outpatient. Exercises designed to facilitate the substitution of alternative strategies to maintain gaze stability as well to improve her static and dynamic balance were added to her program. The patient no longer needed to use a walker, but she had a wide-based gait and had to stop walking before turning around. She had a negative Romberg test but could not perform a sharpened Romberg test. Although her vision improved and she could read if she was sitting quietly, she could not see clearly while in a car and had not resumed driving.

Approximately 2 months later, the patient had a retinal hemorrhage in her left eye. She already had retinal damage in the right eye from her diabetes, which essentially meant that she had only partial visual, vestibular, and somatosensory cues for balance and, as a result, she could no longer keep her balance even in well-lighted conditions. For 1 week she either used a wheelchair or, at home, a walker. Fortunately, her vision recovered and she was again able to walk independently. On her last visit, she reported that she had returned to most activities except driving. Her base of support while walking was more narrow, and her stability while turning had improved. Her Romberg test was clinically normal but she could not perform a sharpened Romberg test with eyes open. She was seeking part-time employment and was waiting for a kidney transplant.

CASE STUDY 2

The patient is a 61-year-old man who was referred by a neurologist for treatment of disequilibrium secondary to BVL. The patient had been hospitalized for a subarachnoid hemorrhage 18 months previously. During his hospitalization, he developed several systemic complications including renal failure, pulmonary infiltrates, and ventriculitis and was treated with two courses of vancomycin, gentamicin, and ceftazidime. The neurologist saw him 7 months after this hospitalization because of the patient's persistent disequilibrium. At that time, the patient complained that he stumbled occasionally and that he had increased difficulty walking on uneven surfaces, in the dark, or when he moved his head quickly. He denied nausea, vertigo, or a rocking sensation, although he did state that he had a feeling of being tilted when he walked. He stated that his disequilibrium began following his hospitalization. He also had bilateral hearing loss but had no complaints of tinnitus or pressure or fullness in the ears. The remainder of his history was noncontributory.

The neurologic examination was normal except for: (1) visual acuity, as assessed using a wall chart, increased from 20/20 with the head stationary to 20/100 during gentle (2-Hz) oscillations of the head; (2) right Horner's syndrome; (3) staircase saccades downward from the midposition; (4) decreased vestibulo-ocular gain based on visualization of the optic nerve head and on the presence of compensatory saccades during rapid head thrusts; (5) mild decrease in vibration sensation in his feet, right more than left; (6) inability to perform tandem walking, sharpened Romberg test or Fukuda's stepping test; and (7) bilateral hearing loss. Quantitative testing of the oculomotor system showed low VOR gain (0.2 and 0.13 to the right and left, respectively) and short time constant (2.2 sec bilaterally) to a 60 deg/sec step rotation and low gain (0.19 and 0.34) and time constants (1.9 and 1.2 sec) to 240 deg/sec rotations. It was concluded that the patient had a bilateral vestibular loss, probably from the gentamicin, and he has referred for vestibular rehabilitation.

TREATMENT

Prior to establishing an exercise program, additional testing was performed. Dynamic posturography showed that the patient had an inability to maintain his balance when both visual and somatosensory cues were altered and a decreased ability to maintain his balance when visual cues were inappropriate (Fig. 15–4). Quantitative visual acuity testing showed that his acuity changed from 20/20 when his head was stationary to 20/40 during 150 deg/sec head movements using a forced-quess paradigm. (The apparent discrepancy between the clinical dynamic visual acuity test, 20/100, and the quantitative dynamic visual acuity test, 20/40, is

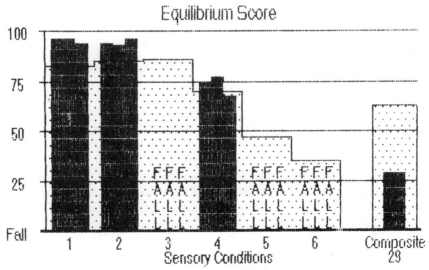

FIGURE 15–4. Results from posturography test in a patient with bilateral vestibular loss. Test conditions were those used in Figure 15–1.

due to the use of a forced-guess paradigm in the latter test.) Quantitative vibration threshold confirmed the moderate loss of vibration perception in his feet. The patient's gait was wide-based, and he frequently side-stepped while walking. He appeared to use excessive visual fixation to maintain his balance during ambulation. The patient was started on a program of exercises designed to (1) enhance his remaining vestibular function, (2) develop alternative mechanisms to improve gaze stability, (3) improve his static balance in the absence of visual cues, and (4) improve his balance while ambulating.

FOLLOW-UP

Six weeks later, the patient's Romberg test was normal, but he still could neither perform a sharpened Romberg test with his eyes open nor perform Fukuda's stepping test with eyes closed. He continued to walk, with a widened base of support. Quantitative testing of the oculomotor system was unchanged from the previous test. Quantitative visual acuity testing showed an acuity of 20/30 during 150 deg/sec head movements, which was a marked improvement over his previous test. The patient wished to return to driving, and we suggested that should he decide to drive, he should start first in local traffic or even in an empty parking lot on a weekend. He was advised that driving at night and high-speed driving would still be hazardous. One month later, the patient reported that he had returned to driving during the day and that he was working part time. He still could not walk in the dark or with his eyes closed without assistance. Several suggestions were made to the patient concerning modifications in his home to assure safety, including emergency lighting that would come on automatically if there were a power failure, railings for all stairways, and safety bars in the bathroom.

SUMMARY

Patients with bilateral vestibular problems can be expected to return to many activities but will continue to have difficulties with balance in situations in which visual cues are absent or diminished. The degree of disability is in part dependent on the degree of the vestibular loss but also reflects involvement of the visual and somatosensory systems. Treatment approaches include increasing the function of the remaining vestibular system, inducing the substitution of alternative mechanisms to maintain gaze stability and postural stability during head movements, and modifications of the home and working environment for safety. Patients should be able to return to work, and most of them will be able to ambulate without the use of a cane or walker, at least when they are in well-lighted environments.

REFERENCES

1. JC: Living without a balance mechanism. N Engl J Med 246:458, 1952.
2. Black, FO, Peterka, RJ, and Elardo, SM: Vestibular reflex changes following aminoglycoside induced ototoxicity. Laryngoscope 97:582, 1987.
3. Esterhai, JL, Bednar, J, and Kimmelman, CP: Gentamicin-induced ototoxicity complicating treatment of chronic osteomyelitis. Clin Orthop Rel Res 209:185, 1986.

4. Brandt, T, Paulus, WM, and Straube, A: Visual acuity, visual field, and visual scene characteristics affect postural balance. In Igarashi, M and Black, FO (eds): Vestibular and Visual Control on Posture and Locomotor Equilibrium. Karger, Basel, 1985, p 93.
5. Bles, W, Vianney de Jong, JMB, and de Wit, G: Compensation for labyrinthine defects examined by use of a tilting room. Acta Otolaryngol 95:576, 1983.
6. Kasai, T and Zee, DS: Eye-head coordination in labyrinthine-defective human beings. Brain Res 144:123, 1978.
7. Baloh, RW, Jacobson, K, and Honrubia, V: Idiopathic bilateral vestibulopathy. Neurology 39:272, 1989.
8. Bronstein, AM and Hood, JD: The cervico-ocular reflex in normal subjects and patients with absent vestibular function. Brain Res 373:399, 1986.
9. Bles, W, Vianney de Jong, JMB, and Rasmussens, JJ: Postural and oculomotor signs in labyrinthine-defective subjects. Acta Otolaryngol (Stockh) 406:101, 1984.
10. Paulus, WM, Straube, A, and Brandt, T: Visual stabilization of posture. Brain 107:1143, 1984.
11. Igarashi, M, et al: Physical exercise and balance compensation after total ablation of vestibular organs. In Pompeiano, O and Allum, JHJ (eds): Progress in Brain Research. Amsterdam, Elsevier, 1988, p 395.
12. Telian, SA, et al: Bilateral vestibular paresis: Diagnosis and treatment. Otolaryngol Head Neck Surg 104:67, 1991.
13. Krebs, DE, et al: Double-blind, placebo-controlled trial of rehabilitation for bilateral vestibular hypofunction: Preliminary report. Otolaryngol Head Neck Surg, 1993, in press.

CHAPTER 16

Assessment and Management of Benign Paroxysmal Positional Vertigo

Susan J. Herdman, PhD, PT

First described by Barany[1] in 1921, benign paroxysmal positional vertigo (BPPV) is characterized by brief periods of vertigo that occur when the subject's head is moved into specific positions, usually with the affected ear down. One of the more common peripheral vestibular disorders, BPPV is particularly amenable to treatment using exercises, and several different treatments have been developed. This chapter describes different treatment approaches for BPPV and discusses the criteria used in choosing the appropriate approach. Case studies are used to illustrate the different treatment approaches.

DIAGNOSIS

As described in Chapter 5, the diagnosis of BPPV is based on patient history and the presence of certain characteristic clinical findings.[1-3] These clinical findings include (1) vertigo induced by moving the patient into a supine position with the head turned to one side and the neck extended so that the affected ear is below the horizontal (see Fig. 13–1); (2) delay in the onset of the vertigo of 1 to 40 seconds after the patient has been placed in the provoking position; (3) the presence of a torsional nystagmus that appears with the same latency as the complaints of vertigo; and (4) a fluctuation in the intensity of the vertigo and nystagmus that crescendo and then decrescendo, disappearing within 60 seconds.

THEORIES OF ETIOLOGY

The characteristics of BPPV can be explained adequately by several different theories. The first theory, *cupulolithiasis*, proposes that degenerative debris from the utricle (possibly fragments of otoconia) adhere to the cupula of the posterior canal making the ampulla gravity-sensitive. This phenomenon was first suggested in 1969 by Schuknecht[4] who found basophilic deposits on the cupula of the posterior canal in patients with a history of BPPV. The increased density of the cupula produces an inappropriate deflection of the cupula of the posterior canal when the head is positioned with the affected ear below the horizon. The result is vertigo, nystagmus, and nausea. The latency to the onset of the vertigo and nystagmus is related to the time needed to displace the gravity-sensitive cupula. The gradual increase in vertigo and nystagmus is related to the increased deflection of the cupula. The gradual decrease in vertigo and nystagmus that occurs if the head-hanging position is maintained is due to adaptation.

The second theory, *canalithiasis*, was proposed by Hall, Ruby, and McClure[5] who suggest that the degenerative debris is not adherent to the cupula of the posterior canal but instead is free-floating in the endolymph (canalithiasis). When the head is moved into the provoking position, the endolymph is moved by the falling otoconia and, in turn, pulls on the cupula, exciting the neurons. The latency of the response is related to the time needed for the cupula to be deflected by the pull of the endolymph. The increase in vertigo and nystagmus that occurs is related to the relative deflection of the cupula. The decrease in vertigo and nystagmus as the position is maintained is due to cessation of endolymph movement. As with the cupulolithiasis theory, the Hallpike-Dix maneuver is most likely to result in vertigo and nystagmus, although symptoms may be provoked by other movements in the plane of the posterior canal. Hall, Ruby, and McClure[5] and others[6] hypothesize that with repeated movement of the head into the precipitating position, some of the debris moves out of the posterior canal thereby reducing the response.

TREATMENT

Several approaches have been developed to treat patients with BPPV. One treatment approach is based on the idea that the debris embedded in the cupula of the posterior canal can be dislodged by repeatedly moving the patient into the position that provokes the vertigo.[7] Two alternative approaches involve single maneuvers of the patient—one maneuver is designed to dislodge debris from the cupula of the posterior semicircular canal while the other single treatment takes the patient through a series of positions to float the debris out of the long arm of the posterior canal.[8-10] A fourth approach, suggested by Norre and De Weerdt[11] and Tangeman and Wheeler,[12] is based on the concept of habituating the central nervous system (CNS) response to movement-provoked vertigo.

Treatment 1: Brandt-Daroff Habituation Exercises

Proposed by Brandt and Daroff[7] this treatment approach requires the patient to move into the provoking position repeatedly, several times a day. The patient first sits

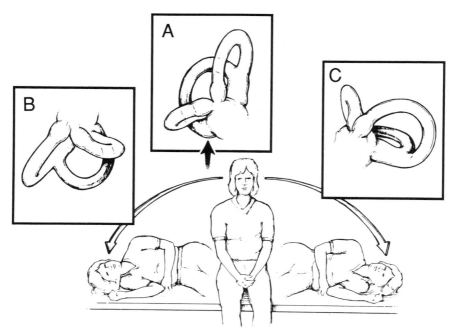

FIGURE 16-1. Brandt's exercises. The patient moves quickly from sitting (*A*) into the side-lying position that produces vertigo (*B*). The patient then stays in that position until the vertigo stops plus an additional 30 seconds and then sits up again (*A*). The patient remains in the upright position for 30 seconds and then moves rapidly into the mirror-image side-lying position (*C*), stays there for 30 seconds and then sits up. The entire maneuver is repeated 15 to 20 times several times a day until the vertigo is gone. The position of the right labyrinth is shown for each head position; the posterior canal is shaded. The arrow in (*A*) indicates the location of the cupula of the posterior semicircular canal. (Adapted from Brandt and Daroff,[7] p 485.)

and then is moved rapidly into the position that causes the vertigo (Fig. 16-1). A torsional and/or upbeating nystagmus occurs with the onset of the vertigo. The severity of the vertigo will be directly related to how rapidly the patient moves into the provoking position. The patient stays in that position until the vertigo stops and then he or she sits up again. Usually, moving to the sitting position will also result in vertigo although this "rebound effect" will be less severe and of a shorter duration. Nystagmus, if reoccurring, will be in the opposite direction. The patient remains in the upright position for 30 seconds and then moves rapidly into the mirror-image position on the other side, stays there for 30 seconds, and then sits up. The patient then repeats the entire maneuver until the vertigo diminishes. The entire sequence is repeated every 3 hours until the patient has 2 consecutive days without vertigo. It is not clear why these exercises result in a decrease in the vertigo and nystagmus. One explanation is that the debris becomes dislodged from the cupula of the posterior canal and moves to a location no longer affecting the cupula during head movement. A second possibility is that central adaptation occurs, reducing the CNS response to the signal from the posterior canal. Brandt and Daroff[7] argue against central adaptation as a mechanism for recovery because many patients recover abruptly.

Treatment 2: Liberatory Maneuver

In this single-treatment approach developed by Semont, Freyss, and Vitte,[8] the provoking position again must be identified. Once the side of involvement has been identified, the patient is quickly moved into the provoking side-lying position with the head turned into the plane of the posterior canal and is kept in that position for 2 to 3 minutes (Fig. 16–2). The patient is then rapidly moved up through the sitting position and down into the opposite side-lying position with the therapist maintaining the alignment of the neck and head on the body. (The face is therefore angled down toward the bed). Typically, nystagmus and vertigo reappear in this second position. If the patient does not experience vertigo in this second position, the head is abruptly shaken once or twice, presumably to free the debris. The patient stays in this position for 5 minutes. The patient is then slowly taken into a seated position. He or she must remain in a vertical position for 48 hours (including while sleeping) and must avoid the provoking position for 1 week following the treatment. Unlike the exercises suggested by Brandt and Daroff,[7] Semont's maneuver usually requires only a single treatment. Reportedly, this approach works by floating the debris through the canal system to the common crus but may also dislodge debris adhering to the cupula.

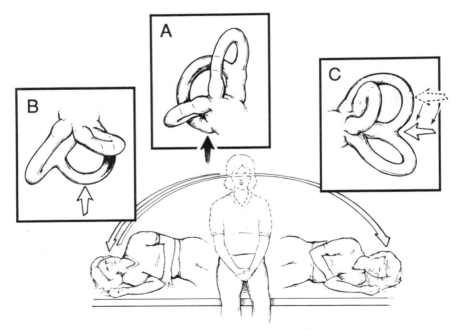

FIGURE 16–2. The Semont maneuver. The patient is moved quickly from sitting (A) into the position that provokes the vertigo (B) and is kept in that position for 2 to 3 minutes. He is then turned rapidly to the opposite ear-down position (C) with the therapist maintaining the alignment of the neck and head on the body. The patient stays in this position for 5 minutes. The patient is then slowly taken into a seated position. He must remain in a vertical position for 48 hours and avoid the provoking position for 1 week. As in Figure 16–1, the position of the right labyrinth is shown for each head position and the posterior canal is shaded. The solid arrow indicates the location of the cupula of the posterior canal; the open arrow indicates the location of debris free-floating in the long arm of the posterior canal during the different stages of the treatment. (Reprinted with permission from Herdman, SJ, et al: Single treatment approaches to benign paroxysmal positional vertigo. Arch Orolaryngol Head Neck Surg 119:450, 1993. Copyright © 1993 American Medical Association.)

Treatment 3: Canalith Repositioning Procedure

Epley[9] has proposed another single-treatment approach in which the patient is also taken through a series of changes in head positions, again to move the head around the debris. In our modification of Epley's treatment, the patient is taken rapidly into the Hallpike-Dix position that provokes the symptoms and is kept in that position for 3 to 4 minutes[10] (Fig. 16–3). The head is then slowly taken through extension (lowering the head even more) and is turned into the opposite Hallpike-Dix position. Epley recommends that the patient be rolled over onto his or her side so that the head is turned toward the floor. The patient remains in this position for another 3 to 4 minutes, then he or she slowly sits up. Like the Semont maneuver, the patient must then remain in an upright position for 48 hours, avoiding bending forward, looking up or down with the head and absolutely not lying down. For 5 more days, the patient is advised not to lie on the affected side. Epley suggests using vibration over the mastoid during the treatment to facilitate the movement of the debris. In our clinic, we have not used vibration, being concerned that more debris could break free from the utricle or other structures to float into the posterior canal. The Epley maneuver is based on the idea that the debris is free-floating in the posterior canal, and the position changes are designed to move the debris out of the posterior canal and into the common crus.

Treatment 4: Habituation

Several different treatments have been advocated for patients who may have BPPV but also complain of disequilibrium associated with head movements in planes other than those that would excite the posterior canal. The exercises of Norre and De Weerdt[11] differ from those described by Brandt and Daroff[7] in that the provoking positions used are specific for each patient and are not limited to the Hallpike-Dix maneuver. In a more recent paper, Norre and Beckers[13] describe the specific movements used to establish the individualized treatments as well as the results of that treatment. Another paper, by Tangeman and Wheeler,[12] describes three phases of treatment. Phase I is similar to the Brandt and Daroff[7] protocol and consists of having the patient move repeatedly into the Hallpike-Dix position; phases II and III include a wide variety of balance exercises that incorporate eye and head movements and seem similar to the Cawthorne-Cooksey exercises advocated for patients with unilateral vestibular hypofunction.[14] The inclusion of specific exercises for balance in these latter approaches is appropriate for the treatment of the postural instability sometimes seen in patients with BPPV (see Chapter 15 on exercises for vestibular hypofunction). In addition, the populations in these studies included patients with vestibular hypofunction or with BPPV plus vestibular hypofunction who would most likely also have balance problems.

TREATMENT EFFICACY

Studies on the efficacy of these treatments indicate that both Brandt's exercises and the Semont and the Epley maneuver facilitate recovery[7–10] (Table 16–1). The results of these studies must be interpreted cautiously, however, because of the high incidence of spontaneous remission that occurs in patients with BPPV. Several authors have reported spontaneous recovery within 3 to 4 weeks,[8,15] although Brandt and Daroff[7] suggest that the vertigo may disappear spontaneously after several months even if left untreated.

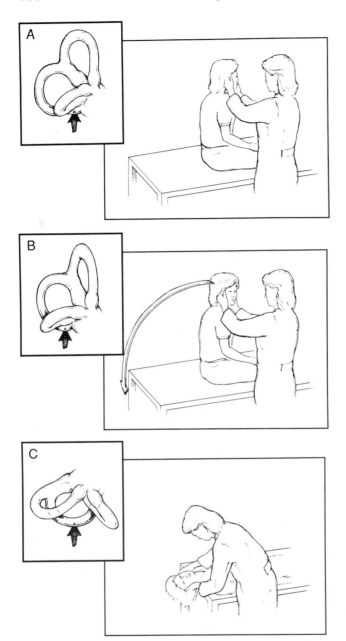

FIGURE 16–3. The modified Epley maneuver. (A–C) The patient is quickly moved into the Hallpike-Dix position with the affected ear down.

Brandt and Daroff[7] studied a series of 67 patients with histories of BPPV of 2 days to 8 month's duration. None of these patients had evidence of other neurologic or neurotologic disease. They reported that 98 percent of the subjects had no symptoms after 3 to 14 days of exercises. The only subject who did not respond to treatment had a perilymph fistula requiring surgical repair. Recurrence was small, affecting only 3 percent of the patients. In our experience with a series of 20 BPPV patients treated with exercises similar to those advocated by Brandt and Daroff,[7] the time until the patients were symptom free (*n* = 12) or had at least a moderate reduction in symptoms (*n* = 7) was more protracted, extending from 1 week to 6 months (this later case being a patient who

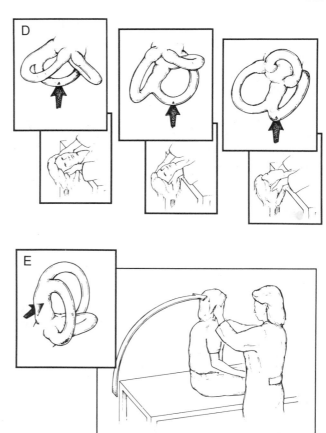

FIGURE 16–3. *Continued.* (D) He is kept in that position for 3 minutes and then the head is slowly moved through extension until the opposite ear is down (opposite Hallpike-Dix position). (E) The patient stays in that position for 4 minutes and then slowly sits up. The patient must then remain with the head in an upright position for 48 hours and must avoid lying on the affected side for 5 days after that. As in Figure 16–2, the position of the right labyrinth is shown for each head position, and the posterior canal is shaded. The arrows point to the presumed location of debris in the canal with each position change. (Reprinted with permission from Herdman, SJ, et al: Single treatment approaches to benign paroxysmal positional vertigo. Arch Otolaryngol Head Neck Surg 119:450, 1993. Copyright © 1993, American Medical Association.)

was afraid to lie down, which extended the treatment course several extra months while he worked at home just to achieve the supine position). Patients in whom there was only partial recovery complained most frequently of an intermittent "swimming" sensation rather than of true vertigo. One patient experienced no change in his vertigo. These patients had histories of BPPV extending from a few days to 35 years. The more

TABLE 16–1 Comparative Efficacy of
Various Treatments for BPPV

Exercise Protocol	No. of Subjects	% Improved or Asymptomatic	Duration of Treatment
Brandt and Daroff[7]	67	98	3 to 14 days
Semont, Freyss, and Vitte[8]	711	84	1 maneuver
Norre and Becker[16,17] Semont's	23	52	1 treatment
Habituation	28	32	1 wk
		100	6 wk
Epley[9]	30	100	Multiple maneuvers in one session
Herdman et al[10]			
Modified Epley	30	90	1 maneuver
Semont	30	90	1 maneuver

protracted the course, the more resistant the BPPV may be to treatment. We also noted that many patients having a more prolonged recovery course had additional CNS disorders that may have compounded the course of recovery.

Semont, Freyss, and Vitte[8] report a series of 711 patients with BPPV treated over an 8-year period. Their paper did not identify if patients had other neurotologic problems. They state only that some of the patients had slightly increased or decreased responses on caloric testing, but their criteria for normal was not given. Statistically significant abnormal responses to caloric testing have been reported to occur in up to 47 percent of patients with BPPV.[3] Semont, Freyss, and Vitte[8] report a "cure" rate of 84 percent after a single treatment and 93 percent after two treatments. Again, recurrence of the symptoms was infrequent (4 percent). We have used the Semont maneuver on a much smaller population. Of 30 subjects treated, the Semont maneuver resulted in remission of symptoms or in significant improvement in 90 percent of patients after a single treatment.[10]

In a randomized study of a series of 60 patients treated with either our modification of the Epley maneuver or with the Semont maneuver, we found that 90 percent were asymptomatic or significantly improved after a single treatment using either maneuver.[10] Patients who had complaints of a swimming sensation but who did not have true vertigo or nystagmus and patients who stated they had significant relief from symptoms but who still had some residual nystagmus, were considered to be "improved" rather than cured.

Norre and Beckers[16,17] compared the efficacy of Semont's technique with habituation exercises. For the habituation treatment, patients repeated the positional changes five times and performed two to three sessions each day. In the series of 23 patients treated with Semont's technique, 52 percent were free of vertigo after one treatment. Only 32 percent of the 28 patients treated with habituation exercises were free of vertigo at the end of 1 week, but the remaining subjects reported a decrease in their symptoms. By the end of 6 weeks, all 28 of the patients treated with habituation exercises had no vertigo. In addition, those patients treated with Semont's technique who did not improve with a single treatment were switched to the habituation paradigm and all but one was free of vertigo at the end of 6 weeks. They concluded that the two treatments were equally effective in the treatment of BPPV.

In summary, comparison of studies of the different treatment approaches for BPPV would suggest that there is similar success with all treatments. Not all treatment approaches are suitable for all patients. However, we can design treatments suited to individual patients with the confidence that the final outcome will be similar.

POSTURAL DISTURBANCES

Several studies have shown that patients with BPPV may also complain of disequilibrium and have abnormal postural responses. Black and Nashner[18] found decreased postural stability in BPPV patients and suggested that they rely excessively on visual cues to maintain balance as indicated by low equilibrium scores on tests 3 and 6 (Fig. 16–4). Unfortunately, Black and Nashner do not report how many of the 11 patients showed this pattern of increased reliance on visual cues. Of a group of 19 patients with BPPV studied by Voorhees,[19] 37 percent had abnormal posturography tests (see Fig. 16–4). He found that these BPPV patients could not use vestibular cues (tests 5 and 6) effectively to maintain balance but did not find the increased reliance on visual cues

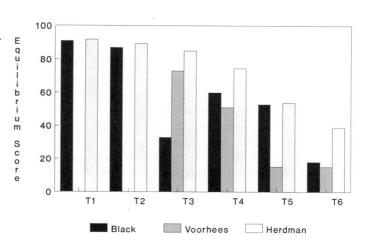

BPPV Patients

FIGURE 16–4. Results of posturography tests on BPPV patients in studies by Black and Nashner,[18] Voorhees,[19] and Herdman et al.[15] Note the differences among the studies for test conditions 3, 5, and 6. Peak to peak AP sway is expressed as an equilibrium score, from 0 = loss of balance to 100 = perfect stability, and are compared with normal values for all ages combined. See Figure 15–1 for test conditions.

suggested by Black and Nashner. We have also studied postural stability in patients with BPPV without any other neurologic findings. When compared with normal data across all ages, our subjects appear to have normal postural stability (see Fig. 16–4). When we compared our subjects with an age-matched group, however, we found that BPPV patients had abnormal anterior-posterior sway when either visual or somatosensory feedback was altered and when both visual and somatosensory feedback were altered. Unlike Voorhees,[19] we did not find a decreased ability to use vestibular cues in our patients (Test 5).

The postural instability of patients with BPPV may not be related to debris in the posterior canal itself. Many patients with BPPV have a history of head injury or have horizontal canal hypofunction as well as positional vertigo. Either of these factors could result in postural instability. Assessment of postural stability, therefore, would be an important part of the assessment of these patients in order to develop an appropriate treatment plan.

ASSESSMENT

The diagnosis of BPPV is usually made by a neuro-otologist or neurologist who would then refer the patient for physical therapy. The physical therapist should assess the patient to determine: (1) what positional changes produce the vertigo, (2) in what ways horizontal canal hypofunction is contributing to the patient's problems, (3) whether there are any balance problems associated with the BPPV, and (4) what other conditions coexist that may affect treatment (i.e., neck pain).

Provoking Positions

Tests to determine the provoking positions are important in order to develop the appropriate treatment protocol and to monitor the progress of the patient. Measurement of the latency and the duration of the vertigo as well as the intensity (scaled 1 to 5 or 1 to 10) should be kept for each of the position changes (see Table 13–4). The positional changes should be performed quickly to provoke a response. Testing must be performed consistently because a decreased response, obtained when the positional change is made too slowly, may imitate improvement. Although nystagmus may be observed in room light, using Frenzel glasses, which prevent the patient from using visual fixation to suppress the nystagmus and also magnify the patient's eyes for the observer, is best. The direction and duration of the nystagmus should be noted. In determining which positions result in vertigo or disequilibrium, care must be taken to distinguish between motion-induced dizziness and position-induced dizziness. For example, if the patient has vestibular hypofunction, movement, but not the final position itself, may result in disequilibrium. Also note that some of the position changes listed in Table 13–4 should not result in vertigo or nystagmus in patients with BPPV because the movements would not excite the posterior canal. They may result in complaints of dizziness, however, in patients with vestibular hypofunction.

Vestibular Hypofunction

Patients can have both BPPV and lateral canal hypofunction. The anterior vestibular artery supplies the ampulla of the lateral and anterior canals and the utricle, whereas the posterior vestibular artery supplies the ampulla of the posterior canal and the saccule. An infarct in the distribution of the anterior vestibular artery would result in lateral canal hypofunction and in degeneration of the macula of the utricle with the subsequent release of debris. If the debris from the utricle floats into the posterior semicircular canal, which is still intact because it receives a different blood supply, the patient will also develop BPPV.

Vestibular hypofunction can often be identified on clinical examination by the otolaryngologist or neurologist. Abnormal findings would include the observed movement of the optic disc using an ophthalmoscope while the head is gently moved, corrective saccades during rapid head thrusts, and changes in visual acuity during head movements and head shaking–induced nystagmus. Caloric or rotational tests and electronystagmography are also performed to determine the side of the lesion (caloric test), the extent of the deficit, and whether the lesion is central or peripheral. These test results can then be used to design an appropriate exercise program.

Balance

Balance should also be assessed in these patients, especially if they also have vestibular hypofunction. Many different clinical tests can be used for assessing postural stability (Table 16–2). These tests are not specific for the vestibulospinal system but are simply ways of assessing postural stability. Assessment of balance should include tests of static (quiet stance) and dynamic (moving) stability under conditions that stress balance, such as decreasing the base of support or requiring head movement, and under conditions that assess the patient's ability to maintain balance using only certain sensory cues. Normal values by age are available for many of these tests. Among the tests are the Romberg and sharpened or tandem Romberg tests, and measurement of one-legged standing balance, all with eyes open and eyes closed. Patients can be required to

TABLE 16-2. Tests for Postural Stability

Romberg: Patient is positioned within 1.5 m of a wall and is asked to stand with feet together and arms placed across the chest. Ability to maintain this position first with eyes open and then with eyes closed is timed for a maximum of 30 sec each. Test can also be performed on foam surface to alter somatosensory cues, with and without visual cues.

Sharpened Romberg (tandem): Patient is positioned as in the standard Romberg, but the feet are in the tandem position. Patient performs test with eyes open and with eyes closed. It does not matter which foot is placed in front.

Stand on one leg: Patient is asked to stand on one leg. Arms do not have to be crossed, but patient should be instructed that he or she is not to brace one leg against the other. Patient performs this test with eyes open and then with eyes closed.

Walk on floor (tandem walk): Patient is asked to walk placing the heel of one foot directly in front of the toes of the other foot for 10 steps. Arms should be placed across the chest. Patient is asked to perform this with eyes open and, if possible, with eyes closed.

Fukuda's stepping test: Patient is asked to march in place for 50 steps. Patient holds arms out in front at 90 degrees of shoulder flexion with elbows straight. Test is performed first with eyes open and then with eyes closed. Test is scored by measuring forward progression and degree and direction of turning.

Gait analysis: Patient is asked to walk at normal speed and cadence. Standard gait analysis is performed with special attention to rotation through trunk and neck and to whether patient uses excessive visual fixation to maintain balance. Patient can also be asked to turn head repeatedly while walking to perturb balance.

maintain balance with eyes open and eyes closed while standing on foam to distort somatosensory feedback. Postural stability can be assessed under more dynamic conditions by observing the patient's ability to perform tandem walking (walk-on-floor-eyes-closed test), the Singleton test, and Fukuda's stepping test. The patient might also be asked to walk while turning the head from side to side, because such movements frequently result in ataxia.

Balance can also be assessed using a force platform. With a force platform, quantifying anterior-posterior and lateral sway while the patient is standing on a stationary surface (static posturography) is possible. A system is also available from Neurocom International, Inc. that quantifies the patient's ability to maintain balance when visual and/or somatosensory cues are either absent or inappropriate. Some force platform systems measure automatic postural responses to sudden translations or rotations of the support surface. Translational (linear) perturbations could include horizontal movements of the support surface in either a fore-aft or a side-to-side direction. Rotational (angular) perturbations would move the support surface so that the toes go up or down (pitch).

GUIDELINES TO TREATMENT OF BPPV

For most patients, any of the various treatments can be used effectively. The following factors should be considered, however:

1. Patients, especially those with long histories of BPPV, may have anxiety about moving into the provoking position. Brandt's exercises may be modified so that the patient has more control over the position change and gradually becomes less fearful of provoking the vertigo and nausea. Also, patients may be more comfortable per-

forming the exercises on the floor rather than on the bed because they know they will not fall. The anxious patient, however, may tend to move out of the provoking position too quickly when attempting to do the exercises on his or her own. The extent of anxiety patients can experience should not be underestimated; one patient with a long history of BPPV became so fearful of provoking the vertigo that he tied one arm down at night to keep from rolling over onto the "bad side."

Patients who are especially fearful of the sensation of the vertigo may be unwilling to perform exercises in which they must repeatedly provoke the vertigo. These patients may be successfully treated using the single-treatment approaches (Semont's and Epley's), recognizing that they will only experience the vertigo one or two times.

2. Patients may not wish to stay in the upright position for the 48 hours required by Semont's and Epley's maneuvers. Furthermore, some patients may have difficulty avoiding bending over (e.g., parents with small children, certain work-related activities). For these patients, Brandt's exercises would be appropriate.

3. The success of Brandt's exercises is dependent on the compliance of the patient. Some improvement may occur within a few days after initiating the treatment, but treatment may have to be continued for extended periods. Weekly clinic visits may help improve the compliance of the patient, but in patients with poor compliance, Semont's or Epley's maneuvers may be the more appropriate choice.

4. The patient must perform the exercise even though it may provoke vertigo and nausea. Usually the vertigo and nausea disappear quickly when the patient is moved out of the provoking position. Repeated positional changes, as would occur with Brandt's exercises, may cause a prolonged and generalized disequilibrium with persistent nausea. The disequilibrium and nausea may be disturbing enough that the patient stops the exercises. Patients should be warned that this may occur but is only a temporary effect. Usually all that is needed is to modify the exercises (e.g., decrease the repetitions for a while) or regulate the time during the day when the exercises are performed. Medication, such as Phenergan, may be taken $\frac{1}{2}$ hour before the exercises are performed. Brandt's exercises are usually performed with the eyes closed to minimize the visuovestibular conflict contributing to the nausea. Opening the eyes may result in an increase in the nausea but may also facilitate adaptation and therefore recovery.

5. Cervical and back pain may preclude the use of Semont's or Epley's maneuvers or may be aggravated by the repeated positional changes of Brandt's exercises. Older patients may be less tolerant of Semont's or Epley's maneuvers, especially if they move cautiously because of other conditions such as arthritis. The positional changes used in Brandt's exercises may be modified to enable the patient to perform them, but the other maneuvers cannot be modified.

6. There is a slight risk of neck injury when performing Semont's or Epley's maneuvers. This risk is small, however, because the head is supported at all times. We have had no neck injuries associated with these procedures. Care should be taken, however, in using any of these procedures in patients with osteoporosis or with previous neck injury or surgery.

7. Semont's and Epley's maneuvers usually are not used in patients with bilateral BPPV because each side must be treated separately. Bilateral BPPV, like BPPV affecting the labyrinth unilaterally, has been reported in idiopathic cases and after head injury.[20]

8. Patients with BPPV and horizontal canal hypofunction are given exercises for both disorders. If the Semont's or the Epley's maneuver is used, delaying initiation of the

vestibular adaptation exercises until after the BPPV is treated is probably better. In this way, there is less risk that the patient may move the head inappropriately during the BPPV treatment. If Brandt's exercises are used, vestibular adaptation exercises may be used concurrently. Exercises to improve postural stability in these patients must be considered.

CASE STUDY 1

A 45-year-old man suffered severe head trauma with facial fractures when he was mugged 5½ months ago. Approximately 3 weeks after the mugging, he noticed that when he rolled over to either side he developed vertigo accompanied by nausea. The vertigo would last for 30 seconds regardless of whether he stayed in the precipitating position or moved onto his back. Presently, he could induce the vertigo by lying down, rolling over, tilting his head up, or sitting up quickly. Between these episodes, he had no vertigo or disequilibrium. However, he had not been able to return to work or to full social activities because of the frequency of the episodes.

ASSESSMENT

Full extraocular movements except for a left cranial nerve VI paresis. Pursuit, saccades, and vestibulo-ocular reflex (VOR) to slow and rapid head movements were within normal limits. Under Frenzel lenses, he was without spontaneous, tragal pressure–induced, or head shaking–induced nystagmus. He developed a torsional nystagmus with left gaze. When moved into the right Hallpike-Dix position, he developed a torsional nystagmus with the fast phases counterclockwise, which did not change with eye position. The nystagmus was accompanied by vertigo and lasted approximately 20 seconds. When he sat up, a torsional nystagmus with the fast phases clockwise appeared for a few seconds. When moved into the left Hallpike-Dix position, he developed a torsional nystagmus with the fast phases clockwise. This was again accompanied by vertigo and lasted for 20 seconds. He stated that the vertigo was more intense in the left Hallpike position than in the right.

DISCUSSION

The diagnosis in this patient was based on the presence of vertigo with torsional nystagmus with a latency to onset, duration, increasing intensity, and fatigability that are characteristic of BPPV. Although the patient showed a torsional nystagmus usually associated with BPPV, the nystagmus did not become upbeating as would be expected with change in eye position in orbit. This has been reported in other cases of BPPV. Bilateral BPPV is reported to occur in 15 percent of patients,[18] and BPPV secondary to head trauma is well-documented.[3] Although bilateral BPPV could easily be treated using Brandt's exercises, the patient decided he would rather use the single-treatment approach than to perform exercises several times a day that would make himself dizzy. The vertigo he experienced a few minutes after the treatment on one occurrence is not unusual with this treatment or with the Semont maneuver. Theoretically, it may be due to the sudden movement of the cupula if there is a sudden release of debris. For this reason, we keep patients under observation in the clinic for 15 to 30 minutes after the treatment.

The patient was treated first using our modification of Epley's maneuver for his left BPPV. He tolerated the treatment well and when re-tested 2 weeks later had no nystagmus and no vertigo. He was then treated, using the same method, for his right BPPV. He tolerated the treatment well, although he did report a brief period of nausea and vertigo a few minutes after the end of the treatment. When he was reassessed 2 weeks later, he still had no vertigo or nystagmus when moved into the left Hallpike-Dix position, although he complained of a brief swimming sensation. When moved into the right Hallpike-Dix position, he developed a torsional nystagmus and complained of vertigo. The treatment was then repeated to the right. When reassessed 1 week later, he had only two beats of nystagmus and a brief period of vertigo. The treatment was repeated for a third time. On reassessment 9 months later, the patient reported he had only one brief episode of vertigo that occurred when he stood up quickly. He had experienced no further vertigo when lying down, rolling over, or bending over.

CASE STUDY 2

A 56-year-old obese man reported that several months ago he had a sudden episode of vertigo that lasted for 10 minutes. This resolved but was followed by a second episode $\frac{1}{2}$ hour later. These episodes continued, and he went to the emergency room during an episode that lasted for several hours. Currently, he states that he has visual blurring and disequilibrium whenever he moves his head. He denies falls but does stumble. He has used meclizine and scopolamine without relief. Laboratory tests showed left vestibular hypofunction and left positional nystagmus. Past medical history is significant for two myocardial infarcts in the past 4 years and hypertension. Social history includes smoking $1\frac{1}{2}$ packs per day over 20 years and occasional alcohol.

ASSESSMENT

The patient had normal extraocular movements, normal pursuit, normal saccades, and VOR to slow head movements. With rapid head movements to the left, the patient used corrective saccades to maintain fixation on a stationary visual target. VOR to rapid head movements to the right was normal. Under Frenzel lenses, the patient was without spontaneous or gaze-evoked nystagmus. Following horizontal head shaking, the patient developed a horizontal nystagmus with fast phases to the right that lasted for 5 seconds. There was no nystagmus induced by vertical head shaking. When the patient was moved into the left Hallpike-Dix position, he developed a torsional nystagmus that became upbeating when he looked toward the right. Concurrent with the onset of the nystagmus, he complained of vertigo. The latency and duration were consistent with BPPV. When moved into the right Hallpike-Dix position, the patient also developed vertigo with a counterclockwise fast phase that lasted for 7 seconds. This was followed by a second burst of counterclockwise nystagmus lasting 10 seconds. Approximately

5 seconds later, he again developed a torsional nystagmus with a strong down-beating component.

DISCUSSION

The right-beating nystagmus induced by horizontal head shaking as well as the corrective saccades to maintain visual fixation during rapid head thrusts to the left are consistent with left vestibular hypofunction. This patient's vascular history supports the possibility of a vascular insult in the distribution of the superior vestibular artery affecting the anterior and horizontal canals and the utricle. Posterior canal and saccular function are spared. Presumably, debris from the infarcted tissue floats into the posterior canal producing the left BPPV. The nystagmus when the patient was moved into the right Hallpike-Dix position might also be due to positional vertigo with the down-beating component being one of the less common presentations or it could indicate a central lesion.[3] This patient had a secondary phase of nystagmus that has been reported by several authors.[3]

This patient was treated with exercises for both his vestibular hypofunction and the bilateral BPPV. For his vestibular hypofunction, he was taught exercises designed to increase the gain of the vestibular system (X1 and X2 viewing, see Chapter 15) using foveal and full-field stimuli. The patient performed these exercises with the stimulus placed both near and far and was to perform them both in sitting and standing positions. Brandt's exercises were used to treat the bilateral BPPV. Brandt's exercises were chosen because the patient could begin the vestibular adaptation exercises at the same time.

SUMMARY

BPPV is a common disorder that results in what can be disabling episodes of vertigo. There are several different treatments that can be used to relieve the patient's symptoms and enable the patient to return to normal activities. Which treatment is used depends on many factors, such as the presence of other vestibular deficits and the willingness of the patient to make himself or herself dizzy. Given the different treatments available, however, patients should no longer be told that they must "learn to live with vertigo."

REFERENCES

1. Barany, R: Diagnose von Krankheitserscheinungen im Bereiche des Otolithenapparatus. Acta Oto-Laryngol 2:434, 1921.
2. Dix, MR and Hallpike, CS: Pathology, symptomatology and diagnosis of certain disorders of the vestibular system. Proc Soc Med 45:341, 1952.
3. Baloh, RW, Honrubia, V, and Jacobson, K: Benign positional vertigo: Clinical and oculographic features in 240 cases. Neurology 37:371, 1987.
4. Schuknecht, HF: Cupulolithiasis. Arch Otolaryngol 90:765, 1969.
5. Hall, SF, Ruby, RRF, and McClure, JA: The mechanisms of benign paroxysmal vertigo. J Otolaryngol 8:151, 1979.
6. Epley, JM: New dimensions of benign paroxysmal positional vertigo. Otolaryngol Head Neck Surg 88:599, 1980.
7. Brandt, T and Daroff, RB: Physical therapy for benign paroxysmal positional vertigo. Arch Otolaryngol 106:484, 1980.
8. Semont, A, Freyss, G, and Vitte, E: Curing the BPPV with a Liberatory Maneuver. Adv Oto-Rhino-Laryngol 42:290, 1988.

9. Epley, JM: The canalith repositioning procedure: For treatment of benign paroxysmal positional vertigo. Otolaryngol Head Neck Surg 107:399, 1992.
10. Herdman, SJ, et al: Single treatment approaches to benign paroxysmal positional vertigo. Arch Otolaryngol Head Neck Surg 119:450, 1993.
11. Norre, ME and De Weerdt, W: Positional (provoked) vertigo treated by postural training vestibular habituation training. Agressologie 22:37, 1981.
12. Tangeman, PT and Wheeler, J: Inner ear concussion syndrome: Vestibular implications and physical therapy treatment. Top Acute Care Trauma Rehabil 1:72, 1986.
13. Norre, ME and Beckers, A: Vestibular habituation training: Exercise treatment for vertigo based upon the habituation effect. Otolaryngol Head Neck Surg 101:14, 1989.
14. Hecker, HC, Haug, CO, and Herndon, JW: Treatment of the vertiginous patient using Cawthorne's vestibular exercises. Laryngoscope 84:2065, 1974.
15. Gyo, K: Benign paroxysmal positional vertigo as a complication of postoperative bedrest. Laryngoscope 98:332, 1988.
16. Norre, ME and Beckers, A: Exercise treatment for paroxysmal positional vertigo: Comparison of two types of exercises. Arch Otorhinolaryngol 244:291, 1987.
17. Norre, ME and Beckers, A: Comparative study of two types of exercise treatment for paroxysmal positioning vertigo. Adv Oto-Rhino-Laryngol 42:287, 1988.
18. Black, FO and Nashner, LM: Postural disturbance in patients with benign paroxysmal positional nystagmus. Ann Oto Rhino Laryngol 93:595, 1984.
19. Voorhees, RL: The role of dynamic posturography in neurotologic diagnosis. Laryngoscope 99:995, 1989.
20. Longridge, NS and Barber, HO: Bilateral paroxysmal positioning nystagmus. J Otolaryngol 7:395, 1978.

CHAPTER 17

Vestibular Rehabilitation in Traumatic Brain Injury

Anne Shumway-Cook, PhD, PT

This chapter discusses the confounding influence of traumatic brain injury (TBI) on the assessment, treatment, and recovery of function in patients with peripheral vestibular system pathology. The vestibular pathologies associated with TBI are similar to those commonly found in most neuro-otologic practices. What distinguishes the TBI patient from other patients with peripheral vestibular disease is the mechanism of vestibular injury and the high incidence of other neurologic deficits complicating the recovery process.

Recognizing and treating symptoms of vestibular dysfunction, including dizziness and imbalance, is an essential part of TBI rehabilitation. Many therapists involved in rehabilitating the TBI patient are familiar with approaches to treating imbalance but lack strategies to treat complaints of dizziness. As a result, therapists often try to avoid provoking dizziness when treating TBI patients. However, avoiding the movements that provoke dizziness can actually delay recovery from vestibular system dysfunction, resulting in persisting symptoms that complicate recovery and contribute to long-term loss of functional independence.[1-5]

This chapter discusses mechanisms of traumatic injury producing peripheral vestibular system pathology in TBI. Strategies for assessing and treating symptoms of peripheral vestibular system dysfunction are reviewed. In addition, the effect of central neural injuries producing central sensory, motor, and cognitive deficits on strategies for treating the TBI patient are addressed.

VESTIBULAR PATHOLOGY IN TRAUMATIC BRAIN INJURY

As many as 30 to 65 percent of TBI patients suffer symptoms of traumatic vestibular pathology at some point during their recovery.[4-9] Symptoms of peripheral vestibular system dysfunction can include vertigo, eye-head discoordination, and disequilibrium.[10]

The specific constellation of symptoms found in individual patients will vary depending on the type and extent of injuries to both vestibular and central neural structures. Understanding peripheral vestibular pathology and its effect on gaze, postural, and perceptual functions is essential because treatment varies according to the patient's symptoms and diagnosis.[11]

Mechanism of injury and resulting vestibular pathologies reported to occur frequently in TBI are summarized below.

Concussion

Inner-ear concussion injury is the most common vestibular sequela of TBI.[8,12,13] Symptoms of concussive-type vestibular injury can include high-frequency sensorineural hearing loss, benign paroxysmal positional vertigo (BPPV), lack of postural control, and gait ataxia. BPPV in TBI is believed to occur because of the intense acceleration of the utricular otolithic membrane resulting in displacement of otoconia to the posterior semicircular canal. Displaced otoconia, adhering to the cupula or free-floating in the long arm of the posterior canal, may result in displacement of the cupula in response to gravity in specific positions.[14]

Fracture

Traumatic fractures of the temporal bone can produce unilateral or bilateral vestibular system dysfunction. Transverse fractures account for approximately 20 percent of all temporal bone fractures and are reported to result most frequently from blows to the occiput.[12,15] Transverse fractures of the temporal bone produce a unilateral loss of vestibular function that can be either partial or complete. Functional effects of a unilateral loss of vestibular function include spontaneous nystagmus (acute stage only) and provoked vertigo, problems with gaze stabilization, and disequilibrium.[16]

Longitudinal fractures account for approximately 80 percent of all temporal bone fractures and are associated primarily with blows to the parietal and temporal regions of the skull.[12,15] Anatomic damage associated with longitudinal fractures is primarily to middle-ear structures, leading to conductive hearing loss; any associated vestibular symptoms are considered secondary to a concussive injury to the membranous labyrinth.

Intracranial Pressure and Hemorrhagic Lesions

Changes in intracranial pressure can produce ruptures in the round or oval window and a perilymph fistula (PLF) between the middle and inner ear.[8,11,17–19] PLF can result in fluctuating hearing loss, episodic vertigo, and gait and balance disturbances. In addition, patients with PLF may have a number of cognitive symptoms, including memory, concentration, and attentional deficits.[20] The incidence of PLF in head-injured patients is uncertain.[18,20,22,23]

Vascular injuries, including hemorrhage into the membranous labyrinth, can injure the endolymphatic system producing a posttraumatic hydrops or "Ménière-type" syndrome, with corresponding symptoms.[8,11]

Central Vestibular Lesions

Traumatic head injury can also produce damage to central vestibular structures.[3,13,21] Multiple petechial hemorrhages in the brain stem that damage central vestibular structures have been reported in head-injured patients with both mild (no loss of consciousness) and moderate damage. Symptoms include spontaneous nystagmus and oculomotor problems, including ocular dysmetria, cogwheeling during smooth-pursuit eye moments, and marked optokinetic asymmetries. Spontaneous and/or provoked vertigo may or may not occur in the patient with central vestibular lesions.

VESTIBULAR REHABILITATION IN TRAUMATIC BRAIN INJURY

Vestibular rehabilitation is a comprehensive approach to assessing and treating symptoms of vestibular system pathology.[22-24] Evaluation involves assessment of vertigo, control of eye–head coordination for stabilizing gaze, and musculoskeletal and neural components of postural control underlying functional independence in sitting, standing, and walking. Treatment relies on exercises to facilitate central nervous system (CNS) compensation for vestibular pathology, thereby alleviating symptoms.

Assessment

TBI produces a variety of sensory, motor, and cognitive impairments. This constellation of impairments makes assessment of the TBI patient with vestibular system pathology a complex process involving the evaluation of multiple functions and systems. The goal of assessment is to ascertain the patient's functional problems and the many sensory, motor, and cognitive limitations contributing to loss of functional independence. Because functional deficits following TBI are usually due to a combination of these factors, sorting out the relative contribution of vestibular system pathology to overall loss of function is difficult.

VERTIGO

When assessing vertigo, the therapist notes whether dizziness symptoms are spontaneous or provoked and determines the situations and conditions that precipitate complaints of dizziness.[22,23,25] Characteristics of vertigo are noted, such as onset latency, duration, intensity, and effect of repeating the movement. Associated autonomic symptoms, such as nausea, sweating, and pallor, are noted, and presence of nystagmus is recorded.

The TBI patient with partial loss of vestibular function in the acute stage will experience both spontaneous and provoked vertigo. Often by the time the TBI patient enters a rehabilitation program, spontaneous complaints have resolved, but movement-provoked vertigo lasting seconds to minutes persists. Vertigo in the patient with BPPV lasts 30 to 45 seconds and is provoked by placing the patient in the Hallpike position. Patients with BPPV may also show transient vertigo when leaning over, when looking up on a diagonal plane, or when turning their heads quickly during gait.[26,27]

EYE–HEAD COORDINATION

Eye movements from both the visual and vestibular systems used to keep gaze stable during voluntary and involuntary movements of the head are examined.[23] Testing is done with the patient seated, standing unsupported, and walking. Visually generated eye movements, including smooth-pursuit and saccadic eye movements, are assessed. The patient's ability to maintain a stable gaze during horizontal, vertical, and diagonal head motions of varying speed is examined. Finally, the patient's ability to keep gaze fixed on an object moving in phase with the head is used to test visual suppression of vestibular-driven eye movements. Subjective complaints of dizziness, blurred vision, or oscillopsia are noted. Episodes of staggering and disequilibrium are recorded during a variety of walking tasks, such as walking with brisk head movements, walking with pivot turns, and during abrupt stops. In the TBI patient, eye–head discoordination can result from (1) damage to the vestibular system disrupting vestibulo-ocular reflex (VOR) function; (2) deficits within the visual system including loss of ocular motility, visual acuity or field deficits, or visual perceptual deficits; (3) orthopedic injuries limiting cervical motion; and (4) damage to cerebellar structures resulting in loss of visual suppression of VOR.[28,29]

POSTURAL CONTROL UNDERLYING STABILITY

Stability is defined as the ability to maintain the center of body mass within limits determined principally by the extent of the support base.[30] Stability requires a continuous interaction between the individual and the environment and involves many bodily subsystems collectively referred to as the postural control system (see Chapter 2 for more detail).

Assessment of stability determines the constellation of constraints contributing to instability in each TBI patient. Constraints are defined as limitations within the individual that restrict sensory and motor strategies for postural control.[31] As shown in Figure 17–1, constraints on stability in the TBI patient can be musculoskeletal, neuromuscular, sensory-perceptual, or cognitive. Procedures for assessing constraints on stability in the TBI patient have been described in detail elsewhere and so will only be briefly reviewed here.[31,32]

Musculoskeletal Constraints

Musculoskeletal constraints such as decreased joint range of motion, muscle contractures, and loss of flexibility are common in TBI patients. Musculoskeletal constraints may be the result of prolonged immobilization following orthopedic injuries or the effects of excessive muscle tone.

Neuromuscular Constraints

Neuromuscular constraints affect the patient's ability to generate and coordinate the muscular forces necessary to control posture. Clinically, multijoint coordination for balance is qualitatively assessed by the therapist while the patient assumes and maintains a fixed posture, recovers a posture when perturbed, and maintains an appropriate posture during an ongoing movement, such as gait. Although not performed routinely in the clinic, electromyography and kinematic analysis of associated body movements can be used to quantify discoordination in stance and gait and improvements during the course of recovery.

Weakness, particularly hemiparesis, is frequently a primary neuromuscular con-

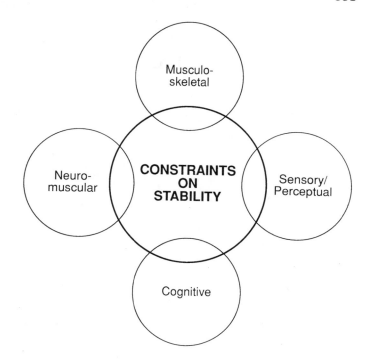

FIGURE 17–1. Categories
of constraints on stability following traumatic brain injury.

straint on balance in the TBI patient. Traumatic injury to the cerebellum or deep
hemorrhagic lesions in the basal ganglia can affect the timing and scaling of muscles
working synergistically for postural control. Clinical indicators of muscular discoordination during postural tasks include asymmetric use of limbs for movement control;
excessive movements at the joints, including excessive flexion of the hip; and loss of knee
control.

Sensory Constraints

The primary focus of assessment of sensory constraints is to determine the patient's
ability to remain oriented under different sensory conditions and to assess whether
perceptions relevant to stability are accurate.[22,23]

Moving platform posturography is one approach to examining the organization and
selection of senses for postural control.[33] Posturography uses a moving force plate in
conjunction with a moving visual surround to determine the patient's ability to correctly
select from among visual, somatosensory, and vestibular inputs, the most appropriate
sense for orientation (see Chapter 2).

Alternatively, the Clinical Test for Sensory Interaction in Balance (CTSIB) tests the
patient's use of alternative sensory cues for orientation, using procedures similar to those
of posturography.[34] A modified Japanese lantern placed over the head is used to minimize the effectiveness of visual cues for postural orientation. Compliant foam (medium-
density Sunmate foam) is used to reduce the effectiveness of support surface somatosensory inputs for orientation. The six sensory conditions are shown in Figure 17–2.
Procedures for administering the CTSIB are detailed elsewhere.[35]

Sensory constraints affecting orientation in the TBI patient can result from pathology within the peripheral vestibular system or within central structures that organize
sensory information for postural orientation. While both posturography and the CTSIB

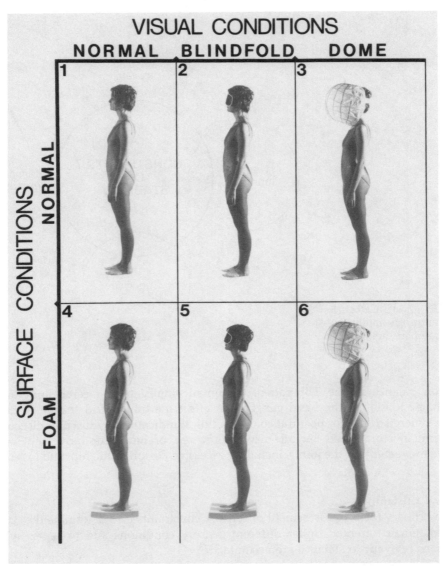

FIGURE 17–2. The six positions used to test sensory interaction in balance. (From Shumway-Cook and Horak.[34] Reprinted from PHYSICAL THERAPY with the permission of the American Physical Therapy Association.)

can identify and quantify functional problems in selecting sensory inputs for postural control, they cannot determine the anatomic location of injury producing these functional problems.

Treatment

Strategies for treating vestibular system dysfunction are individualized to each patient's problems. Strategies focus on both remediating underlying constraints and improving functional skills. Major areas of exercise are head exercises for habituation of dizziness, exercises to recover eye–head coordination for improved gaze stabilization, and sensorimotor retraining to remediate postural dyscontrol in sitting, standing, and walking.[22,23]

Modifying a vestibular exercise program for the TBI patient usually involves providing:

1. Physical assistance because of movement problems
2. Increased supervision because of cognitive and behavioral problems
3. Progressing the patient more slowly because of a multiplicity of problems

VERTIGO

Habituation exercises to decrease dizziness involve repeating the positions and movements that provoke vertigo. Five repetitions of the habituation exercises are incorporated into twice-daily physical therapy treatments, usually at the end of each exercise session.

Habituation exercises are routinely modified to accommodate both movement and cognitive limitations in the TBI patient. Written exercise sheets are used, and patients are provided logs to record exercise sessions. Because of the high frequency of behavioral and cognitive problems, including attention and memory deficits, closer supervision and physical assistance are more often required when treating vestibular dysfunction in the TBI patient then in other types of patients.

In our facility, the liberatory movement[36] (see Chapter 16) to cure BPPV is rarely used with TBI patients because the strict requirements for avoiding head movements following the procedure are not realistic for many patients in a rehabilitation environment.

EYE–HEAD COORDINATION

Exercises to improve gaze stabilization during head movements include visual tracking tasks with head still, visual tracking tasks during progressive head movements, and exercises to improve visual modulation of VOR (see Chapter 14).[16,24,37] The patient repeats these exercises first in supported sitting and progresses to standing and walking.

Treatment of cervical complaints is essential to recovery of function in many TBI patients, particularly those with whiplash. Vestibular rehabilitation exercises combined with physical modalities and orthopedic manual skills have produced excellent results.[38]

POSTURAL CONTROL

Treatment of stability involves remediating constraints and improving sensory and motor strategies for stability.[22,23,31] Biomechanical limitations and movement disorders are a particular concern in patients with vestibular pathology because they limit a patient's ability to move in ways that are necessary for compensation.

Treatment of biomechanical limitations includes physical modalities, such as heat and ultrasound, as well as exercises to improve range of motion, joint flexibility, and body alignment.[39] Treatment of neuromuscular problems varies depending on the nature of the problem. Strengthening exercises are used to improve impaired force generation. Therapy for muscular discoordination includes functional electrical stimulation, electromyographic biofeedback, and neuromuscular facilitation exercises.

Exercises to improve sensory function for orientation require the patient to maintain balance during progressively difficult movement tasks while the therapist varies the availability and accuracy of one or more senses for orientation.[22,23] For example, during exercises to decrease sensitivity to visual motion cues, the patient performs balance and movement tasks when visual cues are reduced or absent (eyes closed or while wearing blinders or a blindfold) or inaccurate for orientation (prism glasses, optokinetic stimuli, and within a large moving visual surround).[40] During these exercises, accurate orientation cues from the surface are essential.

In contrast, exercises to improve use of vestibular inputs for postural control in the patient with partial loss of vestibular function involve decreasing the availability of *both* visual and somatosensory input for orientation. An example would be asking the patient to reach for an object while wearing blinders and standing unsupported on a piece of foam.

Patients who have had a complete bilateral loss of vestibular function are taught to rely on visual and or somatosensory cues for postural control. Because these patients have no residual vestibular function available to them, the goal of therapy is sensory substitution rather than enhancement of remaining vestibular function.

In summary, treatment of postural dyscontrol in the TBI patient with associated vestibular system pathology is directed at helping the patient to reestablish effective sensorimotor strategies for balance control. Therapy is focused on practicing functional tasks, such as sitting and standing unsupported and moving from sit to stand. In addition, treatment seeks to remediate specific deficits in musculoskeletal and sensorimotor systems underlying poor postural control.

Expected Recovery Period

The time required for recovery from a traumatic vestibular lesion may be longer than that required for vestibular lesions of other causes.[41] In the TBI patient with vestibular system pathology, concomitant CNS lesions impair the compensatory process itself. As a result, recovery from traumatic vestibular lesions is often protracted. Pfaltz and Kamath[41] compared recovery in patients with a unilateral loss of vestibular function due to various pathologies including trauma, Ménière's disease, labyrinthectomy, and other diseases. At 6 months, only one third of the patients with unilateral loss due to trauma were symptom-free, whereas the majority of other patients had achieved compensation and were symptom-free. At 18 months, many of the trauma patients continued to show persisting symptoms of vestibular system pathology.

Berman and Fredrickson[3] studied 321 patients with mild and moderate head injuries and vestibular system pathology. Vertigo was reported in 34 percent of patients with mild head injuries, and 50 percent in patients with moderate head injuries. Of those patients with central vestibular dysfunction, 60 to 70 percent had persisting symptoms 5 years postinjury. Almost half of these patient never returned to work.

These and other studies suggest that the typical time course for recovery from vestibular system pathology in TBI patients is protracted, requiring one to three times longer than in patients with vestibular system pathology due to other causes. Usually, many patients with traumatic vestibular dysfunction show persisting symptoms of dizziness and disequilibrium several years following trauma. The degree to which specific exercise interventions can influence the time course of recovery from vestibular system dysfunction in the TBI patient is an important theoretic and clinical question currently under study.

CASE STUDY

The following case study illustrates the applications and results of a rehabilitation approach to assess and treat vertigo and postural dyscontrol in a traumatically brain-injured patient with vestibular system pathology.

SD is a 31-year-old man admitted for rehabilitation 1 month following a closed head injury. SD fell 40 feet, striking the left side of his head, and experienced a brief (less than 5 minute) loss of consciousness. He was admitted to the hospital with a Glasgow Coma Score of 13. Computed tomography showed multiple left parietal–occipital cerebral contusions. Associated trauma included three fractured ribs and a contusion of the left hip. There was no previous history of medical or neurologic problems.

Otologic evaluation included both a clinical examination and electronystagmography, including tests for gaze and positional nystagmus; oculomotor function (saccade, smooth pursuit, and optokinetics); and VOR function using rotational chair testing. Results from this examination indicated the presence of a posttraumatic BPPV. Other test results were within normal limits, suggesting no evidence for vestibular hypofunction or a central vestibular lesion.

ASSESSMENT

Rehabilitation assessment determined the following problems:

Functional Problems

1. Decreased independence in stability skills
2. Decreased independence in mobility skills, including transfers and gait (patient used a cane and required standby assistance
3. Decreased independence in activities of daily living (ADL) skills requiring balance
4. Decreased independence due to cognitive and behavioral problems

Sensorimotor Constraints

1. Positional vertigo in the left Hallpike position, as well as vertigo during gait with vertical head motions
2. Postural dyscontrol including:
   a. Right hemiparesis and dyscoordination
   b. Limitation of range in right ankle
   c. Asymmetries in weight-bearing, primarily in stance and during gait
   d. Difficulty organizing sensory inputs for balance and effectively using vestibular inputs for orientation in the absence of visual and somatosensory cues

Other Problems

1. Pain due to fractured ribs and contusions on the left hip
2. Moderate cognitive impairments including memory and attention deficits
3. Decreased awareness of his limitations raising a number of safety issues

TREATMENT AND RATIONALE

Treatment included:

1. Vertigo habituation exercises
   a. A modified Hallpike-Dix maneuver for decreasing positional vertigo
   b. Progressive head-movement exercises in the vertical plane in standing and walking
2. Balance retraining
   a. Exercises to increase strength and coordination in the right extremities
   b. Postural sway biofeedback to reduce weightbearing asymmetries in standing and to improve range of center of mass movements over the hemiparetic leg
   c. Manual cues and feedback to improve joint coordination at the knee and hip while the patient practiced voluntary sway about the ankles in stance, moving from sit to stand, and during gait
   d. Balance and ADL exercises while standing on foam, with blinders, or with eyes closed to increase use of vestibular inputs for postural control; practice maintaining balance in standing and during stepping in place during optokinetic stimulation

Following 5 months of rehabilitation (2 months as an inpatient, 3 months as an outpatient), the patient had no complaints of vertigo on lying down but had very brief nystagmus and minimal vertigo (intensity 2, lasting 10 seconds) in the left Hallpike position. In addition, mild vertigo (intensity 3) persisted during gait with head motions; however, this was not associated with ataxia.

Postural control underlying stability in sitting, standing, and walking had improved, and the patient was transferring and walking independently and no longer needed a cane to walk. Results of posturography testing examining sensory and motor aspects of postural control in SD prior to and following rehabilitation are shown in Figures 17–3 and 17–4.

A. 1 mo Post-TBI

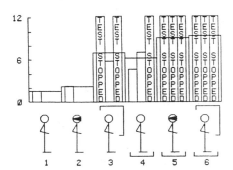

B. 6 mos Post-TBI

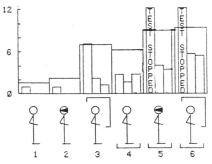

FIGURE 17–3. Recovery of sensory organization aspects of postural control is shown by comparing body sway during altered sensory conditions at 1 month and 6 months post-TBI. See text for details.

A. 1 mo Post-TBI

B. 6 mos Post-TBI

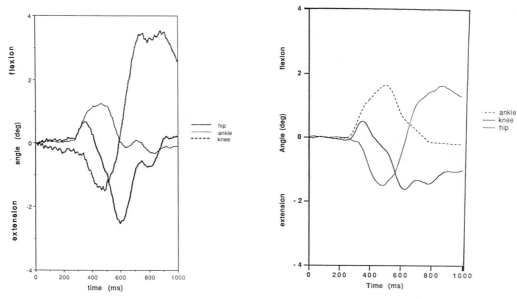

FIGURE 17–4. Recovery of motor coordination aspects of postural control is shown by comparing kinematic changes at the ankle, knee, and hip during corrections for a forward loss of balance at 1 month and 6 months post-TBI. See text for details.

Figure 17–3 compares performance on balance tasks under altered sensory conditions at 1 month and 6 months post-TBI. Peak-to-peak center-of-gravity angle, in degrees, is plotted for individual trials in the six conditions; conditions 3 through 6 have three trials each (see Chapter 2 for a complete description of sensory conditions). Encompassing individual trials is a larger histogram that shows the upper limits of normality, established using the 95th percentile from 250 normal controls ages 8 to 70.[42] At 1 month, SD lost balance (indicated in Figure 17–3 by "test stopped") when either visual or surface cues for orientation were reduced or inaccurate (conditions 3, 4, 5, and 6). At 6 months postinjury, he fell on the first trial only when deprived of both visual and surface cues simultaneously (conditions 5 and 6).

Figure 17–4 compares kinematic changes at the ankle, knee, and hip during corrections for a forward fall. At 1 month post-TBI, SD had problems coordinating the ankle, knee, and hip joint in the right leg during movements to correct for forward loss of balance. Compared to kinematic data from normal subjects,[32] SD demonstrated increased hip flexion, delays in the reversal of ankle joint motion from dorsiflexion to plantarflexion, and an increase in total net angular displacement of the knee. Multijoint dyscoordination was associated with asymmetric torque traces and increased center-of-mass displacement. Figure 17–3B shows kinematic data from the same joints at 6 months post-TBI. Improvements can be seen in decreased hip flexion, quicker reversal from ankle dorsiflexion to plantarflexion, and less motion at the knee. Kinematic changes were associated with more symmetric torque traces and smaller center-of-mass displacement.

SUMMARY

Assessment and treatment of vestibular system pathology are essential parts of rehabilitating the TBI patient. However, in the TBI patient, injuries to other parts of the CNS can complicate recovery from vestibular system pathology in several ways: (1) associated trauma can produce pain and restrict movements; (2) musculoskeletal and neuromuscular problems can affect the patient's ability to move in ways that are necessary to CNS compensation; (3) damage to visual and somatosensory systems may limit the availability of these senses as alternatives to lost vestibular inputs; and (4) cognitive and behavioral problems make compliance to a vestibular exercise program difficult.

Finally, intracranial injury can damage neural structures important to the compensatory process, resulting in persisting symptoms and a protracted recovery.

A comprehensive treatment plan that incorporates vestibular rehabilitation exercises modified to adjust for the above limitations is an effective way to gain functional independence and minimize persisting and disabling symptoms of vestibular system pathology in TBI patients.

REFERENCES

1. Igarashi, M, Ishikawa, M, and Yamane, H: Physical exercise and balance compensation after total ablation of vestibular organs. Prog Brain Res 76:395, 1988.
2. Lacour, M and Xerri, C: Vestibular compensation: New perspectives. In Flohr, H and Precht, W (eds): Lesion Induced Neuronal Plasticity in Sensorimotor Systems. Springer-Verlag, New York, 1981.
3. Berman, J and Fredrickson, J: Vertigo after head injury — A five year follow-up. J Otolaryngol 7:237, 1978.
4. Barber, HO: Head injury: Audiological and vestibular findings. Ann Otol Rhinol Larngol 78:239, 1969.
5. Pearson, BW and Barber, HO: Head injury: Some otoneurologic sequelae. Arch Otolargyngol 97:81, 1973.
6. Griffith, MV: The incidence of auditory and vestibular concussion following minor head injury. J Laryngol Otol 93:253, 1979.
7. Gibson, W: Vertigo associated with trauma. In Dix, R and Hood, JD (eds): Vertigo. John Wiley and Sons, New York, 1984.
8. Healy, GB: Hearing loss and vertigo secondary to head injury. N Engl J Med 306:1029, 1982.
9. Toglia, JU, Rosenberg, PE, and Ronis, ML: Vestibular and audiologic aspects of whiplash injury and head trauma. J Forensic Sci 14:219, 1969.
10. Baloh, RW: Dizziness, Hearing Loss and Tinnitus: The Essentials of Neurotology. FA Davis, Philadelphia, 1984.
11. Black, FO: Vertigo. Curr Ther Otolaryngol Head Neck Surg 4:59, 1990.
12. Nelson, JR: Neurootologic aspects of head injury. In Thompson, RA and Green, JR (eds): Advances in Neurology, vol 2. Raven Press, New York, 1979.
13. Karnik, PP, et al: Otoneurologic problems in head injuries and their management. Internat Surg 60:466, 1975.
14. Schuknecht, HF: Mechanism of inner ear injury from blows to the head. Ann Otorhinolaryngol 78:253, 1969.
15. Lindsay, JR and Heminway, WG: Postural vertigo due to unilateral sudden partial loss of vestibular function. Ann Otol 65:692, 1956.
16. Herdman, SJ: Treatment of vestibular disorders in traumatically brain-injured patients. J Head Trauma Rehabil 5:63, 1990.
17. Jacobs, GB, et al: Post traumatic vertigo: Report of three cases. J Neurosurg 51:860, 1979.
18. Glasscock, ME, McKennan, KX, and Levine, SC: Persistent traumatic perilymph fistulas. Laryngoscope 97:860, 1987.
19. Lehrer, JF, et al: Perilymphatic fistula — A definitive and curable cause of vertigo following head trauma. West J Med 141:57, 1984.
20. Grimm, RJ and Black, FO: Perilymph fistula syndrome: Defined in mild head trauma. Acta Otol (suppl)464:1, 1989.
21. Ylikoski, J, Palva, T, and Sanna, M: Dizziness after head trauma: Clinical and morphologic findings. Am J Otol 3:343, 1982.
22. Shumway-Cook, A and Horak, F: Vestibular rehabilitation: An exercise approach to managing symptoms of vestibular dysfunction. Semin Hearing 10:196, 1989.

23. Shumway-Cook, A and Horak, F: Rehabilitation strategies for patients with vestibular deficits. Neurol Clin 8:441, 1990.
24. Herdman, SJ: Assessment and treatment of balance disorders in the vestibular deficient patient. In Duncan, P (ed): Balance, Proceedings of the APTA Forum. APTA, Alexandria, 1989.
25. Norre, ME, and De Weerdt, W: Positional (provoked) vertigo treated by postural training. Vestibular habituation training. Agressologie 22:37, 1981.
26. Epley, J: New dimensions of benign paroxysmal positional vertigo. Otolaryngol Head Neck Surg 88:599, 1980.
27. Shumway-Cook, A: Unpublished material, 1990.
28. Louis, M: Visual field and perceptual deficits in brain damaged patient. Crit Care Update 8:32, 1981.
29. Stanworth, A: Defects in ocular movement and fusion after head injury. Br J Ophthalmol 58:266, 1974.
30. McCollum, G and Leen, TK: Form and exploration of mechanical stability limits in erect stance. J Motor Behav 21:225, 1989.
31. Shumway-Cook, A and McCollum, G: Assessment and treatment of balance deficits in the neurologic patient. In Montgomery, P and Connoly, B (eds): Motor Control: Theoretical Framework and Practical Application to Physical Therapy. Chattanooga Corp, Cattanooga, 1991.
32. Shumway-Cook, A and Olmscheid, R: A systems analysis of postural dyscontrol in traumatically brain-injured patients. J Head Trauma Rehabil 5:51, 1990.
33. Nashner, LM: Adaptation of human movement to altered environments. Trends Neurosci 10:358, 1982.
34. Shumway-Cook, A and Horak, F: Assessing the influence of sensory interaction on balance. Phys Ther 66:1548, 1986.
35. Horak, F: Clinical measurement of postural control in adults. Phys Ther 67:1881, 1987.
36. Semont, A, Freyss, G, and Vitte, E: Curing the BPPV with a Liberatory Maneuver. Adv Otorhinolaryngol 42:290, 1988.
37. Zee, DS: Vertigo. In Johnson, RT (ed): Current Therapy in Neurological Disease, BC Decker, Philadelphia, 1985.
38. Shumway-Cook, A and Myers L, Unpublished observations, 1991.
39. Shumway-Cook, A, Anson, D, and Haller, S: Postural sway biofeedback: Its effect on reestablishing stance stability in hemiplegic patients. Arch Phys Med Rehabil 69:395, 1988.
40. Bles, W, de Jong, JMB, and deWit, G: Compensation for labyrinthine defects by use of a tilting room. Acta Otolaryngol (Stockh) 95:576, 1983.
41. Pfaltz, CR and Kamath, R: Central compensation of vestibular dysfunction: (I) Peripheral lesions. Adv Otorhinolaryngol 30:335, 1983.
42. Peterka, R, Black, FO, and Schoenfoff BS: Age-related changes in human postural control: Sensory organization tests. J Vestibular Res 1:73, 1991.

CHAPTER 18

Treatment of Vestibular Deficits in Children with Developmental Disorders

Georgia A. DeGangi, PhD, OTR, FAOTA
Mary McCandless Goodin, MEd, OTR
Shirley Wietlisbach, MS, OTR

The vestibular system develops early and is the predominant sensory system functioning at birth. Investigators of fetal development have found that the vestibular nerve myelinates at 28 weeks gestational age. In utero, the fetus receives constant vestibular stimulation from movement of the amniotic fluid as well as the mother's own body movements, and the vestibular system enables the fetus, and later the infant, to receive and respond to specific movement stimuli. Because the vestibular system assists the infant in orienting in space and in initiating exploratory and adaptive movements, this system, along with the tactile system, are particularly critical for development of basic functions in the young infant.[1] As a result, individuals with vestibular deficits occurring during development are believed to have problems in refinement of motor skills, visuospatial and language abilities, hand dominance, and motor planning.[2,3]

One of the major difficulties in identifying vestibular deficits in children is that the traditional tests of vestibular function, such as the rotary chair or the caloric test, are rarely performed to confirm the presence of a vestibular deficit. Labeling specific problems, such as difficulties with language and visuospatial skills, as being due to a vestibular deficit is often theoretic. Nevertheless, a number of treatment approaches have been proposed based on the presumed role of the vestibular system in developmental disorders. This chapter explores different types of problems that have been attributed to the vestibular system. Assessment strategies are discussed, including a brief review of instruments available to test vestibular dysfunction in infants and children. Symptoms observed during infancy through childhood that are believed to be due to vestibular deficits are presented with case examples. Lastly, treatment approaches to address the various types of vestibular dysfunction are described. When possible, reference will be made to data that support the role of the vestibular system and the rationale for treatment.

DEVELOPMENTAL DEFICITS ATTRIBUTED TO THE VESTIBULAR SYSTEM

The most common sensory-based developmental and learning problems in infants and children involve the processing of tactile and vestibular information, coordination of movements between the two body sides, and sequencing and planning of movements.[5,6] These problems may be from deficits in the central processing of vestibular, propriocep-tive, or tactile sensory inputs and their integration with higher cortical functions.

Symptoms that are believed to indicate vestibular dysfunction in infants are often puzzling. These symptoms may include sleep difficulties, poor self-calming, very low or high activity level, atypical muscle tone with slowness in attaining motor milestones, and either an underresponsiveness or overresponsiveness to movement stimulation.[7,8] The problem usually becomes more definitive in the preschool years when delays in fine and gross motor skills, balance, motor planning, and coordination become more evident.[9] Distractibility, defensiveness to touch, and problems with language and visuospatial skills may also be evident.[6] Problems that have been attributed to the vestibular system in the school-aged years include dysgraphia, dyslexia, attention deficits, and reading disabilities.[10]

DOCUMENTATION OF VESTIBULAR DEFICITS

Although the methods of documenting vestibular dysfunction vary considerably across studies, vestibular processing deficits have been observed among children with learning disorders and motor incoordination[2,11-13] and in autistic children.[14-17] Contro-versy has arisen regarding the existence of vestibular-proprioceptive deficits, largely due to disagreements concerning the validity of clinical measurement procedures.[4,18] Empiri-cal evidence suggests that vestibular disorders should be identified using a meaningful cluster of test scores and clinical observations rather than a single measure used in isolation.[12] Ayres[19] initially documented the incidence of vestibular-based problems to be 50 percent of children identified as learning-disabled. Further refinement is needed in measures of vestibular dysfunction, however, before confidence can be placed in these findings.

In children with autism and schizophrenia, vestibular dysfunction is often evi-denced by decreased nystagmus in response to galvanic, caloric, and rotational stimula-tion.[15,16] Likewise, deficits in equilibrium and certain postural responses have been observed in conjunction with depressed vestibulo-ocular reflexes (VOR) and related autonomic reactions such as dizziness or nausea following movement stimulation.[17] Some autistic children crave spinning, whereas others prefer to look at spinning objects such as fans and wheels, suggesting differences in the processing of vestibular informa-tion within a given population.[20-23] In the former case, the child is apparently trying to stimulate the vestibular system through direct movement, while in the latter, the stimula-tion occurs through the optokinetic system.

Early manifestations of vestibular dysfunction have also been examined. Infants who are hypersensitive to movement stimulation show early problems with sleep, state control, and mood regulation.[7] At 8 to 11 months of age, these infants showed intolerance for low-to-ground positions (e.g., prone or supine), a strong preference for upright postures, low muscle tone, slowness in developing motor skills, delayed balance, and/or fear of irregular or unexpected movement. These infants continued to display sensory integrative difficulties at 4 years of age.[8,24] Although the sample was small (9 regulatory disordered and 11 normal 8- to 11-month-old children), infants who demonstrated hyperreactivity to vestibular stimulation continued to demonstrate this problem as preschoolers. Other associated problems in the sample at 4 years of age included high activity level and short attention span, tactile hypersensitivities, and motor planning difficulties.

ASSESSMENT OF VESTIBULAR PROCESSING PROBLEMS IN CHILDREN

Infants and children who are suspected of having vestibular dysfunction should be referred to an occupational or physical therapist experienced in sensory integration assessment in children. Formal assessment should include examination of vestibular reactivity and functioning, postural control and muscle tone, balance, motor planning, and bilateral motor coordination. Not only should the assessment evaluate the child's performance in sensorimotor processes affecting functional learning and behaviors, but it should also incorporate behavioral observations of how the child functions within the home and school environment. Clinical observations of the child in natural play contexts are very useful (i.e., observations of child on playground equipment or mobile and suspended equipment) to substantiate standardized testing. Presenting concerns, symptoms, and test findings should be integrated when making clinical decisions about a child's vestibular difficulties. A single sign of vestibular dysfunction does not constitute a disorder and should be interpreted with caution.

Clinical Assessment

INFANCY

An assessment tool that can be used to assess vestibular processing with infants is the Test of Sensory Functions in Infants (TSFI).[25] It is a 24-item test developed to measure sensory processing and reactivity in infants. It focuses on evaluation of responses to tactile deep pressure, visual-tactile integration, adaptive motor skills, ocular motor control, and reactivity to vestibular stimulation. It was constructed as a criterion-referenced test and has been validated on developmentally delayed and regulatory-disordered infants from 4 to 18 months of age. The vestibular subtest focuses on the infant's responses to being moved in space by the examiner or parent in a systematic rough-housing routine, and therefore measures the infant's reactivity to movement in space.

The TSFI does not offer a comprehensive measure of vestibular functioning in infancy. It is intended to be used in combination with neuromotor assessments that include observations of muscle tone, reflex maturation, and postural mechanisms. The

TABLE 18–1 Assessment of Vestibular Dysfunction in Infants

Vestibular Function	Assessment Tool
Processing of movement in space	Test of Sensory Functions in Infants[24]
Muscle tone, reflex maturation, and postural mechanisms	Chandler Movement Assessment of Infants[41]
Functional motor skills	Infant Neurological International Battery (INFANIB)[42]
	Bayley Scales of Infant Development, Motor Scale[43]
	Peabody Developmental Motor Scale[44]

infant's motor skills should be assessed as well. Table 18–1 presents some of the tests that can be used for these purposes.

PRESCHOOL YEARS

Once the child reaches the preschool years, there are several assessment instruments that can be used. The DeGangi-Berk Test of Sensory Integration (TSI)[26] can be used with pre–school-aged children with mild motor handicaps. The test, a criterion-referenced test, was designed to measure overall sensory integration in 3- to 5-year-old children with delays in sensory, motor, and perceptual skills or for children suspected of being at risk for learning problems. Its focus is primarily on the vestibular-based functions and includes subtests measuring postural control, bilateral motor integration, and reflex integration. The TSI should be administered in conjunction with measures of functional motor performance (e.g., Peabody Developmental Motor Scales). The domains of vestibular-based functions assessed by the TSI are presented in Table 18–2.

In addition to the TSI, Dunn[27] developed a guide to testing clinical observations in kindergartners for 5- to 6½-year-olds. It contains a set of clinical observations for postural mechanisms, postural security, balance, and basic motor planning. There are also some clinical observations of attention, social interaction, and sensory reactivity that accompany the Miller Assessment for Preschoolers,[28] although these have not been standardized.

SCHOOL-AGED YEARS

Once the child reaches school age, more definitive testing of sensory integrative functions can be conducted. The Sensory Integration and Praxis tests[29] were designed to identify sensory integrative disorders involving form and space perception, praxis, vestibular-bilateral integration, and tactile discrimination. The tests are primarily intended for 4- to 8-year-olds with learning disabilities. These tests are particularly useful in delineating areas of treatment for children with sensory integrative disorders.[6]

Lastly, a clinical test that is often used to measure vestibular functioning is the Southern California Postrotary Nystagmus Test (SCPNT).[3] The SCPNT is designed to measure the normalcy of postrotary nystagmus in 5- to 9-year-old children. It can be administered in a short time; however, the examiner must be very experienced in its administration and knowledgeable about conditions that may affect test results (e.g., visual fixation, arousal level, and lighting).[17] The examiner must also have a great deal of

TABLE 18-2 DeGangi-Berk Test of Sensory Integration

Subtest	Task	Behaviors Assessed
Postural control	Monkey task	Antigravity flexion
	Side sit co-contraction	Co-contraction of upper extremities and trunk
	Prone on elbows	Co-contraction of neck
	Wheelbarrow walk	Stability of neck, trunk, and upper extremities
	Airplane	Antigravity extension
	Scooter board-co-contraction	Co-contraction of upper extremities
Bilateral motor	Rolling pin activity	Symmetric bilateral control of arms, trunk rotation, crossing midline
	Jump and turn	Bilateral control of lower extremities, trunk rotation
	Diadokokinesis	Bilateral motor control and motor planning of hands
	Drumming	Bilateral coordination in alternating pattern
	Upper extremity disassociation, task crossing midline	Motor accuracy, trunk control in drawing arm
Reflex integration	Asymmetric tonic neck reflex (ATNR)	Integration of ATNR in quadruped
	Symmetric tonic neck reflex (STNR)	Integration of STNR in quadruped
	Diadochokinesis	Associated reactions

experience in the interpretation of test results. The test results may be confounded by examiner's reaction time, movement of the subject's head during rotation of the board, and inaccuracies in observing the onset and cessation of nystagmus.[30,31] The SCPNT can be used with children with learning disabilities, autism, or mental retardation as well as children with vestibular dysfunction who are able to follow the test directions and maintain the test position. Test results of autistic and mentally retarded children should be interpreted with caution since there are no reliability studies on these populations. Since 20 percent of the normative sample is likely to demonstrate hypo- or hyperreactive nystagmus, it is important to administer other measures of vestibular function in conjunction with the SCPNT to make a definitive diagnosis of vestibular dysfunction.

Clinical Observations

Clinical observations may be useful in screening a child for vestibular dysfunction (Table 18-3). The list may be used to make observations or they may be administered in a questionnaire format to the parents or teacher. The areas covered include symptoms of over- or underresponsiveness to movement, and problems in motor control and motor planning. Most normal children will display a few symptoms in any one category; however, persistent difficulties that interfere with function differentiate the child with vestibular dysfunction. Any child who displays three or more symptoms in any one category should be referred to an occupational or physical therapist for further testing.

TABLE 18–3 Screening a Child for Vestibular
Hypersensitivity or Hyposensitivity

Vestibular Hypersensitivity

1. Easily overwhelmed by movement (i.e., car sick).
2. Strong fear of falling and of heights.
3. Does not enjoy playground equipment and avoids rough-housing play.
4. Is anxious when feet leave ground.
5. Dislikes having head upside down.
6. Slow in movements such as getting onto therapy bench.
7. Slow in learning to walk up or down stairs, relies on railing longer than other children same age.
8. Enjoys movement that she or he initiates but does not like to be moved by others, particularly if the movement is unexpected.
9. Dislikes trying new movement activities or has difficulty learning them.
10. Tends to get motion sick in a car, airplane, or elevator.

Vestibular Hyposensitivity

1. Craves movement and does not feel dizziness when other children do.
2. Likes to climb to high, precarious places. No sense of limits or controls.
3. Is in constant movement, rocking or running about.
4. Likes to swing very high and/or for long periods.
5. Frequently rides on the merry-go-round while others run around to keep the platform turning.
6. Enjoys getting into an upside-down position.

TREATMENT APPROACHES TO VESTIBULAR PROBLEMS IN CHILDREN

General Principles

The major principle underlying treatment of vestibular problems is the importance of improving the child's ability to organize and process vestibular input occurring during movement, thus allowing the child to produce an adaptive response to the environment. Treatment of children with vestibular-based problems needs to be directed toward normalizing the child's responses to sensory input and toward developing more adaptive and functional motor skills. The child's ability to actively control the sensory stimulation while simultaneously engaging in purposeful motor activity is essential to the intervention process. Because many children with vestibular dysfunction also exhibit emotional problems, these also need to be addressed in the therapeutic process.

Sensory integrative therapy uses vestibular stimulation to influence balance, muscle tone, oculomotor responses, movements against gravity, postural adjustments, and activity level. Linear movement activities (e.g., walking, jumping) are believed to assist the child in acclimating to the environment, facilitating the development of an understanding of the body position and body movement in space, whereas rotary and irregular movement activities (e.g., spinning, accelerating and decelerating, playing in unusual positions) are believed to provide powerful input to the system for arousal and alerting.

A major premise of sensory integrative therapy is that movement activities should be self-initiated to elicit adaptive responses (Table 18–4). For example, because children with severe tonal disturbances often have considerable difficulty self-initiating adaptive

TABLE 18–4 Guidelines for Vestibular Stimulation Activities

1. The child should always be actively involved (e.g., Pushing himself or herself on equipment, or telling the therapist when to stop or start the motion).
2. Vestibular stimulation should always be provided within the context of the child's movement problems (e.g., postural control, bilateral integration, or better attention and self-calming).
3. Without a purpose, vestibular stimulation can be extremely disorganizing.
4. Activities should be selected that provide ocular input, because the vestibular system works optimally in conjunction with visual input and with proprioceptive input (e.g., the lights may be dimmed while the child navigates through a tunnel on a scooter board with a flashlight).
5. Proprioceptive input may be enhanced through the use of weighted objects, firm pressure to joints, movement against gravity, traction, or resistive activities.
6. In order for responses to vestibular stimulation to be adaptive, the movement should be provided in all planes and in all directions of movement. Vestibular input may also be varied in terms of speed, frequency, and timing.

movement, opportunities for active, purposeful movement need to be provided via mobile surfaces (i.e., water beds, large foam mattress "clouds").

There is no set prescription for therapy for a child with vestibular dysfunction. Because each child brings a unique combination of characteristics, these must be addressed in the therapy process. Therapeutic activity should involve the child's choice of activity guided by his or her own interest and skill. Play is the medium through which therapy is adapted. For example, the child may develop an imaginary game where he or she is flying through space like "flight man." The therapist seeks to structure the environment to facilitate the child's responses.

As with any sensory stimulation, the child's responses should be watched carefully to assure that the stimulation is perceived as pleasurable and useful to the child as he or she learns new skills. Autonomic responses such as increased respiration, flushing or pallor, sweating, nausea or yawning, or severe dizziness and loss of balance should be observed. They may not always occur immediately during or after the stimulation. Instead the child may become disorganized or ill later in the day or after additional vestibular stimulation (i.e., ride home) loads the system to its maximum toleration level. Slow rocking with firm pressure on the abdomen, use of firm tactile input, and cognitive games such as counting or singing will help the child to regroup if the input has been too intense.

Specific Problem: Gravitational Insecurity and Intolerance of Movement

Postural or gravitational security seems to play an important role in the development of emotional stability as well as balance, postural mechanisms, and spatial perception.[32,33] Children hypersensitive to movement are usually overwhelmed by intense movement stimuli, such as spinning, frequent changes in direction and speed, or unusual body positions (e.g., inverted). Typically they are fearful about leaving the earth's surface and are thus called gravitationally insecure.[34] Often they will display considerable autonomic responses (dizziness, nausea) during and after any type of vestibular stimulation. Thus, the gravitationally insecure child demonstrates an extreme fearfulness of moving in space. Children with gravitational insecurity typically have a strong preference for upright positions, avoid rotational movement patterns such as transitional movements, prefer close-to-ground positions (i.e., W-sitting posture), "lock" the body and neck in rigid postures to avoid movement stimulation, and tend to avoid movement activities. Not only are they fearful of body movement in space, but they resist any change in their body that may be perceived as threatening. Imposed movement is particularly upsetting to the child. The emotional response accompanying gravitational insecurity is associated with a sudden change of head position, a displacement in the body's center of gravity, or the feet suddenly leaving the ground. As a result of insecurities in moving in space, children with gravitational insecurity tend to be very emotionally unstable. They frequently display fearfulness of new situations, rigidity, and a resistance to change. Fisher and Bundy[32] believe that gravitational insecurity may be due to poor modulation of otolithic inputs.

CASE STUDY 1

HISTORY

Emily was a $4\frac{1}{2}$-year-old with low muscle tone, fearfulness in new movement activities, and poor balance. She fell frequently at school and avoided any playground activities. Although her fine and gross motor skills were at age level, she had difficulty with dynamic balance. Emily was a very shy and withdrawn child. When presented with motor tasks, Emily tended to cry silently even during very appealing activities. At table-top tasks, Emily was very anxious, sitting with her shoulders in a tense, elevated posture. Emily was not sensitive to touch; in contrast, she would seek close proximity with the examiner or her mother whenever she was required to move.

ASSESSMENT

Emily demonstrated weakness in postural control (e.g., inability to lift her body up against gravity in either a flexed or extended body posture). She would sit in a W-sitting posture and preferred close-to-ground activities. Low muscle tone was observed in her winged scapula and rounded trunk posture when standing upright. She often yawned and complained of feeling tired. Her movement quality was stiff, awkward, and lacked fluidity. Emily was very slow and deliberate in her movement patterns. When placed in a sitting position on the therapy ball, Emily clung to the examiner and was extremely fearful. In addition to definite indicators of gravitational insecurity, Emily showed some evidence of motor planning difficulties. She displayed much fear and anxiety when approached with a new motor challenge, particularly sequenced, unfamiliar movement patterns such as galloping.

TREATMENT

The child with gravitational insecurity needs a slow, gradual approach to introducing movement. This child responds best when movement is linear such as forward-back or side to side, because gravitational insecurity is hypothesized to be the result of poor modulation of otolithic input. The reason that this type of input is so calming and easy to accept is that it does not involve any rotary movements or large movement displacements of the head in space. Orbital spinning (modified spinning with face remaining in one direction) is usually accepted as well. Coupling movement activities with firm deep-pressure activities helps the child to organize the movement experience through the sense of touch. The child needs a very gradual approach, starting with activities that are close to the ground. If vestibular stimulation is imposed or forced on the child, it can be more disorganizing than integrating. Therapy must be carefully graded to challenge the child, yet within the confines of what the child can tolerate and integrate. The child should be moved slowly and in a rhythmic fashion. Maintaining close body contact with the child helps him or her to learn to tolerate any movement, thus providing inhibition through the tactile sense. Helping the child to anticipate where his or her body is moving in space by providing visual or auditory cues also helps the child to know where he or she is about to move. Activities should be selected that are first close to the ground (i.e., a sit-'n-spin or T-stool). The child may need to be enticed to just touch moving equipment or to put a favorite toy on the swing in the first weeks of treatment. In this way, the child may gradually learn to tolerate the visual component of watching the movement before he or she is expected to move in space. If the child is allowed to decide on a movement and then enact the movement, it helps to modulate the vestibular input.

Specific Problem: Hyporeactivity to Movement in Space

When children have a high tolerance for vestibular input (hyporeactivity to movement), the behavioral repertoire is different. These children may seek movement experiences and yet do not seem to profit from them. One may see explosive movement quality, poor judgment in starting and stopping movement activities, or difficulty with transitional movements. Children with vestibular problems typically exhibit low muscle tone and may not be able to move against gravity easily enough to stimulate the vestibular system in a variety of movement planes. As a result, poverty of movement provides fewer opportunities for developing vestibular output for postural control and balance. Individuals with hyporeactivity to movement often display short mean durations of postrotary nystagmus[29] and demonstrate reduced or absent velocity storage.[12] Children who are hyporeactive to movement usually crave movement and do not display any evidence of autonomic responses, such as dizziness, associated with movement.

CASE STUDY 2

HISTORY

As an infant, Fred would scream whenever lying down, and he experienced carsickness. He liked to swing very high and for long periods of time, liked fast-moving carnival rides, and never became dizzy. He only liked movement that he could initiate and resisted being moved by others. Fred enjoyed vibration created by power saws and drills, although he was sensitive to their noise. At age $5\frac{1}{2}$

years, Fred had been seeing a psychologist for several months because of significant behavioral problems at home and school. The psychologist believed that an impasse had been reached in treatment and that a new approach might be necessary for continued progress to occur. Fred's kindergarten teacher reported that he was very bright and knew all the answers. However, he did not do what was asked of him in school, did not finish assignments, had difficulty sitting still, and frequently jumped around. In addition, he sometimes got stuck on one activity and had difficulty making transitions to new activities. His mother's concerns centered around his tendency to fight her about everything all day long, his aggressiveness with other children, and his destructive nature. She also was worried about his poor judgment regarding his own safety. For example, he would jump off the top of the shed and would jump out the car window unless restrained in a car seat. Fred preferred to play alone at home rather than with other children in the neighborhood.

ASSESSMENT

During the occupational therapy evaluation, Fred showed normal postural reactions, good balance, and very slight motor planning problems. Gross and fine motor skills were well developed. In this one-to-one situation, Fred could sit still for 45 minutes and showed good attention to the various activities presented to him. Fred's activity level increased dramatically, however, when he was permitted to play on the suspended equipment (i.e., swings). On the swing, he continually asked to go faster and higher, then would suddenly jump or dive off. He exhibited no fear of any activity or piece of equipment. In addition to these observations, Fred exhibited depressed nystagmus on the postrotary nystagmus test.

The results of the evaluation suggested that Fred was having difficulty processing and appropriately using vestibular input. His vestibular system appeared to be underresponsive to many forms of vestibular sensory stimulation, compelling him to seek dangerous thrills and to overlook the consequences of his actions. It is likely that problems in this area were affecting his ability to develop appropriate behavioral limits and social interactions. He also seemed overly sensitive to being moved by others, suggesting that he was both underresponsive and overresponsive to vestibular stimulation. By responding aggressively, he could control situations and therefore avoid unexpected movement by others.

TREATMENT

The child who is hyporeactive to movement in space often craves spinning and will seek fast-moving, rough kinds of games. This type of child may disorganize very rapidly and without warning. Vestibular stimulation needs to be carefully directed and combined with purposeful, goal-directed activities so that the child learns to control the sensory stimulation and modify his or her responses accordingly. Movement stimulation activities that are very intense and stimulating should be coupled with inhibitory or calming ones. Rotary (spinning, rolling down a ramp) and irregular, fast-moving input that requires the eyes to constantly adapt to a new visual focus are typically used in treatment for this type of child. Inverted body positions (upside down) are also highly stimulating because they involve a complete displacement of the head.

TABLE 18–5 Common Symptoms Associated
with Vestibular-Postural Deficits

1. Poor equilibrium reactions due to lack of centering of the trunk
2. Extraneous body movements when attempting to hold stable body postures with weak muscle co-contraction
3. Fixations in the neck, trunk, and shoulders during skilled motor activities (i.e., drawing)
4. Low muscle tone and poor joint stability
5. Weakness of the trunk and neck in assuming antigravity postures (i.e., prone extension and supine flexion)
6. Poor distal prehension with lack of fine fingertip prehension and controlled wrist rotation
7. Lack of integration of primitive reflexes
8. Ocular-motor problems including poor eye convergence and quick localizations of the eyes
9. Shortened duration of postrotary nystagmus

Specific Problem: Vestibular-Postural Deficits

Vestibular-postural problems are among the most common type of vestibular-based deficits (Table 18–5). The neck and trunk muscles provide stability in movement, and their development provides the foundation for postural control. If the proximal musculature is not well developed, the child is often unstable in maintaining body postures, has poor balance, and may have poor fine manipulation and locomotor skills. Frequently children with minor neurologic impairments have difficulty with postural reactions including balance, ocular-motor control, and visuospatial skills.[35] Children with severe emotional and behavioral problems have also been reported to display deficient equilibrium and postural responses, decreased postrotary nystagmus, and an absence of autonomic responses such as dizziness and nausea following vestibular stimulation.[36]

TREATMENT

Intervention directed toward improving postural mechanisms should focus on improving muscle tone, developing antigravity postural control, improving muscle co-contraction, and developing righting and equilibrium reactions. Intervention should first be directed toward improving muscle tone and developing antigravity postural control. Through the use of basic antigravity postures combined with vestibular stimulation and functional activities, muscle tone may be improved. Sometimes specialized handling techniques may be required to increase tone in the low-tone child. For example, compression over the shoulders while the child is placed in a prone extension posture will increase tone. A variety of materials such as stretchy ropes, resistive therapy bands, or heavy weighted toys help to stimulate tone as well.

Postures that require the child to assume total body flexion against gravity should be emphasized first. In the flexor feeding pattern, the trunk and neck flex while the extremities move toward the body midline. This heavy work pattern involves the abdominals and neck flexors together with the proximal limb muscles. Because the arms and legs move toward the body midline, this pattern is closely associated with feeding, power grip of the hands, and eye–hand coordination at the body midline. This position also facilitates convergence of the eyes at close range and grip in the hands. Because the flexors of the body are mobilizers, they are also critical for initiation of movement and consequently play a part in motor planning. Climbing and jumping activities are two examples of how this pattern is observed in everyday activity. The pattern may be stimulated in activities such as holding onto a suspended tire in a flexed position, pulling up on a chin-up bar, or putting together pop beads or some other resistive toy. The pattern that one observes in the arms is a coming together toward the midline in a bilateral symmetric movement.

The next major postural pattern that should be emphasized in treatment is total body extension against gravity. Extension against gravity should be stimulated following flexion activities in a treatment session. In this pattern, extensor tone in the neck and trunk develops, which is necessary for stability of the trunk, neck, and extremities. Both the pivot-prone and prone-extension patterns are used in treatment. Extension against gravity is important for proximal stability in holding postures such as sitting, holding of the arms in space during reach, and in balance. There is a high correlation between holding of extensor postures and vestibular function.[17]

Extension against gravity can be easily elicited through the use of vestibular stimulation activities. For example, placing the child prone in a hammock swing while throwing a ball into a receptacle will elicit an extended body posture while the arms are required to hold in space. Because the pivot-prone and prone-extension patterns elicit bilateral scapular and trunk activity, bilateral-symmetric and alternating upper-extremity movements help to enhance the pattern. For example, stepping on alternating arms in a wheelbarrow walking pattern facilitates prone extension while developing bilateral alternating arm movements. Generally, fast-accelerating movement and swinging in a linear movement plane elicit the prone-extension pattern. For example, acceleration down a ramp while riding prone on a scooter board will result in the child lifting his or her body up into the pivot-prone pattern. While lying prone on equipment (i.e., therapy balls, scooter boards), the child should be engaged in activities that motivate the child to lift and hold his or her body up. Usually, this involves requiring the child to reach upward in tasks such as putting magnets on a wall, throwing a ball into a basket, or pushing a rolling pin up a ramp.

Developing muscle co-contraction of the neck, trunk, and extremities is an important next step in treatment. Co-contraction is evidenced when the flexors and extensors contract simultaneously in a coordinated manner. Co-contraction allows for smooth, steady coordinated movements while working against gravity. Co-contraction of the neck is especially important for the development of visual perception inasmuch as neck stability is essential before the eyes become stabilized. It is also important for balance. Activities whereby alternating resistance is applied help to facilitate co-contraction (i.e., resist trunk and extremities of child in a game where the child "freezes" like a statue). Functional activities that require co-contraction are carrying weighted boxes or pushing furniture.

Specific Problem: Vestibular-Bilateral Integration

Vestibular dysfunction is often observed in combination with bilateral integration problems, particularly in children who have postural deficits. Bilateral motor integration involves the ability to coordinate the two body sides and develop lateralization.[37] Children with problems in this area frequently do not establish a hand dominance by school age. Frequently, the child will interchange hands with no consistent preference for one hand. Bilateral assistive skills where one hand acts as a specialized hand and the other as an effective stabilizer are difficult. For example, simple tasks such as buttoning and cutting with scissors are delayed. Reciprocal bilateral movements such as skipping, jumping, or alternating the hands in a drumming pattern are difficult. Oftentimes the child lacks precision in hand function and cannot sequence hand movements. The child may lack symmetry and control in gross motor movements. As a result, the child is often very clumsy and stiff in gross motor tasks such as rolling and walking, because these movements require coordination of the two body sides. The child lacks flexibility in rotating the trunk, and there is also a strong resistance in crossing the body midline. Consequently, the child may turn the entire body when required to cross the midline rather than rotating the trunk.

TREATMENT

Bilateral integration consists of several components: crossing the body midline, coordination of the two body sides in symmetric and alternating movements, and differentiation of one body side from the other in skilled movements. Table 18–6 presents a list of sequential techniques to improve bilateral integration.

An important aspect of both postural control and bilateral integration is the development of trunk rotation. It allows for the refinement of equilibrium reactions as well as crossing midline functions of the arms and hands. It is not until the child has a secure basis for movement against gravity that trunk rotation can develop. It first emerges with

TABLE 18–6 Techniques to Improve Bilateral Integration

Function	Emphasis in Treatment
Convergence in body midline	Bringing extremities to midline body position; activities that require power grip (i.e., squeezing a toy) or that involve maintaining the hands and/or feet in a controlled midline position (i.e., flexed body position)
Crossing midline activities	Combine with trunk rotation activities; crossing midline in skilled activities (e.g., reaching up and across body for object held in space)
Coordination of the two body sides	Symmetric body movements, sides first followed in bilateral symmetric tasks by alternating movements. These should be stimulated in conjunction with postural patterns of flexion or extension (e.g., rolling pin activities, jumping on a trampoline, throwing a large ball into a basket, or pushing oneself from a wall surface while swinging in a hammock).
Contrasting the two body sides in alternating movement	Activities that require alternating hands or feet in a reciprocal pattern (e.g., drumming the hands in rhythms, propelling a bicycle, or walking on hands in a wheelbarrow walk)
Differentiation of the two body sides	Contrast two body sides, then develop one side of the body in skilled actions while the other side acts as the stabilizer. Use of bilateral assistive upper extremity tasks (e.g., buttoning, scissor cutting, stringing beads, or handwriting or lower extremity tasks such as skilled ball sports [i.e., soccer])

segmental rolling and is important for smooth, graded movements requiring trunk rotation. Therapists work specifically on trunk rotation in activities that require the child to reach out to the body side to obtain a large toy with two hands. Trunk rotation may be stimulated by resisting diagonal movements against gravity (i.e., sitting up from inverted back-lying position using trunk rotation or resistive rolling up a ramp).

Specific Problem: Vestibular-Based Motor Planning Problems

Developmental dyspraxia, also known as a motor planning disorder, is a sensory processing deficit which, in part, may be related to the vestibular processing disorder. Some types of developmental dyspraxia are related to tactile processing problems. The problem lies not so much in the processing of sensory input or the ability to produce the movement skill but in the intermediary process of planning the movement. The child with developmental dyspraxia has significant problems in planning and directing goal-directed movement and skilled or nonhabitual motor tasks. As a result, the dyspraxic child is often vulnerable to distraction because he or she lacks the internal organization to focus behavior.[38] The distinct types of motor planning problems are presented in Table 18–7. Children with vestibular dysfunction may exhibit any of these types of dyspraxia.[39,40]

Some of the common symptoms of the child with dyspraxia are delays in dressing and delays in fine and gross motor skills involving imitation, sequenced movements (i.e., lacing, skipping), and construction (i.e., building from a block model). Poor accuracy of movement is observed, and skilled hand movements such as handwriting are typically very difficult for the dyspraxic child. Movement quality of dyspraxic children may be explosive with poor judgment of force, speed, and aim. Speech articulation may be poor because this is also a planned, skilled motor activity. Nonhabitual tasks are most difficult for the dyspraxic child; therefore, he or she prefers routines and strongly resists changes. Transitions from one activity to the next may cause behavioral upset.

Initiation of new movement sequences or new organized plans of behavior are difficult. For instance, the child may not be able to tell the therapist what he or she plans to do because the child lacks an internal plan. As a result, one may see the dyspraxic child as becoming either very disruptive and aggressive, particularly when there is no external structure to organize the child, or the child may become very passive and prefer repetition of certain favorite activities, resisting new and different tasks. One may

TABLE 18–7 Types of Motor Planning Problems

Postural dyspraxia	Inability to plan and imitate large body movements and meaningless postures
Sequencing dyspraxia	Difficulty making transitions from one motor action to another and in sequencing movements (e.g., thumb-finger sequencing)
Oral and verbal dyspraxia	Inability to produce oral movements on verbal command or in imitation, a skill that affects speech articulation
Constructional dyspraxia	Inability to create and assemble three-dimensional structures (e.g., block bridge)
Graphic dyspraxia	Inability to plan and execute drawings
Dyspraxia involving	Inability to use objects, symbolic actions, symbolically

observe tantrums, aggressive behavior, poor play skills with peers, frustration, and a strong resistance to change. Some children become very controlling and manipulative because of their inability to control and impact their environment. Poor self-concept is a major problem of the dyspraxic child.

TREATMENT

There are three primary processes that must occur in treatment for the child with developmental dyspraxia. These include (1) developing the conceptual organization of the skill or task; (2) developing a plan or program of action; and (3) executing the plan. It is rare for a child to have a motor planning problem without difficulty in the tactile or vestibular system. Treatment for children with vestibular-based motor planning problems should first focus on vestibular awareness; therefore, vestibular stimulation activities should precede motor planning tasks in a therapy session. Postural and other motor problems associated with the vestibular-based motor planning problem should be addressed in the treatment process as well.

Ideation is the first stage of motor planning. During this stage, the child with vestibular-based dyspraxia will have difficulty initiating purposeful movement. The child needs to link the feeling of enacting the motion or action with the concept of what actions lead to task completion. The therapist may move the child through the action while describing what is happening. By using vestibular stimulation in a very specific way, the child can attach meanings to the action. For example, a child may not be able to plan the motor sequence of how to push himself on a scooter board. The therapist may hold the child's hands and contrast fast and slow movement on a scooter board in a game, then vary other task characteristics, such as holding a hoop versus the therapist's hands, or riding down a ramp or inside a tunnel. Each of these variations of the same action will help the child to conceptualize the motor action that is required to propel through space on the scooter board. Motor planning activities should be varied according to sequence, ordering, position, and timing.

The child may not be able to choose a motor task at first because the child does not have a concept of what he or she is able to do with the different toys and materials. The therapist may select a simple planning task and then model how to do it. For example, the therapist may demonstrate jumping off a platform into a large bin of balls, a task that offers both challenge and success. If the child shows fear or is unable to complete the action required, the task should be modified to assure that the child can succeed. Sometimes children are more interested to try a difficult task if they have experienced moving through the motions. Once the child has engaged in the task successfully a few times, it is important to then vary the task demands slightly to present a new challenge. In this way, the child must learn to self-correct and to execute new movement patterns.

Before the child can plan out what he or she wants to do, the child must be prepared to act. The young patient needs to be motivated to do the action; therefore, it is important to find activities that excite the child and solicit his or her interest and involvement. The first step in learning to plan an action is to be able to experience it and to verbalize or conceptualize what needs to happen. Once the child has enacted the action with a model or the therapist's assistance, he or she needs to understand what the end goal will be and how to get there. Selecting activities that give sensory feedback throughout the sequence helps the child to construct a plan. For example, if an obstacle course is used, the child may crawl through an opening in a large foam tunnel, then pull herself or himself on the scooter board by holding a resistive rope, and lastly, swing while pushing over the large sandbag person. Each of these would have distinctly different sensory inputs that would help the child mark each event in time and space.

Verbal mediation is an important aspect of learning to plan motor activities. The therapist may help the child to articulate what he or she is doing to help the child link language with motor actions. Verbal commands from the therapist while the child engages in a sequenced task help to organize the sequence for the child. Once the child has consolidated his or her actions with verbal guidance from the therapist, the child should then be helped to articulate what he or she is going to do next.

VESTIBULAR-BASED DYSPRAXIAS

The most common types of motor-planning disorders observed in children with vestibular-based problems are related to postural, sequencing, bilateral motor coordination, motor planning, constructional, and praxis to verbal commands.[39] Treatment should focus on the ability to plan whole-body movements in space and to combine the body with objects. Through the use of postural patterns of flexion and extension against gravity, trunk rotation, and diagonal rotary patterns, the child can learn to map simple body movements in space. These postural patterns should always be combined with functional activities so that the movement pattern has a purpose for the child. The body flexors are the mobilizers, and the extensors are the stabilizers; therefore, flexion is often needed in children who have troubles learning how to initiate movement patterns. These whole-body patterns should be used first before small skilled movements are attempted (i.e., cutting a "play dough" snake with scissors). Activities should use vestibular-proprioceptive sensory stimulation in combination with a strong visual component to help the child to see what he or she is doing in space and to visualize the effect his or her actions have on objects. For example, having the child sit in a hammock and swing to kick over a tower of cardboard blocks will give the child vestibular, proprioceptive, and visual feedback to consolidate the motor plan of kicking over the tower. The major emphasis is therefore placed on relating the body in space in relation to objects. Activities involving motor accuracy (i.e., throwing Velcro balls at a target), bilateral motor coordination, and sequencing of fine and gross motor movements (i.e., skipping, cutting out a triangle) should follow treatment directed toward basic postural patterns.

SUMMARY

The vestibular system is complex in its neural connections. As a result, it impacts the individual's ability to detect motion, differentiate motion within the visual field, develop a body scheme, attend and modulate arousal, develop muscle tone and postural control, and develop motor coordination including bilateral motor control. When vestibular dysfunction is present, it may be manifested in a number of ways. The most common types of vestibular-based problems include gravitational insecurity, underresponsiveness to movement in space, intolerance of movement, vestibular-postural deficits, bilateral integration problems, and motor planning problems associated with the underlying vestibular disorder. These underlying vestibular-based deficits can have a profound effect on learning and emotion regulation. Although a variety of assessment strategies have been developed that evaluate the various vestibular-based functions, continued instrument development is needed to refine measures, particularly for infants and young children. Research is also needed to determine the effects of vestibular stimulation on improving postural mechanisms, attention, learning, motor planning, and emotion regulation in different populations.

REFERENCES

1. Naunton, R (ed): The Vestibular System. Academic Press, New York, 1975.
2. Ayres, AJ: Sensory Integration and Learning Disorders. Western Psychological Services, Los Angeles, 1972.
3. Clark, DL: The vestibular system: An overview of structure and function. Phys Occup Ther Pediatr, 5:5, 1985.
4. Ayres, AJ: Southern California Postrotary Nystagmus Test Manual. Western Psychological Services, Los Angeles, 1975.
5. Clark, F, Mailloux, Z, and Parham, D: Sensory integration and children with learning disabilities. In Pratt, PN, and Allen, AS, (eds): Occupational Therapy for Children, 2nd ed. CV Mosby, St. Louis, 1989, p 457.
6. Fisher, AG, Murray, EA, and Bundy, AC: Sensory Integration Theory and Practice. FA Davis, Philadelphia, 1991.
7. DeGangi, GA and Greenspan, SI: The development of sensory functions in infants. Phys Occup Ther Pediatr 8:21, 1988.
8. DeGangi, GA: Assessment of sensory, emotional, and attentional problems in regulatory disordered infants. Infants Young Child 3:1, 1991.
9. DeGangi, GA, Berk, RA, and Larsen, LA: The measurement of vestibular-based functions in preschool children. Am J Occup Ther 34:452, 1980.
10. DeQuiros, JB and Schrager, OL: Neuropsychological Fundamentals in Learning Disabilities, rev ed. Academic Therapy Publications, Novato, California, 1979.
11. DeQuiros, J: Diagnosis of vestibular disorders in the learning disabled. J Learning Disabil 9:50, 1976.
12. Fisher, AG, Mixon, J, and Herman, R: The validity of the clinical diagnosis of vestibular dysfunction. Occup Ther J Res 6:3, 1986.
13. Horak, FB, et al: Vestibular function and motor proficiency in children with impaired hearing, or with learning disability and motor impairments. Dev Med Child Neurol 30:64, 1988.
14. Maurer, RG and Damasio, AR: Vestibular dysfunction in autistic children. Dev Med Child Neurol 21:656, 1979.
15. Ornitz, E: Vestibular dysfunction in schizophrenia and childhood autism. Comparative Psychiatry 11:159, 1970.
16. Ornitz, EM: The modulation of sensory input and motor output in autistic children. J Autism Childhood Schizophrenia 4:197, 1974.
17. Ottenbacher, K: Identifying vestibular processing dysfunction in learning disabled children. Am J Occup Ther 32:217, 1978.
18. Polatajko, HJ: The Southern California Postrotary Nystagmus Test: A Validity Study. Can J Occup Ther 50:119, 1983.
19. Ayres, AJ: The Effect of Sensory Integrative Therapy on Learning Disabled Children. Center for the Study of Sensory Integrative Dysfunction, Pasadena, 1976.
20. Allen, DA: Autistic spectrum disorders: Clinical presentation in preschool children. J Child Neurol 3(suppl): S48, 1988.
21. Ayres, AJ and Tickle, LS: Hyper-responsivity to touch and vestibular stimuli as a predictor of positive response to sensory integration procedures by autistic children. Am J Occup Ther 34:375, 1980.
22. Bauman, M and Kemper, TL: Histoanatomic observations of the brain in early infantile autism. Neurology 35:866, 1985.
23. Grandin, T and Scariano, MM: Emergence: Labeled Autistic. Arena, Novato, California, 1986.
24. DeGangi, GA, Porges, SW, Sickel, RZ, et al: Four-year follow-up of a sample of regulatory disordered infants. Infant Mental Health Journal, in press.
25. DeGangi, GA and Greenspan, SI: Test of Sensory Functions in Infants. Western Psychological Services, Los Angeles, 1989.
26. Berk, RA and DeGangi, GA: DeGangi-Berk Test of Sensory Integration. Western Psychological Services, Los Angeles, 1983.
27. Dunn, W: A Guide to Testing Clinical Observations in Kindergartners. American Occupational Therapy Association, Rockville, Maryland, 1981.
28. Miller, LJ: Miller Assessment for Preschoolers. Foundation for Knowledge in Development, Littleton, Colorado, 1982.
29. Ayres, AJ: Sensory Integration and Praxis Tests. Western Psychological Services, Los Angeles, 1989.
30. Cohen, H and Keshner, EA: Current concepts of the vestibular system reviewed: 2. Visual/vestibular interaction and spatial orientation. Am J Occup Ther 43:331, 1989.
31. Cohen, H: Testing vestibular function: Problems with the Southern California Postrotary Nystagmus Test. Am J Occup Ther 43:475, 1989.

32. Fisher, AG and Bundy, AC: Vestibular stimulation in the treatment of postural and related disorders. In Payton, OD, et al (eds): Manual of Physical Therapy Techniques. Churchill Livingstone, New York, 1989, p 239.
33. Matthews, PBC: Proprioceptors and their contribution to somatosensory mapping: Complex messages require complex processing. Can J Physiol Pharmacol 66:430, 1988.
34. Ayres, AJ: Sensory Integration and the Child. Western Psychological Services, Los Angeles, 1979.
35. Steinberg, M and Rendle-Short, J: Vestibular dysfunction in young children with minor neurological impairment. Dev Med Child Neurol 19:639, 1977.
36. Ottenbacher, KJ: Vestibular processing dysfunction in children with severe emotional and behavioral disorders: A review. Phys Occup Therapy Pediatr 2:3, 1982.
37. Magalhaes, LC, Koomar, JA, and Cermak, SA: Bilateral motor coordination in 5- to 9-year-old children: A pilot study. Am J Occup Ther 43:437, 1989.
38. Ayres, AJ, Mailloux, ZK, and Wendler, CL: Developmental dyspraxia: Is it a unitary function? Occup Ther J Res 7:93, 1987.
39. Ayres, AJ: Developmental Dyspraxia and Adult Onset Apraxia. Sensory Integration International, Torrance, California, 1985.
40. Conrad, K, Cermak, SA, and Drake, C: Differentiation of praxis among children. Am J Occup Ther 37:466, 1983.
41. Chandler, L, et al: Chandler Movement Assessment of Infants. Rolling Bay, Washington, 1988.
42. Ellison, PH, Horn, JL, and Browning, CA: Construction of an Infant Neurological International Battery (INFANIB) for the assessment of neurological integrity in infancy. Phys Ther 65:1326, 1985.
43. Bayley, N: Bayley Scales of Infant Development. Psychological Corporation, New York, 1969.
44. Folio, MR and Fewell, RR: Peabody Developmental Motor Scales. DLM Teaching Resources, Allen, TX, 1983.

Index

An "f" following a page number indicates a figure; a "t" indicates a table.

W

X